CHANGING SUBSTANCE ABUSE THROUGH HEALTH AND SOCIAL SYSTEMS

CHANGING SUBSTANCE ABUSE THROUGH HEALTH AND SOCIAL SYSTEMS

Edited by

William R. Miller

University of New Mexico
Albuquerque, New Mexico

and

Constance M. Weisner

University of California, San Francisco
San Francisco, California

Kluwer Academic / Plenum Publishers
New York, Boston, Dordrecht, London, Moscow

ISBN 0-306-47256-2

233 Spring Street, New York, New York 10013

http://www.wkap/nl/

10 9 8 7 6 5 4 3 2 1

A C.I.P. record for this book is available from the Library of Congress

Printed in the United States of America

Contributors

Robert Anderson, Department of Psychology, University of New Mexico, Albuquerque, New Mexico 87131

Melanie E. Bennett, Department of Psychiatry, University of Maryland School of Medicine, Baltimore, Maryland 21201

Joyce Bittinger, Department of Psychology, University of New Mexico, Albuquerque, New Mexico 87131

Michelle Boycott, Department of General Practice, University of Wales, College of Medicine, Cardiff CF3 7PN, Wales, United Kingdom

Andraé Brown, Department of Professional Psychology and Family Therapy, Seton Hall University, South Orange, New Jersey 07079

Faye J. Calhoun, National Institute on Alcohol Abuse and Alcoholism, National Institutes of Health, Bethesda, Maryland 20892

Mikyta Daugherty, Department of Psychology, University of New Mexico, Albuquerque, New Mexico 87131

Ernest J. Dole, Department of Pharmaceutical Care, Lovelace Health Systems, Albuquerque, New Mexico 87108

Alan J. Flisher, Department of Psychiatry and Mental Health, University of Cape Town, Cape Town, Republic of South Africa

Sonja Frison, Behavioral Medicine Unit/Division of Preventive Medicine, University of Alabama, Birmingham, Alabama 35294

Nancy S. Handmaker, Department of Psychology, University of New Mexico, Albuquerque, New Mexico 87131

Robert B. Huebner, Division of Clinical and Prevention Research, National Institute on Alcohol Abuse and Alcoholism, National Institutes of Health, Bethesda, Maryland 20892

William H. James, College of Education, University of Washington, Seattle, Washington 98195

Denise Laframboise, Department of Psychology, University of New Mexico, Albuquerque, New Mexico 87131

Craig T. Love, Center for Alcohol and Addiction Studies, Brown University, Providence, Rhode Island 02912

A. Thomas McLellan, Department of Psychiatry, University of Pennsylvania School of Medicine, Philadelphia, Pennsylvania 19106

Robert J. Meyers, Center on Alcoholism, Substance Abuse, and Addictions, University of Mexico, Albuquerque, New Mexico 87106

Jesse B. Milby, Department of Psychology, University of Alabama, Birmingham, Alabama 35294

William R. Miller, Department of Psychology, University of New Mexico, Albuquerque, New Mexico 87131

Wanjirû Mukoma, Department of Psychiatry and Mental Health, University of Cape Town, Cape Town, Republic of South Africa

Judith K. Ockene, Division of Preventive and Behavioral Medicine, University of Massachusetts Medical School, Worcester, Massachusetts 01655

Lori Pbert, Division of Preventive and Behavioral Medicine, University of Massachusetts Medical School, Worcester, Massachusetts 01655

Stephen Rollnick, Department of General Practice, University of Wales College of Medicine, Cardiff CF3 7PN, Wales, United Kingdom

Paul M. Roman, Center for Research on Behavioral Health and Human Services Delivery, University of Georgia, Atlanta, Georgia 30682

Susan J. Rose, Helen Bader School of Social Welfare, University of Wisconsin, Milwaukee, Wisconsin 53201

Carol R. Schermer, Department of Surgery, University of New Mexico Health Sciences Center, Albuquerque, New Mexico 87131

Natasha Slesnick, Center on Alcoholism, Substance Abuse, and Addictions, University of New Mexico, Albuquerque, New Mexico 87106

Jane Ellen Smith, Department of Psychology, University of New Mexico, Albuquerque, New Mexico 87131

Constance Weisner, Department of Psychiatry, University of California, San Francisco, California 94143

Allen Zweben, Helen Bader School of Social Welfare, University of Wisconsin, Milwaukee, Wisconsin 53201

Foreword

The National Institute on Alcohol Abuse and Alcoholism (NIAAA) of the National Institutes of Health in the United States was pleased to co-sponsor this international conference on the treatment of addictive behaviors. This conference provided an opportunity to understand how integrating alcohol prevention and treatment interventions into existing health and social service systems can be effective in reducing the economic burden of alcohol and other drug misuse on society. The topics addressed were critical to the health of the people not only in Africa but in the world, critical to the economies, to the quality of the workforces, to the quality of life, and to the effectiveness of health care systems for all countries.

In the United States it is estimated that 100,000 people die each year from alcohol-related causes. Problematic drinking is a costly matter. Studies of the prevalence of patients screening positive for alcohol abuse indicate that the adverse consequences of alcohol use are a burden to society and to its health care systems. A recent report on the economic costs of alcohol abuse in the United States estimated that alcohol-related problems cost approximately $185 billion a year. Alcohol problems cost more and cause more deaths than all illegal drugs put together. Alcohol abuse and risky drinking patterns lead to alcohol-related problems for otherwise productive citizens. Internationally, much effort has been spent in documenting and discussing the consequences of alcohol abuse and alcohol. In addition to alcohol-related automobile accidents, homicides, on-the-job accidents, risky sexual behavior, and failure to fulfill major work or home responsibilities there is a litany of medical, social, legal, financial, and spiritual (actions while intoxicated or alcohol seeking that betrays an individual's own values) problems and consequences that occur. While fully effective treatments that provide consistent, positive results for all patients continue to elude us, much progress can be made from integrating techniques into our current system of care that have been found to have high potential.

We do understand that issues related to the global problems of alcohol abuse and dependence and alcohol control are complex. Policies in addressing the consequences of abuse and the prevention of abuse and alcoholism must often be balanced by understanding the economic benefits to a country from its sale and distribution. Also, most people use and enjoy alcohol responsibly and without consequence. It is a complex set of issues indeed. Although alcohol can harm body tissues, there are studies to suggest that low levels of consumption may have some protective effects in some people. Studying the protective effects of small or moderate doses of alcohol, therefore, is also an important area of research. The risks and benefits are different for different people and different for different stages of life. It is complex indeed. Clearly, these factors must be considered in thinking about our research agenda and judging the adaptability of research-based intervention strategies.

Our work in supporting and organizing this conference reflects the mission of our Institute and our interest in establishing working relationships with researchers in Africa and other countries around the world. The NIAAA is one of 18 Institutes in the National Institutes of Health in the United States. The mission of the NIH is to improve health through the conduct of research. To that end, NIAAA conducts and supports biomedical and behavioral research on the effects of alcohol on the human mind and body, on prevention and treatment of alcohol abuse and alcoholism, and on the epidemiology of alcoholism and alcohol-related problems. We do not provide services, but we conduct health services research targeted to improve services. During NIAAA's history, researchers have made much progress in understanding why some people develop a pathological appetite for alcohol. A benchmark in the history of alcoholism research was the demonstration that for many people, susceptibility to alcoholism is inherited. Population-based studies, twin and adoption studies, and animal studies all confirm that there is a genetic component in the risk for alcoholism. But environment plays a role—maybe a great or even greater role—and these factors interact. In addition, many individuals who are not clinically alcohol dependent have many alcohol-related problems. Interventions for these problems that bring individuals into contact with health and social service systems were the focus of the conference, and became the focus of this book.

NIAAA-supported research has led to many advances in what we know about causes, consequences, treatment, and prevention of alcohol abuse and alcoholism. We now have a more complete understanding of the toxicology of alcohol in the brain, heart, liver, marrow, and, especially in the developing fetus. We now know from our controlled trials in prevention that establishing mutually reinforcing community interventions can significantly reduce nighttime traffic accidents and visits to the emergency room. This is significant because many countries, including the United States, have spent vast amounts of money on prevention programs developed mostly by intuition and plausibility and frequently accomplishing little. Moreover, we now know from our treatment research efforts that behavioral interventions for alcohol problems, among them Motivational Interviewing; Cognitive Behavioral Therapy; Brief Intervention; and Twelve-Step Facilitation, can result in meaningful reductions in alcohol problems. Finally, we now know from our work on the organization and financing of alcohol services—conducted under the auspices of our health services research program—that protocols for identifying and treating alcohol problems *can* be successfully integrated into medical settings—especially in emergency rooms and in the offices of primary care physicians.

This meeting brought some of the leaders in alcohol research and treatment from the U.S. and other countries. The meeting helped to exchange information, gain a perspective, and further the knowledge base in addressing alcohol abuse and dependence. We certainly realize that what has been found to be effective and appropriate in the United States may not be acceptable or appropriate in other countries. In fact, one of the values of international exchanges of information is in the fact that the U.S. is not a homogenous population and what works in other countries may inform our approaches to sub-populations and cultures within America. This has certainly been the case in addressing fetal alcohol syndrome and the results of prenatal alcohol exposure. In collaborating, we have learned of many similarities and differences in effects and benefitted from the discussion of potential solutions to the problems. We believe it is important to move forward in addressing practical and feasible approaches to alcohol abuse and alcoholism in our international community so that we might free global resources and energies for use on other pressing health concerns.

This conference was the fourth trip for NIAAA staff and scientists to South Africa since 1996 to conduct the business of the Institute in furthering collaborative research efforts and exchanging information. Teams of research scientists and clinicians and practitioners have planned and conducted research projects and prevention and treatment workshops in South Africa and interacted with the researchers and clinicians. So the Institute has been collaborating and we certainly hope, much to our mutual benefit.

There is much work to be done to address the consequences of alcohol abuse, alcohol misuse and alcohol dependence. Alcohol is the number one substance of abuse in the world. The solutions to the alcohol-related problems that we have as a global community can best be addressed by a concerted effort to exchange information, to adapt successful strategies to our individual cultures and environments, and to benefit from the results of collaborative studies. This volume is an important step in that direction.

Faye J. Calhoun, D.P.A., M.S.
Director, Office of Collaborative Research

Robert B. Huebner, Ph.D.
Deputy Director, Division of Clinical and Prevention Research

National Institute on Alcohol Abuse and Alcoholism
National Institutes of Health, Bethesda, Maryland

Preface

The presence of addictive behaviors in health and social systems is a topic of worldwide concern. The scope of alcohol and other drug problems far exceeds the reach of specialist systems, even in countries where such systems are well developed. As this book documents, alcohol and drug problems are related to numerous health and social problems that bring individuals into contact with health care, spcoa, welfare, and criminal justice systems. In addition, individuals with substance use problems are found in such institutions as schools and the workplace. This raises the important practical opportunity of addressing these problems "where they are." Further, it is far more difficult to treat more severe problems of addiction than those which are less advanced. Often before an individual's problems become severe enough to treat within a specialty system, he or she has had numerous alcohol-and-drug related contacts with health and social service systems.

The book focuses on key strategies to address addictive behaviors effectively and efficiently through existing health and social service institutions. The chapters of this book also reflect a commitment to the application of evidence-based practice across the various settings addressed. The book was also shaped by the challenge of developing culturally relevant community level interventions for a wide array of indigenous organizations. Chapters in the first section discuss the scope of alcohol and drug problems across community institutions and question traditional paradigms of what treatment is, where it should be located, and how it should be evaluated. The remaining chapters discuss the inter-relationship of alcohol and drug problems with other health, mental health, and social agencies. They address both organizational and clinical issues, including opportunities and barriers related to developing appropriate screening, assessment, and interventions across a wide range of formal and informal community services.

This book arose from an international conference, and benefited from the quality of the discussions, as well as the diversity and collective energy of the participants. The authors reworked conference presentations into chapters of an integrated volume, reflecting the exchange of international information that occurred. It is clear that the field has far to go in developing mainstream approaches which address alcohol and drug problems where they naturally occur. However, we see it as one of the most pressing issues for the field, and one that needs to draw from the experiences of individuals working and conducting research in culturally relevant settings. This book is an important step in stimulating that collaboration. Alcohol and drug problems are indeed addressable in diverse settings around the world, and it is exciting and crucial that we begin to learn from each other and develop new paradigms that help us to think about treatment, where to locate it, and ultimately how to assess and evaluate its effectiveness.

Constance Weisner, Dr. P.H. and
William R. Miller, Ph.D.

Acknowledgments

This collection of papers by experts in alcohol and drug studies was developed for the Ninth International Conference on Treatment of Addictive Behaviours (ICTAB), September 21–25, 2000, in Cape Town, South Africa. Contributors from around the world gathered to discuss the theme "Addressing Addictive Behaviors through Health and Social Systems." Substance abuse is a field of growing importance to sub-Saharan Africa, as well as other regions of the world. That the setting was South Africa, a county facing critical substance abuse-related issues with enthusiasm and new approaches, helped keep the focus on "real life" issues faced by community professionals and agencies. Conference presenters and attendees came from Africa, Europe, Asia, and the U.S. From South Africa, representatives from government agencies, universities, specialty alcohol and drug treatment agencies, the welfare system, the criminal justice system, and the health system attended.

The conference was organized by the University of New Mexico Center on Alcoholism, Substance Abuse, and Addictions (CASAA). It was supported and co-sponsored by the U.S. National Institute on Alcohol Abuse and Alcoholism (NIAAA). The government of South Africa was represented through its Ministry of Health. We are grateful, too, to conference co-chairs, Dr. Stephen Rollnick of the University of Wales, and Dr. Solomon Rataemane of the University of the Free State, South Africa. All royalties from this book are being donated to the South African National Council on Alcoholism and Drug Dependence.

Contents

CHANGING SUBSTANCE ABUSE THROUGH HEALTH AND SOCIAL SYSTEMS

PART A

Three Questions

This is likely to be a controversial book. The authors collectively argue, in essence, that while there is a role for addiction treatment settings, it is hopeless to rely on specialist treatment as a primary remedy for these complex societal problems. It is noteworthy that the authors include clinicians who have been prominent in developing and evaluating addiction treatment methods. This volume represents something of a turning point in thinking about social approaches for addressing substance abuse and dependence.

This first section consists of three chapters that set the stage for the rest of the book. Each raises a broad question, reviewing research findings that point to answers. In Chapter 1, Editor Constance Weisner examines the daunting international scope of health and social problems related to alcohol, tobacco, and other drug use. So broad is the impact that, aware of it or not, virtually all health and social service systems are already working with substantial levels of substance abuse and dependence among those they serve. This is particularly so in health care and criminal justice systems.

Editor William Miller then asks, in Chapter 2, whether "treatment" is actually the right way of thinking about how to address alcohol/drug problems. He integrates research on natural history, treatment outcomes, and psychosocial correlates of substance use problems, to question the conception that the appropriate way to address addictions is by treating them as an individual disorder.

Finally, Thomas McLellan compares the course and treatment of drug addiction to that of chronic diseases such as hypertension, diabetes, and cancer, making the case that society's expectations for drug abuse programs have been inordinately high and broad. He compares the merits and costs of treatment with those of other possible societal responses such as incarceration, and questions whether acute treatment is a viable model for addressing addictions.

CHAPTER 1

What is the Scope of the Problem and its Impact on Health and Social Systems?

CONSTANCE WEISNER

INTRODUCTION

Throughout the world, alcohol and drug problems are costly to societies and the health and social functioning of their citizens. In the early 1980's, the World Health Assembly identified problems related to alcohol consumption as "among the world's major public health concerns" (Jernigan, Monteiro, Room & Saxena, 2000). Since then, alcohol and drug use has increased in both developed and developing countries. As an introduction for the chapters which follow, this chapter provides a brief overview of the scope and cost of alcohol and drug problems in various parts of the world, discusses the limited capacity of specialty alcohol and drug agencies to treat them, and presents a case study which illustrates the impact of alcohol and drug problems on community agencies. A very sensible approach, emphasized throughout this book, is to implement prevention and treatment interventions within health and social agencies where individuals with these problems are naturally found, rather than focusing scarce resources in specialty settings that see far fewer individuals. Primary health care and criminal justice agencies deserve particular attention in this regard.

THE EXTENT AND COST OF PROBLEMS

Much of the work assessing the nature and extent of problems internationally has come from studies or workgroups convened by the World Health

CONSTANCE WEISNER • Department of Psychiatry, University of California, San Francisco, California 94143

Organization (WHO). WHO's study on the Global Burden of Disease found that 3.5% of world-wide loss of disability-adjusted life-years was attributable to alcohol, 2.6% to tobacco, and another .6% to illegal drugs (Jernigan et al., 2000, Murray & Lopez, 1996). A ranking of countries by 1996 per capita alcohol consumption found that developed countries, particularly Europe and the U.S., had generally the highest levels of consumption (Hurst, Gregory & Gussman, 1997).

However, the production and distribution of alcohol have become a global industry. The increased consumption of developing countries (Hurst et al., 1997, Jernigan et al., 2000), when considered with the high consumption of already developed countries is an indication that substance abuse problems may increase sharply as countries develop (Riley & Marshall, 1999). An analysis of trends in Asia, Central and South America, and sub-Saharan Africa found that economic development increased buying power, and that was associated with increased alcohol consumption and harm (Jernigan et al., 2000). The report identified Latin America as the developing region most at risk, with alcohol problems related to almost 10% of the disability-adjusted life years lost (Jernigan & Indran, 1999). Rates in Mexico, Peru, Chile, Venezuela were almost as high as the U.S.

Illicit drug use has traditionally been a large problem in Europe, the U.S., and Asia (WHO Expert Committee on Drug Dependence, 1998). It has been studied most comprehensively in Europe and the U.S. Cannabis has been, and continues to be, the particular substance most available and most used in the European Union and United States (National Institute on Drug Abuse, 1989). In the European Union amphetamines and ecstasy are the drugs next most commonly used, with cocaine and heroin use rising (European Monitoring Centre for Drugs and Drug Addiction, 2000). In the U.S., use of cannabis, cocaine, hallucinogens, and nonmedical use of psychotherapeutics are most common, with large variations across regions of the country. For example, methamphetamine use has had higher prevalence on the west coast and cocaine in the eastern cities (National Institute on Drug Abuse, 1989). In Asia, opiates have traditionally been considered a larger problem than alcohol. Currently, there are alarming trends in non-medical use of psychotherapeutics, such as benzodiazepines (WHO Expert Committee on Drug Dependence, 1998).

The estimates of overall costs of substance abuse to society are high. For example, in the U.S. the cost of alcohol, drugs, and smoking was estimated to be $428 billion in 1995 (Rice, 1999). In Latin America, in 1996, WHO and the World Bank estimated that alcohol accounted for 9.6% of the total cost burden of all disease (Medina-Mora, Carlini-Cotrim & Madrigal, 2000). For South Africa, estimates of alcohol-related costs (not including drugs) have been over 2% of the GNP, or around $1.7 billion per year (Parry & Bennetts, 1999).

Consumption rates and alcohol-related problems also vary within countries. A 1985 study in China found rates of alcohol dependence to range from 5% to 35% across provinces (Yanyi, 1992). A recent WHO study examined consumption patterns in eight countries: Brazil, India, Malaysia, Mexico, Nigeria, Papua New Guinea, South Africa, and Zimbabwe. It found increased availability of alcohol and increased consumption with related problems in all these countries over the last decade. Significantly, diverse population groups have been affected (Marshall & Riley, 1999). For example, in Zimbabwe, alcohol consumption by women has greatly increased, and of particular concern is increased consumption by young people (Jernigan, 1999). South Africa represents a common trend; men continue to have the highest levels of consumption and problems, but women's consumption is also rising, as is that of youth, of those in specific occupations, such as the mining industry, and those living in urban areas (Parry & Bennetts, 1999). Studies of secondary students in Zimbabwe found problems with alcohol, cannabis, tobacco, and inhalants, though there were important differences between urban and rural students, and also differences by socio-economic and cultural group (Eide & Acuda, 1995, 1996). In sub-Saharan Africa, Asia and India, new health problems are developing, and new populations are using alcohol and drugs (Hao & Young, 2000, Jernigan & Indran, 1999, Saxena, 2000, Yanyi, 1992).

Critical social and health problems are increasingly attributed to substance use, including HIV-AIDS, hepatitis B, hepatitis C, tuberculosis, neonatal defects, violence and other crime, homelessness, and welfare dependency (Bennett, Campillo, Chandrashekar & Gureje, 1998, European Monitoring Centre for Drugs and Drug Addiction, 2000, National Institute on Alcohol Abuse and Alcoholism, 1997, Weisner, Mertens, Parthasarathy & Moore, 2001). The health sector bears a main burden of handling problems. In South Africa, 25–30% of hospital admissions are estimated to be associated with alcohol and drug use (Albertyn & McCann, 1993 cited in Parry & Bennetts, 1999), for general trauma cases, rates of 38% were found in urban areas and 49% in rural (Parry & Bennetts, 1999). Rates of fetal alcohol syndrome are also rising (Parry & Bennetts, 1999). In Zimbabwe health problems related to consumption are becoming more prominent the WHO study found drinkers to have higher rates of sexually transmitted diseases (STD's), work related injuries, and traffic accidents (Chinyadza et al., 1993 cited in Jernigan, 1999). Chinyadza and colleagues' survey (Jernigan, 1999) also showed frequent heavy drinking among those using primary care centers.

Increased health and other problems are also of concern in Asian countries. In India, rates of health problems related to substance use, including cancer, accidents and injuries, neuropsychiatric disorders, toxicities from impurities and adulterants, nutritional deficiencies, and infections (including alarming rates of increase of HIV) have increased (Saxena, 2000). Thus, with consumption increasing in many countries, and the relation of heavy consumption and drug use to health and social functioning, important questions arise as to whether the substance abuse specialty system is the most efficient and effective community response.

THE CAPACITY OF TREATMENT SYSTEMS: WHERE SHOULD TREATMENT BE PLACED?

Given the extent of the problem across countries, it is almost impossible to provide sufficient treatment with specialty services. The largest capacity and broadest range of services are found in Western Europe and the U.S. (Klingemann, Takala & Hunt, 1992), but even there, services are inadequate. In developing countries, specialty treatment systems are small and often located only in urban areas. It is unrealistic to think that they can serve the large numbers of people needing services (World Health Organization Programme on Substance Abuse, 1993b,c).

Although the prevalence of alcohol and drug-related problems is high, not many people are finding, or seeking, specialty treatment (European Monitoring Centre for Drugs and Drug Addiction, 2000, WHO Expert Committee on Drug Dependence, 1998, World Health Organization Programme on Substance Abuse, 1993a). Rather, because of the relationship between alcohol and other health and social problems, problem drinkers are found across a variety of community agencies (Institute of Medicine, 1990).

When we look at the agencies and institutions where these health and social problems are taking individuals, we have a strong argument for placing substance abuse screening and intervention services in health, criminal justice and social welfare agencies, in occupational settings and educational settings, and in non-governmental organizations and voluntary agencies (Gureje, 2000, World Health Organization Programme on Substance Abuse, 1993c). The WHO's Regional Committee for Europe developed a European Alcohol Action Plan as a possible model for other regions. Its goals were: "To ensure accessibility of effective treatment and rehabilitation services, including those integrated into primary health care settings, with trained personnel, for people with hazardous, harmful and dependent alcohol consumption and members of their family" and "To enhance the capacity for society to deal with alcohol through the training of professionals in different sectors such as those of health, social welfare, education and the judiciary, along with the strengthening of community development and leadership" (Jernigan et al., 2000).

In many countries it will be a challenge to accommodate alcohol and drug services in community agencies. Countries such as India use the primary care system to treat the broad spectrum of health problems, including alcohol and drugs, but their clinicians lack training in substance abuse and are overburdened with treating other medical problems. Alcohol-related problems remain largely unaddressed across most countries (Saxena, 2000, WHO Expert Committee on Drug Dependence, 1998). Despite these difficulties, a number of factors call for us to take a community perspective in addressing the rapid increase in alcohol and drug problems in most of the world. Treatment availability is generally inadequate, especially in developing countries, and there are population groups who have limited access in all countries. Everywhere, alcohol and drug problems are associated with many other health and social problems which are addressed in a variety of community agencies and institutions. The following case study, as well as the WHO studies discussed above, illustrate the importance of broadening our perspective where treatment should be placed, and of investinging treatment resources within these agencies.

A CASE EXAMPLE

The case study is from the Community Epidemiology Laboratory (CEL) in a northern California county (Weisner & Schmidt, 1995a). In the United States a county is a subdivision of a state, and health and social services are usually organized at the county level. The northern California county was selected because of its diversity in population characteristics, its mix of rural and urban areas, and it generalizability to other U.S. counties on the relationship between alcohol consumption and problems. Importantly, it was the U.S. site in the World Health Organization's Study of Community Response to Alcohol-Related Problems (Roizen, 1983). The county has a population of about 900,000, is heterogeneous in its urban/rural and ethnicity characteristics, and has a typical array of health and social services (Greenfield & Weisner, 1995, Schmidt, Weisner & Wiley, 1998, Weisner, 1992, Weisner & Schmidt, 1995a).

The project studied community agency systems where prior research had identified the presence of people with alcohol and drug problems (Institute of Medicine, 1990, Weisner, 1987). It studied alcohol and drug agencies (Caetano & Weisner, 1988, Weisner, 1988), mental health agencies (Schmidt & Roizen, 1988), emergency rooms (Cherpitel, 1988), primary health care clinics (Cherpitel, 1989), welfare agencies (Schmidt, 1991), and criminal justice agencies (Roizen, 1991). The project sampled these systems at their entry points; i.e. in the welfare study the sample included the seven district agencies where applications for welfare are taken, and the criminal justice system was sampled at the one facility where arrest "bookings" were processed and through which individuals entered other parts of the system. The studies used a two-stage design: the first level of sampling in each system covered the full spectrum of eligible publicly owned or contracted services; the second level covered all consecutive new admissions, or every "nth" admission. In-person, structured interviews were conducted by trained interviewers independent of the agencies, by the third day for residential services and by the third visit for outpatient services. This analysis is based on the public agencies only. In addition, a county population survey was conducted (Trocki & Roizen, 1993, Weisner & Schmidt, 1995a). It was a two-stage area probability sample of households in the county in which census blocks were the first selection stratum and households the second. Each study included in-person structured interviews by trained interviewers independent of the agencies.

The project used a core of comparable measures across studies. Problem-drinking status was defined as meeting two of the following criteria during the previous year: drinking 5 or more drinks per day at least once a month, at least one serious alcohol-related social consequence, and at least one alcohol dependence symptom (dependence measured by DSM-III-R alcohol dependence criteria). Problem drug status was defined as weekly drug use, which was measured by the use of any one type of drug (out of nine) at least weekly during the previous year. The operationalization of the criteria are described in several publications; for example, problem drinking (Weisner & Schmidt, 1995a), alcohol dependence (Weisner, 2001), and weekly drug use (Weisner & Schmidt, 1995b). Data within each sample are weighted to adjust for the sampling fraction, response rate, and fieldwork agency for a 24-week period in each agency (Tam, 1997).

Prevalence of Alcohol and Drug Problems within Community Agencies

Table 1 presents the proportion of problem drinkers, alcohol dependent individuals, and drug users in the general population, and entering each agency system. The general population and health agency samples have similar rates of 15% or less. The welfare, mental health, criminal justice, and drug treatment samples have relatively high proportions of problem drinkers (ranging from 24% to 53%). Although rates for alcohol dependence are understandably lower than for problem drinking, the distribution across systems is similar to that for problem drinking. Rates for weekly drug use for the welfare sample are higher than for the alcohol measures, but otherwise they fall between the two measures and follow a similar pattern across agencies.

Prevalence of Alcohol and Drug Problems within a Community Context

Although Table 1 illustrates the "burden" of alcohol and drug disorders within each system, it does not show which community institutions bear the largest overall burden of problems in the community. To do this, weights were also developed to adjust for variation in sampling fractions across the samples; they adjust each sample to represent its respective population of the problem

Table 1 Prevalence of new admissions[1] of selected problem measures across general population and community agency caseloads (in %)

	Problem Drinking[2]	Alcohol Dependence[2]	Weekly Drug Use[3]
General Population	11	2	6
Agency Samples			
Primary Care	15	8	13
Emergency Room	30	14	N/A
Criminal Justice	50	18	44
Welfare	24	11	27
Mental Health	33	17	27

[1] Data are weighted to adjust each sample for variation in agencies sampling fraction, rate, and fieldwork duration.
[2] Data from Weisner, C. "The provision of services for alcohol problems: a community perspective for understanding access" *Journal of Behavioral Health Services Research* 2001;28(2): 130–142.
[3] Data from Weisner, C. and Schmidt, L. (1995) "Expanding the Frame of Health Services Research in the Drug Abuse Field," *Health Services Research* 30(5): 707–726.

being measured (i.e., problem drinking) in the context of the county's community institutions. Thus, in Table 2, data are weighted to appropriately represent problem drinking (or alcohol-dependence or weekly drug use), taking the prevalence of the problem and each system's size into consideration (Tam, 1997). For most systems, the contrast is striking. For example, in examining the total group (gender differences will be described later), while Table 1 showed that public primary health clinics had problem drinking rates of 15% for individuals coming for services, Table 2 shows that they provided services to fully 42% of the problem drinkers entering services in the county during that time. Only about 13% of the county's problem drinkers were entering alcohol or drug treatment agencies.

The question could be asked whether the proportion of problem drinkers in specialty treatment was low because their problems were not sufficiently severe to require those services. The table also examines the more severe cases (those who met criteria for DSM-III-R alcohol dependence) who might be expected to be entering treatment. For these dependent individuals, although more are entering alcohol and drug treatment agencies relative to other types of agencies than was the case for problem drinkers (9% versus 4%), the numbers remain relatively small. The same is true for weekly drug use. The distribution of weekly drug users across systems indicates that only about 7% were in substance abuse specialty agencies. The ordering of community systems for both alcohol dependence and weekly drug use is remarkably similar to that for problem drinking. For those who were alcohol dependent, the proportion in primary care (56%) was substantially higher than in criminal justice (24%) agencies. Fairly equal numbers were in primary care and criminal justice agencies. However, the differences between primary care and criminal justice were not as large for weekly drug use (43% versus 39%). Overall, primary health

Table 2 Distribution of new admissions[1] of selected problem measures[2] in individuals across community agency systems (in %)

	Problem Drinking			Alcohol Dependence			Weekly Drug Use		
	Men	Women	Total[3]	Men	Women	Total	Men	Women	Total[4]
Primary Care	35	60	42	47	73	56	29	64	43
Criminal Justice	51	19	41	31	9	24	54	16	39
Welfare	6	12	8	7	6	7	9	20	11
Alcohol Treatment	5	4	4	10	6	9	3	2	3
Drug Treatment	2	4	2	3	1	2	3	2	3
Mental Health	2	5	3	2	5	3	2	4	3

[1] Data weighed for design effects, non-response, and to a common fieldwork duration so that each agency system sample is shown proportionate to its size.
[2] Problem drinking, alcohol dependence, and weekly drug use rates are calculated over a base of their respective rates across all agency systems.
[3] Data from Weisner, C. "The provision of services for alcohol problems: a community perspective for understanding access" *Journal of Behavioral Health Services Research* 2001;28(2):130–142.
[4] Data from Weisner, C. and Schmidt, L. (1995) "Expanding the Frame of Health Services Research in the Drug Abuse Field," *Health Services Research* 30(5): 707–726.
Percents do not always add to 100 due to rounding error.

and criminal justice handled the largest proportion of individuals with alcohol and drug disorders entering services in the county (over 40% each), while specialty alcohol and drug treatment agencies saw a far lower proportion.

Gender Differences as an Example of Variation in Population Characteristics

These data suggest that it would make sense to screen for substance abuse problems in primary care and criminal justice agencies. However, as discussed earlier, there are indications that important differences exist by gender. We find that in this U.S. county as well. Table 2 shows that problem drinking men are most likely found in the criminal justice system (51%), followed by primary care (35%), while women are most likely to be found in primary health care clinics (60%), followed by criminal justice (19%), and welfare (12%). The results for those who were alcohol-dependent followed the same pattern as for women, with the vast majority (73%) in primary care agencies. Alcohol dependent men were also more likely to be found in primary care settings, but the differences were not so large (47% in primary care and 31% in criminal justice agencies).

For the gender distribution of weekly drug use across community institutions, differences were again large, with primary care handling most of the women (64%) and the criminal justice system most of the men (54%). For women, welfare agencies were second (20%) and criminal justice agencies were third (16%). Almost one-third of the men (29%) were found in primary care clinics. Less than 7% of men and 4% of women were entering substance abuse agencies.

Of note is that these findings are not due to our looking at just one "treatment" episode or window of time; other analyses of these data have shown that even lifetime examinations of utilization patterns do not differ greatly (Tam, Schmidt & Weisner, 1996). From these data, it is clear that more individuals would have an opportunity to receive services if they were provided within the context of the larger community response to health and social problems.

LOCATING SUBSTANCE ABUSE INTERVENTIONS IN HEALTH AND SOCIAL SERVICE SYSTEMS

The WHO studies have shown that alcohol and drug problems are of concern throughout much of the world, that they are related to many health and social problems, and that resources to develop specialty treatment systems to meet that need are not available. The California example illustrates that even in a country with a rather extensive treatment system, few individuals with substance abuse problems enter specialty treatment. However, because of their substance abuse-related problems, these individuals encounter a wide range of health and human service organizations.

In light of these real-life conditions across countries, putting the priority on developing specialty substance abuse programs seems daunting and even shortsighted. A more pragmatic approach would be to "mainstream" services, i.e., place services in the institutions where people with such problems are naturally found. Because of the large differences by gender and type of problem, different population groups might be targeted across settings. For example, in the U.S., screening women in primary care appears to be particularly important, while, the reverse is true for men in the criminal justice system. The literature described above suggests that these differences are also found, and perhaps even accentuated, across cultures and countries. Specific patterns will vary, however. For example, Bennett and colleagues in summarizing findings from the eight country WHO study pointed out that screening for alcohol problems among women would be more relevant in Mexico and Nigeria than in India (Bennett et al., 1998). The international literature would suggest that other institutions, such as secondary schools, are important settings for identifying adolescents.

A further benefit of incorporating screening and interventions within health, criminal justice and other institutional settings may be the reduced stigma attached to receiving help. A WHO study found that substance abuse problems were stigmatized across all the countries studied. (Room, Rehm, Trotter, Paglia & Üstün, 2001). The eight-country study found differences in cultural understanding and responses to "dependence" and its symptom criteria (Schmidt & Room, 1999). These studies suggest that screening for inappropriate consumption levels within community settings, rather than focusing on primary disorders, may reduce stigma and avoid cultural barriers in definitions and interpretations. Such an approach increases the potential for reaching individuals earlier, before their problems become more complex and more difficult to treat.

Thus, addressing problems in health and social service systems is practical because that is where individuals with such problems present. It also has a potential for larger social impact. Importantly, the strategies that many countries have developed in adapting services to indigenous institutions need to be taken seriously. These approaches often are targeted toward the larger community rather than individuals. (See examples of services in Bolivia, Peru, Mexico, India, and Sri Lanka (World Health Organization Programme on Substance Abuse, 1993c).

In addition, screening instruments are available for use in primary care, some of which have been developed in a cross-cultural context. For example, the Alcohol Use Disorders Identification Test (AUDIT) was developed and validated in six countries for identification of alcohol problems in primary care settings (World Health Organization Programme on Substance Abuse, 1993a). Developing culturally relevant interventions to follow such screening are important next steps.

Subsequent chapters present an overview of substance abuse treatment and evaluation, and models for screening and interviewing in different community systems. Chapter 2 examines conceptions of alcohol and drug abuse treatment in light of natural history, treatment outcomes, and psychosocial correlates of substance use problems. In so doing, it questions whether the appropriate way to address such problems is by treating them as individual disorders. The following chapter examines ways of evaluating addictions treatment within the context of a chronic disease model. A section on intervening through health care systems follows, with a discussion of linkages of alcohol, tobacco, and other drug abuse to public health problems. The chapters in this section examine intervening through primary care clinics, through emergency and trauma services, through specialist clinics, and pharmacy services. The case of tobacco is considered separately from alcohol and drugs.

Issues related to intervening through mental health services are addressed in the next section, with chapters devoted to the relationship of mental health and substance use disorders and integrating services for dual diagnosis patients. The last section, on intervening through social systems, examines the relationships between substance abuse and other social problems, including social welfare systems, school systems, correctional systems, the workplace, religious organizations, social support networks, and among displaced peoples. The book concludes with a focus on the need for evidence-based policy, prevention and treatment.

ACKNOWLEDGMENTS

Data collection and preparation of this manuscript were supported by National Institute on Alcohol Abuse, National Center Grant AA05595 and R37AA10359. Study directors participating in the Community Epidemiology Laboratory studies were Raul Caetano, M.D. Ph.D.; Cheryl Cherpitel, Dr. P.H.; Denise Herd, Ph.D.; Ron Roizen, Ph.D.; Laura Schmidt, Ph.D.; Karen Trocki, Ph.D.; and Constance Weisner, Dr.P.H. The author wishes to acknowledge Helen Matzger, M.P.H. for programming and literature review work and Agatha Hinman, B.A. for editorial assistance.

Part of the data for Tables 1 and 2 are from: Weisner, C. and Schmidt, L. (1995) "Expanding the Frame of Health Services Research in the Drug Abuse Field," *Health Services Research* 30(5): 707–726, and are reprinted with the permission of the Health Research and Educational Trust, copyright 1995. Data for Tables 1 and 2 are also drawn from: Weisner, C. (2001) *Journal of Behavioral Health Services & Research*, "The Provision of Services for Alcohol Problems: A Community Perspective for Understanding Access, 28(2): 130–142.

REFERENCES

Bennett, L. A., Campillo, C., Chandrashekar, C. R. & Gureje, O. (1998). Alcoholic beverage consumption in India, Mexico, and Nigeria. *Alcohol Health & Research World* 22(4), 243–252.

Caetano, R. & Weisner, C. (1988). Technical report for the study of dimensions of dependence. Alcohol Research Group.

Cherpitel, C. J. (1988). Technical report for Contra Costa County casualty (Emergency Room and Coronor's Office). Alcohol Research Group.

Cherpitel, C. J. (1989). Technical Report for Primay Care Study, Technical Report. Alcohol Research Group.

Eide, A. H. & Acuda, S. W. (1995). Drug use among secondary school students in Zimbabwe. *Addiction* 90, 1517–1527.

Eide, A. H. & Acuda, S. W. (1996). Cultural orientation and adolescents' alcohol use in Zimbabwe. *Addiction* 91(6), 807–814.

European Monitoring Centre for Drugs and Drug Addiction. (2000). *2000 Annual Report on the State of the Drugs Problem in the European Union*. European Monitoring Centre for Drugs and Drug Addiction, Lisbon, Portugal.

Greenfield, T. K. & Weisner, C. (1995). Drinking problems and self-reported criminal behavior, arrests and convictions: 1990 U.S. alcohol and 1989 county surveys. *Addiction* 90(3), 361–373.

Gureje, O. (2000). Alcohol problems and responses: challenges for Africa. *Journal of Substance Use* 5, 56–61).

Hao, W. & Young, D. (2000). Drinking patterns and problems in China. *Journal of Substance Use* 5, 71–78).

Hurst, W., Gregory, E. & Gussman, T. (1997). International survey: alcoholic beverage taxation and control policies. Brewers Association of Canada.

Institute of Medicine. (1990). *Broadening the base of treatment for alcohol problems*. National Academy Press, Washington, D.C.

Jernigan, D. H. (1999). Country profile on alcohol in Zimbabwe. In: *Alcohol and Public Health in 8 Developing Countries* (edited by Riley, L. & Marshall, M.). World Health Organization, Geneva, 157–175.

Jernigan, D. H. & Indran, S. K. (1999). Country profile on alcohol in Malaysia. In: *Alcohol and Public Health in 8 Developing Countries* (edited by Riley, L. & Marshall, M.). World Health Organization, Geneva, 61–73.

Jernigan, D. H., Monteiro, M., Room, R. & Saxena, S. (2000). Towards a global alcohol policy: alcohol, public health and the role of WHO. *Bulletin of the World Health Organization* 78(4), 491–499.

Klingemann, H., Takala, J. P. & Hunt, G. (1992). *Cure, care or control: alcoholism treatment in sixteen countries*. State University of New York Press, Albany, NY.

Marshall, M. & Riley, L. (1999). Introduction. In: *Alcohol and Public Health in 8 Developing Countries* (edited by Riley, L. & Marshall, M.). World Health Organization, Geneva, 5–12.

McCrady, B. S. & Miller, W. R. (1993). Research on Alcoholics Anonymous: Opportunities and alternatives. Rutgers Center of Alcohol Studies, New Brunswick, NJ.

Medina-Mora, M. E., Carlini-Cotrim, B. & Madrigal, E. (2000). Alcohol policies in developing countries: Latin America. *Journal of Substance Use* 5, 47–55.

Mertens, J., Weisner, C. & Sterling, S. (2001). Disparities across treatment settings for the medically indigent: implications for substance abuse screening and interventions. *FrontLines* June, 6;8.

Murray, C. J. L. & Lopez, A. D. (1996). Quantifying the burden of disease and injury attributable to ten major risk factors. In: *The global burden of disease: a comprehensive assessment of mortality and disability from diseases, injuries, and risk factors in 1990 and projected to 2020* (edited by Murray, C. J. L. & Lopez, A. D.) 1. Published by the Harvard School of Public Health on behalf of the World Health Organization and the World Bank, Cambridge, MA, 295–324.

National Institute on Alcohol Abuse and Alcoholism. (1997). Alcohol and health: ninth special report to the U.S. Congress. U.S. Department of Health and Human Services, Rockville, MD.

National Institute on Drug Abuse. (1989). *National Household Survey on Drug Abuse: Population estimates 1988*. National Institute on Drug Abuse, Rockville, MD.

Parry, C. D. H. & Bennetts, A. L. (1999). Country profile on alcohol in South Africa. In: *Alcohol and Public Health in 8 Developing Countries* (edited by Riley, L. & Marshall, M.). World Health Organization, Geneva, 135–156.

Rice, D. P. (1999). Economic costs of substance abuse, 1995. *Proceedings of the Association of American Physicians* 111(2), 119–125.

Riley, L. & Marshall, M. (1999). Alcohol and Public Health in 8 Developing Countries. World Health Organization, Geneva, 179.

Roizen, R. (1983). Alcohol dependence symptoms in cross-cultural perspective: a report of findings from the World Health Organization Study of Community Response to Alcohol-Related Problems, symposium on cross-cultural studies of drinking problems, Farmington, Connecticut.

Roizen, R. (1991). Contra Costa County jail study of the Community Epidemiology Laboratory project: technical report. Alcohol Research Group.

Room, R., Rehm, J., Trotter, R. T. I., Paglia, A. & Üstün, B. (2001). Cross-cultural views on stigma, valuation, parity and societal values towards disability. In: *Disability and Culture: Universalism and diversity* (edited by Üstün, B., Chatterji, S., Bickenbach, J. E., Trotter, R. T. I., Room, R., Rehm, J. & Saxena, S.). Hogrefe and Huber, Seattle, WA, 247–291.

Saxena, S. (2000). Alcohol problems and responses: challenges for India. *Journal of Substance Abuse* 5, 62–70.

Schmidt, L. (1991). Technical report: 1989 Community Epidemiology Laboratory survey of welfare recipients. Alcohol Research Group.

Schmidt, L. & Roizen, R. (1988). Technical Report: Contra Costa County mental health client study of the Community Epidemiology Laboratory Project. Alcohol Research Group.

Schmidt, L. & Room, R. (1999). Cross-cultural applicability in international classifications and research on alcohol dependence. *Journal of Studies on Alcohol* 60(4), 448–462.

Schmidt, L. & Weisner, C. (1993). Developments in alcoholism treatment: a ten year review. In: *Recent developments in alcoholism* (edited by Galanter, M.) 11. Plenum, New York, 369–396.

Schmidt, L., Weisner, C. & Wiley, J. (1998). Substance abuse and the course of welfare dependency. *American Journal of Public Health* 88(11), 1616–1622.

Tam, T. (1997). Technical report on the Alcohol Treatment Utilization Study in Public and Private Sectors: within and across sector weights. Alcohol Research Group, Berkeley, CA.

Tam, T., Schmidt, L. & Weisner, C. (1996). Patterns in the institutional encounters of problem drinkers in a community human services network. *Addiction* 91(5), 657–669.

Trocki, K. & Roizen, R. (1993). Technical Report: The Contra Costa County General Population Survey. Alcohol Research Group.

Weisner, C. (1987). The social ecology of alcohol treatment in the U.S. In: *Recent developments in alcoholism* (edited by Galanter, M.) 5. Plenum, New York, 203–243.

Weisner, C. (1988). Community response to substance abuse problems: a survey of clients in drug treatment programs. Alcohol Research Group.

Weisner, C. (1992). The merging of alcohol and drug treatment: a policy review. *Journal of Public Health Policy* 13(1), 66–80.

Weisner, C. (2001). The provision of services for alcohol problems: a community perspective for understanding access. *Journal of Behavioral Health Services Research* 28(2), 130–142.

Weisner, C., Mertens, J., Parthasarathy, S., Moore, C. & Lu, Y. (2001). Integrating primary medical care with addiction treatment: A randomized controlled trial. *Journal of the American Medical Association* 286(14), 1715–1723.

Weisner, C. & Schmidt, L. (1995a). The Community Epidemiology Laboratory: Studying alcohol problems in community and agency-based populations. *Addiction* 90(3), 329–342.

Weisner, C. & Schmidt, L. A. (1995b). Expanding the frame of health services research in the drug abuse field. *Health Services Research* 30(5), 707–727.

WHO Expert Committee on Drug Dependence. (1998). Thirtieth Report [WHO technical report series, No. 873]. World Health Organization, Geneva, Switzerland, 50 p.

World Health Organization Programme on Substance Abuse. (1993a). *Approaches to Treatment of Substance Abuse [an ex-official publication]*. World Health Organization, Geneva, Switzerland.

World Health Organization Programme on Substance Abuse. (1993b). Factors influencing treatment. In: *Approaches to Treatment of Substance Abuse [an ex-official publication]*. World Health Organization, Geneva, Switzerland, 31–45.

World Health Organization Programme on Substance Abuse. (1993c). Generalist responses to alcohol and other drug problems. In: *Approaches to Treatment of Substance Abuse [an ex-official publication]*. World Health Organization, Geneva, Switzerland, 53–67.

Yanyi, Z. (1992). The alcoholism treatment system in China. In: *Cure, Care or Control: Alcoholism treatment in sixteen countries* (edited by Klingemann, H., Takala, J.-P. & Hunt, G.). State University of New York Press, Albany, NY, 269–275.

CHAPTER 2

Is "Treatment" the Right Way to Think about It?

WILLIAM R. MILLER

THE EXPERT MODEL

I come to this chapter, and to the transition in perspective that it reflects, as a clinical psychologist trained in a traditional scientist-practitioner model. My graduate education and thus my early teaching and research focused on individual pathology and its treatment. Both the program from which I received my Ph.D. training and the one in which I have taught for 25 years are accredited by the American Psychological Association, and reflect its model of clinical training: the psychologist learns to recognize and diagnose psychopathology, to assess its manifestations in the individual, to develop a treatment plan (ideally based on empirically supported methods), and to administer treatment interventions appropriate to remove or ameliorate the identified pathology and deficits. In short, most psychologists are trained to be expert physicians of the psyche. Indeed, in the mid-20th century, a heated battle was fought over whether psychotherapy could be provided *only* by medical doctors.

With the discovery of effective medical treatments, the expert model has worked remarkably well in addressing acute medical problems. When experiencing physical symptoms, one goes to a highly-trained expert who asks questions, diagnoses the problem, and prescribes a curative solution. Differential diagnosis is crucial. Bacterial infections call for an appropriate antibiotic whereas viral infections do not. Cancers warrant specific interventions to cure them, or at least to extend and improve the quality of life, with specific tumors responding differentially to various treatment options. Broken bones are treated differently from muscle sprains, pneumonia from tuberculosis.

WILLIAM R. MILLER • Department of Psychology, University of New Mexico, Albuquerque, New Mexico 87131

These and other health problems, however, are strongly linked to lifestyle, environment, and volitional behavior. Diet and exercise patterns profoundly affect the incidence and course of hypertension, diabetes, and heart disease. Smoking causes a host of disabling diseases and some of the most lingering and painful ways to die. The link to lifestyle and behavior is by no means limited to chronic diseases. Burns and traumatic injuries are associated with risk-taking, drinking, and smoking. These lifestyle-behavioral factors (and our failure to address them) contribute to enormous health and social costs.

The expert model of psychotherapy represents a straightforward extension of the acute care medical model to the management of problems in living. In its most extreme form, the person is removed from the community for a period of time and treated in a specialist environment such as an inpatient ward or residential program. The implication would seem to be that curative or remedial treatment can be administered to the individual apart from his or her normal context, much as a malfunctioning automobile is brought into a garage for repair before being returned to the street. To be sure there are other (e.g., protective) uses of inpatient care, but historically in the treatment of psychosocial problems in general and substance use problems in particular, treatment has been usually thought of as correctively delivered to the individual, or sometimes to the family system.

Certainly such an expert model dominated the treatment of addictive behaviors in many nations during the latter half of the 20th century. Its essential tenets, often implicit and assumed as true, included:

1. *Addictions require formal treatment.* The assumption is that addictions rarely if ever remit if left untreated. U.S. television commercials of the period, advertising inpatient hospital programs, implied that the only alternative to formal treatment was continued deterioration and death.
2. *Loss of control is fundamental.* The problem lies within the individual, who is incapable of making responsible choices, and therefore the person's own wishes and preferences must be over-ridden, often through coerced treatment.
3. *Treatment works.* Treatment must be provided by experts with specialized knowledge of how properly to handle addictions. Only certain approaches are effective, and these differ dramatically from the manner in which other problems can be treated.
4. *Intensity of treatment is crucial.* More is better than less, and the optimal is intensive inpatient or residential treatment for several months or more.

Consider the case of a city in New Mexico, bordering on Indian country, and widely acknowledged as having some of the highest rates of alcohol-related problems, illnesses, violence, and mortality in the nation. Seeking to deal with the problem, the city engaged expert consultants from a distant state to recommend remedies. The costly report in essence recommended ringing the city with specialist inpatient treatment programs, to which affected individuals could be mandated. Great societal problems, it seemed, call for massive expansion of specialist treatment and suspension of normal civil liberties.

PUZZLING FINDINGS

What does research have to say about this expert model of treatment? There are some encouraging findings, to be sure. In both randomized trials and naturalistic studies, people who receive treatment typically fare much better than those who do not. As a rule, the longer people stay in treatment, the better they do. At least in the treatment of alcohol use disorders, the long-term outcomes are rather good: most people show substantial improvement (Miller, Walters & Bennett, 2001). Yet over the course of three decades of treatment research, I have also encountered some consistent findings that troubled me, and have caused me to rethink the expert-technical model in which I was trained.

Natural Recovery

One of these is the prevalence of *natural recovery*, meaning remission without the benefit of formal treatment. We take this for granted with regard to smoking: many people who quit tobacco do so on their own, and those who seek formal treatment for smoking cessation comprise a relatively small and nonrepresentative subset of smokers. The epidemiological data indicate that the same is true for alcohol. Given the sheer number of people with alcohol problems at any given time (usually 9–10% in the U.S.) in relation to treatment admissions, a rather small percentage receive formal treatment. Yet over time, people tend to migrate out of alcohol problems, and do so through a wide variety of routes (Fletcher, 2001). In longitudinal studies, a significant proportion of those with alcohol problems at Time 1 no longer show them at Time 2, and the difference is relatively independent of treatment-seeking (Vaillant, 1995). Research on the transtheoretical model of change indicates that the stages and processes through which people pass in escaping from addictive behaviors are the same in treatment and in natural recovery (Prochaska, DiClemente & Norcross, 1992). There are also sudden, permanent transformational changes that occur in a dramatic moment of insight or epiphany (Miller & C'de Baca, 2001). Such stories of quantum change are often heard in Alcoholics Anonymous meetings, though few seem to occur within the context of formal treatment. All of this underlines the fact that despite the well-documented benefits of treatment, much, even most change in addictive behaviors occurs without formal assistance from a helping professional.

Effective Control Groups

I was also puzzled, in my early clinical trials, by the repeated finding that problem drinkers in our "control" groups, who were given a single session of encouraging advice and some take-home self-help materials, showed about as much improvement as those randomly assigned to receive outpatient treatment (see Miller, 2000 for a review). This led us to explore the literature on brief interventions for alcohol problems, where we found that across many studies conducted in a dozen nations, a session or two of some form of counseling was significantly better than no counseling at all (Bien, Miller & Tonigan, 1993). That is, reductions in drinking and related problems seemed to be triggered by just a brief course of counseling or advice. A little treatment is better than no treatment. The interventions were far too brief to imagine that they were providing significant education, insight, or skill training, let alone personality change. We also noticed, as we collected weekly drinking data during outpatient treatment programs, that most of the change in drinking behavior occurred with the first few sessions (Miller, 2000).

Lack of a Dose Effect

If treatment works, then it is reasonable to expect that more treatment should be better. Not so in clinical trials. Often brief counseling and more extended treatment yield similar outcomes (Bien et al., 1993). Clients randomly assigned to inpatient versus outpatient treatment, or to longer versus shorter treatment typically show very similar benefit (Institute of Medicine, 1990; Miller & Hester, 1986; Project MATCH Research Group, 1997). More expensive treatment methods are generally no more effective, and certainly not more cost-effective, than less costly alternatives (Cisler et al., 1998; Holder et al., 1991, 2000). Client *adherence* does predict treatment outcome. Better outcomes are usually seen in clients who attend more treatment sessions or stay longer in treatment, but the same is true for clients who attend more Alcoholics Anonymous meetings, or who more faithfully take their medication (including placebo) and do their homework. More treatment is not necessarily better treatment, but clients with better adherence are more likely to show change.

Lack of Treatment Differences

Perhaps what it takes is more of the *right* treatment. My training led me to a prescriptive-eclectic perspective that specific treatments would be optimal for different disorders. In fact, the evidence for this is slim. In well-designed randomized trials, treatments designed to differ dramatically in content often yield very similar outcomes, a finding that is common in psychotherapy research more generally. The specific theoretical basis or technical content of treatment typically accounts for a rather small proportion of variance in client outcomes.

Perhaps, then, the secret is to match people with the right treatment, instead of looking for main effects of different approaches. A major U.S. multisite research project was predicated on this perspective, drawing on a set of isolated reports of client-treatment matches in the alcohol literature. In the end, very little evidence was found for the importance of matching, and virtually all of the *a priori* hypotheses based on previously reported client-treatment interactions were not confirmed (Project MATCH, 1997).

Failure of Causal Chains

Perhaps studies of aggregate outcomes are insufficient, and what is needed in order to understand treatment is a careful analysis of the causal chains, the underlying mechanisms by which behavior change occurs. For almost any theory of psychotherapy, it is possible to specify a hypothesized chain of events by which change occurs: Treatment A leads to specific Change B, which in turn results in Outcome C. When a causal chain is confirmed, it supports the assertion that the treatment works for the "right" reason. Here again, psychotherapies old and new have commonly failed to yield the expected result. Systematic desensitization, for example, was based on a very specific theory involving the pairing of successive steps in a fear hierarchy with a counter-conditioning response such as relaxation. While desensitization itself yields excellent results in treating phobias, relative to control conditions, process research soon revealed that neither the successive hierarchy nor the relaxation training was essential to its benefit, and "consistent positive results are obtained despite wide variations in procedural details" (Lang, 1969, p. 189). A more recent example is found in eye-movement desensitization and reprocessing (EMDR). Outcome studies have yielded mixed findings, but the specific hypothesized mechanism of action underlying EMDR—namely, certain eye movements—appears to be unrelated to treatment outcomes (Davidson & Parker, 2001). Morgenstern and Longabaugh (2000) reviewed studies of coping skill training, which has an excellent track record in the treatment of alcohol problems, and found no support for the hypothesized mechanism of change: that people acquire better coping skills and thereby avoid problem drinking. In studies that measured intervening variables, either clients never acquired the target skill, or their level of skill acquisition was unrelated to outcomes. Nevertheless the treatment "works."

Therapist Effects

Another piece of the puzzle is that the "same" treatment can have very different outcomes when delivered by different therapists. My own first exposure to this problem involved a study of behavioral self-control training for problem drinkers in which we found no significant differences among treatment groups of varying intensity (Miller, Taylor & West, 1980). What we did find was large differences in the outcomes of clients based on the therapist who treated them. Clients had been randomly assigned to the nine therapists who were ostensibly delivering the same behavioral treatment in this study. Therapist differences in empathy accounted for two-thirds of the variance in clients' 6-month outcomes, and 25% of variance at 24 months (Miller & Baca, 1983). Another research team working at the same time (Valle, 1981) reported similarly large differences in relapse rates within the caseloads of therapists, predictable from their level of interpersonal functioning (including empathy). Level of therapist education and years of experience, in contrast, seem to have little impact on client outcomes. It appears that the therapist to whom one is assigned makes considerably more difference than the specific substance abuse treatment method employed (Najavits & Weiss, 1994).

Extra-Treatment Determinants

Beyond the influence of therapists, client outcomes appear to be substantially determined by other factors having little to do with the specifics of treatment. Moos and his colleagues (1990) found that drinking outcomes were strongly predicted by client factors, particularly attributes of the post-treatment environment to which the client returned. The specific treatment received was a relatively minor determinant of outcomes after taking into account clients' pre-treatment characteristics and post-treatment environment. This also appears to be true in psychotherapy research more generally (Bohart & Tallman, 1999).

Again, none of this negates the fact that treatment for addictive behaviors is generally associated with demonstrable and substantial benefit. The puzzle is that treatment doesn't seem to work in the ways or for the reasons that we often expect. Even relatively brief counseling can trigger behavior change, and a little treatment sometimes works as well as a lot. Treatment methods that appear to be very different often yield similar outcomes. How clients fare, in fact, may be less influenced by the technicalities of treatment than by the therapist who delivers it, or by the life circumstances that surround them outside of treatment, and a great deal of positive change happens without professional help.

THE DEMISE OF SPECIALIST TREATMENT FOR ADDICTIONS

Addiction treatment in the United States from the 1960s through the 1980s was dominated by a for-profit treatment industry delivering time-limited specialist programs. Inpatient treatment consumed a majority of treatment dollars. Certification and licensure programs arose within medicine, counseling, and psychology to demarcate expert specialists qualified to treat addictions. Gradually treatment systems for alcohol versus other drug problems merged, but still remained largely divorced from health care and mental health systems.

Major changes in health care economics in the U.S. changed all this. Decisions about eligibility and need for treatment were transferred from health care professionals to over-arching and often for-profit managerial systems ("managed care"). These systems dramatically cut reimbursement for inpatient and residential treatment, and many such intensive programs were closed. Large public health care systems (such as the Veterans Administration) all but phased out intensive substance abuse units. To decrease costs, treatment decreased dramatically in duration, and shifted from an individual to group therapy focus. Mental health and substance abuse treatment were combined into a domain called "behavioral health."

There were still more sweeping changes in the provision of behavioral health care. Large health care systems hired less educated (and less expensive) providers, and doctoral-level professionals were slowly edged out of delivering psychotherapy. Psychiatrists, many of whom had entered their speciality because of their interest in people and psychotherapy, were largely restricted to 15-minute (or briefer) medication checks. My own profession of psychology, quickly losing its psychotherapy market, is aggressively lobbying for medication prescription privileges, and may follow the same path as our psychiatric colleagues. It is telling that in many U.S. communities, the only place where one can access long-term individual psychotherapy (other than on a self-pay basis) is in clinics training the next generation of psychotherapists.

There is much to decry in a for-profit system of health care where private earnings are enhanced by cutting services. Yet in light of the above research findings, some of the changes that have occurred so rapidly under managed care were warranted. Costly inpatient and residential care had clearly been overused and abused in the U.S., and a shift of emphasis was needed to outpatient services that can reach a larger number of people. There is no persuasive evidence that doctoral-level professionals as therapists produce better outcomes than masters-level clinicians. Length of treatment is not, in itself, a significant determinant of outcome, and we needed a shock to the system to jolt us out of the model that more is always better. Much can be done with even relatively brief counseling.

The prior isolation of substance abuse treatment from other health care systems also had many undesirable aspects. People who need one type of these services often need the others as well. Clinicians are familiar with the problems of bouncing clients around for addiction treatment in one setting, mental health services in another, medical care in yet another (Shavelson, 2001). The sequencing of care is often arbitrary. People with alcohol and other drug problems are also far more likely to turn up in health care and mental health settings than they are to walk through the door of a specialist treatment program. Very little has been done to screen for and address addictive behaviors within health care settings, where a third to a half of all consultations may be the direct or indirect result of substance use disorders. The separate specialist mentality has fostered a "not our problem" perspective among other health care providers, confusing a continuum of care with referral for specialist treatment. Furthermore, the belief that addiction treatment requires a separate, unique approach and expertise unnecessarily dissuaded health care professionals from attempting to address these problems themselves. Nothing in the outcome literature indicates that recovering professionals are any more (or less) effective than those without a personal history of substance abuse, or that specialists are more effective than generalists in treating addictive behaviors.

BEYOND SPECIALIST TREATMENT

Most of this speaks to the North American context, with a history of specialist addiction treatment. In the developing world, health care resources are sufficiently sparse that a separate specialist treatment system for this one class of problems is understandably rare, except for an economically privileged minority. Indeed, there is little to indicate that the 20th century U.S. system of addiction treatment should be envied or emulated elsewhere.

The affluent and developing worlds, albeit for different reasons, share a pressing need to address addictive behaviors through the generalist systems of medical and mental health care, and of social services. In more affluent nations, the isolation of addiction treatment has had adverse effects on coordination of care, as noted above, without yielding any substantial effect on the population frequency of alcohol and drug problems. In the U.S., for example, the societal prevalence of alcohol use disorders is roughly the same as when epidemiological surveys were begun in the late 1960's (Cahalan, 1970). Similarly, the overall outcomes of alcohol treatment, as reflected in large multi-site studies, have not changed appreciably in three decades (Miller et al., 2001). In the developing world, by contrast, there simply is no viable alternative to working through existing health and social systems. There are few resources to develop a separate specialist system of care, nor is there a compelling reason to do so.

Part of the problem is that, at least in the U.S., we have treated addiction as if it were an acute illness, to be addressed via a time-limited episode of specialist treatment. When behavior change does not maintain after such a treatment episode, it is termed a "relapse" and perhaps regarded as a failure of therapy or (more often) of the client. One receives treatment by going to a specialist office or unit, at a time convenient for the staff. There are often "waiting lists" for treatment, which convey the message that no change is expected (or possible) until expert treatment can be provided. In order to qualify for treatment, clients are often required to show favorable prognostic signs, and any resumed use of the problem drug may be a reason for discharge, perhaps with a prohibition again re-entering treatment for a period of time (Shavelson, 2001).

Yet addiction is not an acute illness. To be sure, there can be acute medical problems associated with certain aspects of addiction, such as detoxification. The course of substance dependence, however, more closely resembles the management of chronic conditions such as diabetes or hypertension. It is not likely to be cured or even dramatically altered by any single episode of treatment, although full remissions do occur. Instead, optimal care is likely to happen within the context of an *ongoing* relationship, in which support and services are provided as needed through the normal ups and downs of life. These days, this is often referred to as "case management." It is attuned to the person's particular social context, network of relationships, and full spectrum of strengths and problems. The *quality* of the relationship also appears to matter. Contrary to popular U.S. notions of the value of confrontation, the optimal interpersonal style seems to be empathic, patient, supportive and respectful (Alcoholics Anonymous, 1976; Miller, 2000).

Where in society does one find such ongoing relationships, where sustained caring and monitoring are feasible? Primary health care is one possibility, wherein a person may see the same physician or team repeatedly for years. People involved in a social service system may see the same social worker, probation officer, or home care nurse over an extended period of time. Pastoral care also provides such a broader relationship context. Pastors, priests and rabbis not only see their parishioners on a regular basis, but also have a role with broad social access, allowing them to make house calls and initiate contact when concerned. Like religious congregations, the Twelve-Step fellowships such as Alcoholics Anonymous can provide a lifelong and pervasive community of support. Unlike acute care specialist treatment, all of these offer the kind of ongoing contact and care that make sense in addressing addictions.

Such considerations have often been relegated to the domain of "aftercare." Implicit in this term is the assumption that the primary and essential intervention is the period of acute specialist treatment, and that changes accomplished during such treatment are then maintained by some kind of ongoing support. The importance of aftercare is supported by the finding that the maintenance of treatment gains is, indeed, associated with the extent to which the individual makes use of aftercare services (Donovan, 1998), and more generally with the degree of support in the post-treatment environment (Moos et al., 1990).

Acute Treatment + Aftercare = Improvement
Acute Treatment with no Aftercare = Poorer Outcome

An alternative explanation of this finding is that continuing care—which has been called "aftercare"—is actually the essential component in effectively addressing addictions, regardless of episodes of acute specialist treatment. Removing acute treatment from the above equations:

Continuing Care = Improvement
No Continuing Care = Poorer Outcome

In this perspective, a period of acute specialist treatment might be considered to be at best "forecare," a prelude to effectively addressing the problem. That is how detoxification is currently regarded: not likely in itself to yield stable behavior change. An acute inpatient treatment episode would not be expected to resolve diabetes, hypertension, or coronary artery disease. Neither should we expect time-limited acute treatment to be necessary and sufficient in resolving substance use disorders.

There is a further disadvantage in sequestering addictive behaviors within specialist treatment programs. Doing so significantly raises the threshold to recognize and address substance use problems. As in most health areas, prevention and early intervention is far easier (and less costly) than the acute treatment of advanced disease. It is much easier to help people cut back on their drinking when they are not alcohol dependent (Miller et al., 1992). In relying on a specialist treatment system, there is little opportunity to reach people before their problems become severe (Institute of Medicine, 1990). Similarly, thinking of addictions as a unique disorder may dissuade productive talk in primary care settings about general health conditions and how addictive behaviors affect them.

Thinking beyond Treatment

Caring for those who are chronically affected is only one aspect of effectively addressing addictive behaviors. It is an important and humanitarian aspect, perhaps analogous to rescuing people who have been washed over a waterfall. Just as important and humanitarian is the prevention and early intervention for addictive behavior problems—analogous to going upstream to find out why people are falling into the river in the first place, or pulling them out well before they reach the rapids and the waterfall.

As with effective treatment, prevention is likely to occur within the context of community. Preventive interventions designed to do something to alter the individual (such as Drug Abuse Resistance Education, or DARE) have a spotty track record at best in primary prevention. Ongoing health and social services offer a promising context for both universal and indicated prevention of addictive behavior problems. Brief interventions by nonspecialists have a well-documented track record in early intervention with problem drinkers (Bien et al., 1993; Heather, 1998). The clinical method of motivational interviewing shows promise as a generic style for behavior change counseling in health and social service settings (Miller & Rollnick, in press; Rollnick et al., 1999). Prevention (like treatment) in such settings permits one to understand and address addictive behaviors within the broader natural context of the person's other concerns, rather than as an isolated and decontextualized problem.

There remains the danger, of course, of still seeing the problem as residing within individuals rather than their environment. A public health perspective calls one to attend not only to contributions of the agent (in this case, specific drugs) and the individual (host), but also of the environment. Jellinek (1960) warned that the American disease model of alcoholism—as an anomaly resident within the person—tends to cause society to become lax in controlling the drug itself and in addressing social factors that increase abuse and dependence. When alcoholism is thought of as a biological abnormality of certain individuals that renders them incapable of self-control, it makes little sense to impose community or society-wide supply-side controls on alcohol, or to attend to environmental influences on drinking decisions.

Toward Integrated Care

The essence of the above discussion is that acute treatment is an extremely limited model for addressing addictions. Whatever the historical reasons, specialist treatment systems for addictions arose in relative isolation from broader health and social service systems in the United States and many other industrialized nations. This was, I believe, an unfortunate mistake. Addictive behaviors contribute to a host of health and social problems, and thus it is no surprise that people with substance use disorders are seen in health and social service systems more often than in specialist treatment programs.

Similarly, those who do come for specialist treatment present with a wide array of broader health and social concerns that are unlikely to be resolved by an exclusive focus on substance use. Perhaps this is why the alcohol treatment methods with strongest evidence of efficacy tend to be those that address broader life functioning (e.g., Meyers & Miller, 2001; Miller & Wilbourne, in press).

The answer, I believe, is not to be found in referral to specialist treatment programs. That has already been tried. Instead we need better integrated models for addressing substance use disorders within the context of existing health and social services. Addictions should be addressed as part of a network of ongoing inter-related concerns, not as isolated individual pathology. This is, in fact, how substance use and abuse arise, as an integral part of an interconnected web of problem behaviors (Jessor & Jessor, 1977). There follow several implications for addressing addictions.

First, health and social service systems should regularly and routinely screen for substance use disorders, much as vital signs are checked and as health workers are screened for tuberculosis exposure. The prevalence rate of alcohol and other drug problems in the general population is high enough in itself to warrant this, and among those visiting most health and social service systems these rates are doubled or tripled. Such screening is effective in identifying the majority of cases that would otherwise be missed, and acceptance of such screening is high among clients and patients.

Second, there should be care maps for managing addictions within the context of health and social services. Referral to a specialist program is often ineffective in getting the person into treatment, and as discussed above, acute specialist treatment is not an optimal model for effectively managing addictions. When screening raises possible concern about substance abuse or dependence, on-site care routines should be triggered. It makes sense to address addictions as a health concern within the context of ongoing care. A stepped care model seems appropriate, beginning with interventions that are less intensive, intrusive, and costly.

Third, the integration and co-location of services facilitates their utilization. The separation of addiction from other health and social services is one that does not serve clients well. An obstacle to overcome here is prejudice among health professionals against seeing and treating people with primary or concomitant substance use disorders.

Finally, training in how to recognize and address addictive disorders must be included in the routine training of health and social service professionals. Medical education often includes far more training in rare diseases unlikely to be seen in practice, than in the management of one of the most common disorders encountered in almost any health care setting. Wherever people with substance use disorders come into regular contact with health or social services, there is an opportunity for effective intervention. Such preparation is not only needed for the most highly-trained health professionals such as psychologists and physicians. It may be more important and realistic to prepare the front-line care providers who are most likely to see and spend time with people who are impaired by or at risk from addictive behaviors.

The need will remain, of course, for professionals with special interest and expertise in caring for people with substance use disorders. Not every health professional is well prepared or favorably inclined to treat addictions, and a negative attitude toward such patients promotes drop-out and poor outcomes. What is needed is the understanding that addressing addictions falls well within the mission of health care and social services, and a general preparation of professionals to be part of a system that, knowingly or not, already cares for people with substance use disorders. The separatist approach of the past permits professionals and systems to effectively shut such people out of health and social services, relegating them to a quarantined treatment program that is often ill-prepared to understand and address their diverse problems and needs. Complex inter-related problems cannot be addressed well by a fragmented system of care. It is time for health and social services to take responsibility for helping people with addiction problems, rather than rejecting and referring them away from the integrated care that they need.

REFERENCES

Alcoholics Anonymous (1976). *Alcoholics Anonymous: The story of how many thousands of men and women have recovered from alcoholism* (3rd ed.). New York: AA World Services.

Bien, T. H., Miller, W. R., & Tonigan, J. S. (1993). Brief interventions for alcohol problems: A review. *Addiction, 88*, 315–336.

Bohart, A. C. & Tallman, K. (1999). *How clients make therapy work: The process of active self-healing.* Washington, DC: American Psychological Association.

Cahalan, D. (1970). *Problem drinkers: A national survey.* San Francisco: Jossey-Bass.

Cisler, R. A., Holder, H., Longabaugh, R., Stout, R., & Zweben, A. (1998). Estimated and actual replication costs of alcoholism treatment modalities: Case study from Project MATCH. *Journal of Studies on Alcohol, 59*, 503–512.

Davidson, P. R. & Parker, K. C. H. (2001). Eye movement desensitization and reprocessing (EMDR): A meta-analysis. *Journal of Consulting and Clinical Psychololgy, 69*, 305–316.

Donovan, D. M. (1998). Continuing care: Promoting the maintenance of change. In W. R. Miller & N. Heather (Eds.) (1998). *Treating addictive behaviors* (2nd ed., pp. 317–336). New York: Plenum Press.

Fletcher, A. M. (2001). *Sober for good: New solutions for drinking problems—advice from those who have succeeded.* Boston: Houghton Mifflin.

Heather, N. (1998). Using brief opportunities for change in medical settings. In W. R. Miller & N. Heather (Eds.) (1998). *Treating addictive behaviors* (2nd ed., pp. 133–147). New York: Plenum Press.

Holder, H., Longabaugh, R., Miller, W. R., & Rubonis, A. V. (1991). The cost effectiveness of treatment for alcoholism: A first approximation. *Journal of Studies on Alcohol, 52*, 517–540.

Holder, H., Cisler, R. A., Longabaugh, R., Stout, R. L., Treno, A. J., & Zweben, A. (2000). Alcoholism treatment and medical care costs and benefits from Project MATCH. *Addiction, 95*, 999–1013.

Institute of Medicine (1990). *Broadening the base of treatment for alcohol problems.* Washington, DC: National Academy Press.

Jellinek, E. M. (1960). *The disease concept of alcoholism.* New Brunswick, NJ: Hillhouse Press.

Jessor, R. & Jessor, S. L. (1977). *Problem behavior and psychosocial development: A longitudinal study of youth.* New York: Academic Press.

Lang, P. J. (1969). The mechanics of desensitization and the laboratory study of human fear. In C.M. Franks (Ed.), *Behavior therapy: Appraisal and status* (pp. 160–191). New York: McGraw-Hill.

Meyers, W. R. & Miller, W. R. (Eds.) (2001). *A community reinforcement approach to addiction treatment.* Cambridge, UK: Cambridge University Press.

Miller, W. R. (2000). Rediscovering fire: Small interventions, large effects. *Psychology of Addictive Behaviors, 14*, 6–18.

Miller, W. R. & Baca, L. M. (1983). Two-year follow-up of bibliotherapy and therapist-directed controlled drinking training for problem drinkers. *Behavior Therapy, 14*, 441–448.

Miller, W. R. & C'de Baca, J. (2001). *Quantum change: When epiphanies and sudden insights transform ordinary lives.* New York: Guilford Press.

Miller, W. R. & Hester, R. K. (1986). Inpatient alcoholism treatment: Who benefits? *American Psychologist, 41*, 794–805.

Miller, W. R., Leckman, A. L., Delaney, H. D., & Tinkcom, M. (1992). Long-term follow-up of behavioral self-control training. *Journal of Studies on Alcohol, 53*, 249–261.

Miller, W. R. & Rollnick, S. *Motivational interviewing: Preparing people for change* (2nd ed.) (in press). New York: Guilford Press.

Miller, W. R., Taylor, C. A., & West, J. C. (1980). Focused versus broad spectrum behavior therapy for problem drinkers. *Journal of Consulting and Clinical Psychology, 48*, 590–601.

Miller, W. R., Walters, S. T., & Bennett, M. E. (2001). How effective is alcoholism treatment? *Journal of Studies on Alcohol, 62*, 211–220.

Miller, W. R. & Wilbourne, P. L. (in press). Mesa Grande: A methodological analysis of clinical trials of treatments for alcohol use disorders. *Addiction.*

Moos, R. H., Finney, J. W., & Cronkite, R. C. (1990). *Alcoholism treatment: Context, process, and outcome.* New York: Oxford University Press.

Morgenstern, J. & Longabaugh, R. (2000). Cognitive-behavioral treatment for alcohol dependence: a review of evidence for its hypothesized mechanisms of action. *Addiction, 95*, 1475–1490.

Najavits, L. M. & Weiss, R. D. (1994). Variations in therapist effectiveness in the treatment of patients with substance use disorders: An empirical review. *Addiction, 89*, 679–688.

Prochaska, J. O., DiClemente, C. C., & Norcross, J. C. (1992). In search of how people change: Applications to addictive behaviors. *American Psychologist, 47*, 1102–1114.

Project MATCH Research Group (1997). Matching alcoholism treatments to client heterogeneity: Project MATCH posttreatment drinking outcomes. *Journal of Studies on Alcohol, 58*, 7–29.

Rollnick, S., Mason, P., & Butler, C. (1999). *Health behavior change: A guide for practitioners.* New York: Churchill Livingstone.

Shavelson, L. (2001). *Hooked: Five addicts challenge our misguided drug rehab system.* New York: New Press.

Vaillant, G. E. (1995). *The natural history of alcoholism revisited.* Cambridge, Massachusetts: Harvard University Press.

Valle, S. K. (1981). Interpersonal functioning of alcoholism counselors and treatment outcome. *Journal of Studies on Alcohol, 42*, 783–790.

CHAPTER 3

Questioning the Effectiveness of Addiction Treatments

*What is the Evidence?**

A. THOMAS MCLELLAN

INTRODUCTION

Some of the most significant economic and social problems facing society are associated with alcohol and drug dependence (National Institute on Drug Abuse, 1991; Merril, 1993). In the United States alone, it has been estimated that alcohol abuse costs approximately $90 billion and that abuse of other drugs costs approximately $67 billion each year (Rice, Kellman, and Miller, 1991). In terms of public health and safety, many studies have shown that one fifth to one fourth of all deaths annually are associated in some way with alcohol, drug or tobacco use (Horgan, 1994). Finally, the social deterioration associated with substance abuse is illustrated by the fact that more than three-fourths of all foster children in the U.S. are the offspring of alcohol and/or drug dependent parents (Childrens Defense Fund Report, 1994).

Given the magnitude and severity of the crime, family disruption, loss of economic productivity and social decay associated with drug abuse, it is not surprising that we regard it as primarily a social problem requiring a social-judicial remedy—rather than a health problem requiring prevention and treatment. Despite some evidence that substance abuse and addiction may be best considered public health problems requiring prevention and treatment efforts

*Supported by Grants from the National Institute on Drug Abuse, the Robert Wood Johnson Foundation, the Office of National Drug Control Policy and the Department of Veterans Affairs.

A. THOMAS MCLELLAN • Department of Psychiatry, University of Pennsylvania, School of Medicine, Philadelphia, Pennsylvania 19106

(O'Brian and McLellan, 1996; McLellan, O'Brien, and Kleber, 2000) there has been widespread skepticism regarding the value of treatments for substance abuse, and whether such treatments are "worth it." A *Wall Street Journal* article questioned the effectiveness and value of substance abuse treatment, saying "... the success rate of treatment programs is highly uncertain" (Wall Street Journal, 1994).

The reluctance to consider public health, medical model or treatment oriented approaches for dealing with problems of substance abuse appears to be multiply determined. First, there is the question of whether alcohol and drug dependence are "real" medical disorders. Doubts are not confined to the general public but extend well into the ranks of physicians and other health care providers. Another reason that treatment options have often been excluded from social policies on substance abuse is the pervasive view that treatment is designed to help the drug user—but it is *not* designed to help society. Why should a society expend resources to help an individual who may have produced many social problems? Moreover, a medical or treatment approach to substance abuse appears to many individuals to convey the message that the addiction and related problems are not the fault of the addicted person; that they "can't help themselves." These are messages that many people find offensive and unfair. The final and possibly most significant issue that diminishes public perception of the value of substance abuse treatment is the less than expected performance of the substance abuse treatment field on its own standard of effectiveness—one year abstinence rates from alcohol and all drugs. It is well known that many persons who have received treatments have returned to alcohol and drug use—sometimes very soon after treatment. In fact, the great majority of treated substance abusing patients return to substance use within one year after treatment (Miller and Hester, 1986; McLellan and McKay, 1998).

While the concepts and arguments underlying the public expectations of substance abuse treatment appear simple, determining the effectiveness or worth of substance abuse treatment is not a simple matter. In the text that follows, I will discuss these factors and present evidence from research studies pertinent to three domains of outcome: reduction in substance use, improvement in personal and social function, and reduction in threats to public health and safety.

PART I: SUBSTANCE DEPENDENCE—MEDICAL DISORDER OR SOCIAL PROBLEM?

Given the impact that substance abuse has upon social and family life, and the expectations from society for an "effective" intervention to reduce these associated social problems, it is reasonable to think that addiction is *primarily* a "social disorder" and that it is not appropriate to expect any form of healthcare intervention to be effective. Are there are any other medical disorders that are similar to substance use disorders in terms of onset, course and response to treatment, and has the healthcare field been "effective" in treating them?

Factors Associated with the Onset of Substance Dependence—It is clear from the outset that many factors combine to initiate a substance dependence disorder. There is now evidence that there is a genetic component to these disorders. For sake of comparability, heritability estimates from twin studies (Williams, Hunt, and Hasstedt, 1991; Fagard, Brguljan, and Staessen, 1995) of hypertension range from 0.25 to 0.50, depending on the sample and the diagnostic criteria used. Twin studies of diabetes offer heritability estimates of approximately 0.80 for type 2 (Kyvik, Green, and Beck-Nielsen, 1995) and 0.30 to 0.55 for type 1 diabetes. (Kaprio et al., 1992) Finally, twin studies (Duffy et al., 1990; Nieminen et al., 1991) of adult-onset asthma have produced a somewhat broader range of heritability estimates, ranging from 0.36 to 0.70.

Several twin studies (Tsuang et al., 1996; Kendler and Prescott, 1998; VandenBree et al., 1998; True and Xian, 1999) have been published in the substance dependence field, all showing significantly higher rates of dependence among twins than among nontwin siblings and higher rates among monozygotic than dizygotic twins. Published heritability estimates include 0.34 for males dependent on heroin, 0.55 for males dependent on alcohol, 0.52 for females dependent on marijuana, and 0.61 for cigarette-dependent twins of both genders (see Tsuang et al., 1996; Kendler and Prescott, 1998; VandenBree et al., 1998; True and Xian, 1999). The evidence suggests significant genetic contribution to the risk of addiction comparable to that seen in other chronic illnesses.

Since the use of any drug is a voluntary action, behavioral control or willpower is important in the onset of dependence. Thus, at some level an addicted individual is "at fault" for initiating the behaviors that led to a dependence disorder. In fact there are many illnesses in which voluntary choice affects initiation and maintenance, especially when these voluntary behaviors interact with genetic and cultural factors. For example, among males, salt sensitivity is a genetically transmitted risk factor for the eventual development of one form of hypertension (Mitchell et al., 1996; Svetkey et al., 1996). However, not all of those who inherit salt sensitivity develop hypertension. This is because the use of salt is determined by familial salt use patterns and individual choice. Similarly, risk factors such as obesity, stress level, and inactivity are joint products of familial, cultural, and personal choice factors (Mitchell et al., 1996; Svetkey et al., 1996). Thus, even among those with demonstrated genetic risk, a significant part of the total risk for developing hypertension can be traced to individual behaviors.

Factors Associated with the Course of Treatment—As has been said from the outset, there is no reliable "cure" for substance dependence. Dependent users of alcohol and other drugs who attempt to become abstinent are likely to have problems abstaining for more than six months at a time, and as many as 80% will return to substance use (Miller and Hester, 1986; Gerstein and Hardwood, 1990; Gerstein et al., 1979; Armor et al., 1976). Studies of abstinence rates at one year following treatment completion indicate that only 20–40% of treated patients have been able to remain completely abstinent throughout that time period (Miller and Hester, 1986; Gerstein et al., 1979; Armor et al., 1976).

Studies of treatment response have uniformly shown that those patients who comply with the recommended regimen of education, counseling and medication that characterizes most contemporary forms of treatment, typically have favorable outcomes during treatment and longer lasting post treatment benefits (Armor et al., 1976; Moos et al., 1990; Simpson and Savage, 1980; Hubbard et al., 1989; DeLeon, 1984). Thus it is discouraging to many in the treatment field that so many substance dependent patients fail to comply with the recommended course of treatment and subsequently resume substance use. Factors such as low socioeconomic class, co-morbid psychiatric conditions and lack of family or social supports for continuing abstinence are among the most important variables associated with lack of treatment compliance in this field, and ultimately to reoccurrence of the disorders following treatment (Babor et al., 1988; Havassy et al., 1995; McLellan et al., 1980; 1983; Rounsaville et al., 1987; Schuckit, 1985; Alterman and Cacciola, 1991; Hesselbrock et al., 1985).

The diseases of hypertension, diabetes and asthma are also chronic disorders, requiring continuing care for most, if not all of a patient's life. At the same time, these disorders are not necessarily unremitting or unalterably lethal, *as long as the treatment regimen of medication, diet and behavioral change are followed.* This last point requires emphasis. Treatments for these recognized medical disorders are heavily dependent upon behavioral change and medication compliance to achieve their potential effectiveness. In a review of over 70 outcome studies of treatments for these disorders, patient compliance with the recommended medical regimen was noted as the most significant determinant of treatment outcome. Fewer than 50% of insulin dependent diabetic patients fully comply with their medication schedule (e.g. Graber et al., 1992), and fewer than 30% of hypertensive or asthmatic patients comply with their medication regimens (e.g. Horowitz, 1993; Dekker et al., 1993).

The problem is even worse for the behavioral and diet changes that are so important for the maintenance of short term gains in these areas of medicine. In the fields of diabetes and hypertension a review of the large number of recent studies indicates that fewer than 30% of patients in treatment for these disorders comply with the recommended diet and/or behavioral changes that are designed to reduce risk factors for reoccurrence of the disorders (e.g. Clark, 1991; Kurtz, 1990). It is interesting in this context that clinical researchers of these disorders have identified the factors of low socioeconomic class, comorbid psychiatric conditions and lack of family support as the major contributors to lack of patient compliance (see Dekker, 1993 for a discussion of this literature). As in the field of substance abuse treatment, lack of patient compliance with the treatment regimen is a major contributor to the reoccurrence of these disorders and to the development of more serious and more expensive "disease-related" conditions. For example, outcome studies indicate that 30–60% of insulin dependent, diabetic patients, and approximately 50–80% of hypertensive and asthmatic patients suffer a reoccurrence of their symptoms each year and require at least restabilization of their medication and/or additional medical interventions to re-establish symptom remission (Graber et al., 1992; Horowitz, 1993; Dekker et al., 1993; Clark, 1991; Kurtz, 1990).

There are of course differences in susceptibility, onset, course and treatment response among all the disorders discussed here. At the same time there are clear parallels among all of them. All these disorders are multiply determined and no single gene, personality variable, or environmental factor can fully account for the onset of any of these disorders. Behavioral choices appear to be implicated in the initiation of each of these disorders and behavioral control continues to be a factor in determining the course of all these conditions. There are no "cures" for any of these disorders, yet there have been major advances in the development of effective medications and behavioral treatments to reduce primary symptoms of each disorder. Because these conditions are known to be chronic it is acknowledged in the treatment of diabetes, hypertension and asthma that maintenance treatments will be needed to insure that symptom remission continues. Unfortunately, other common features of all these conditions are treatment adherence problems and the chronic, relapsing course of these illnesses. In this regard, it was striking that many of the patient characteristics associated with non-adherence were identical across all four disorders considered and the rates of reoccurrence were also similar.

Perhaps the major difference among these conditions lies in the public's perception of diabetes, hypertension and asthma as clearly medical conditions and substance dependence more as a social problem. It is also interesting that despite rather comparable results, at least in terms of compliance and reoccurrence rates, there is no serious argument as to whether the treatments for diabetes, hypertension or asthma should be supported by contemporary health care systems, while this is very much in question with regard to treatments for substance dependence. In the text that follows, we review the existing evidence for substance abuse treatment effectiveness and value as compared with other public policy alternatives.

APPROPRIATE COMPARISONS TO JUDGE THE EFFECTIVENESS OF ADDICTION TREATMENTS

1) *Do Patients Improve Following Treatment?* Perhaps the most basic question that can be asked of treatment is whether patients who enter show significant reductions in the three outcome domains discussed in Part I of the chapter. Perhaps the most commonly used means of addressing these questions has been a simple comparison of patient status, measured on multiple dimensions, at fixed intervals before and after treatment, that is, a standard "Pre-Post" design.

There have been substantial advances over the past decade in the methodologies associated with pre to post treatment comparisons. It is important to point out that minimal standards for pre to post treatment comparisons now include several quality control features. For example, these evaluations must follow an "*intent to treat design*" where a sample of subjects is selected at admission to treatment and fully characterized from that point throughout the course of their treatment and following their discharge. This is a methodological feature that is required by the U.S. Food and Drug Administration in their evaluations of new drugs and devices (FDA, 1980). This type of evaluation design provides effectiveness estimates that are substantially more conservative than evaluations of samples that have completed the full course of treatment.

A second methodological feature of more rigorous evaluations is the performance of all patient interviews and data collection by *independent evaluators*, not associated with the provision of the intervention. This is critical to the reduction of "demand effects," (i.e. "faking good") that are commonly seen when patients report their levels of improvement directly to the clinical staff that treated them. In this regard, it is also advisable for subjective reports of post treatment status to be accompanied by *breathalyzer and/or urine screening tests and/or collateral reports* to validate patient reports, even when collected by independent evaluators.

Finally, it has been recognized that a high rate of patient follow-up contact is necessary to insure representative information from the treated sample. Again, the Food and Drug Administration requires *a minimum of 70% contact at follow-up* in their studies (FDA, 1980). It has been shown by LaPorte et al. (LaPorte et al., 1981) and by others (Moos, 1974) that those patients who are more difficult to find at follow-up typically have worse outcomes. Studies reporting contact rates that are less than 70% are likely to overestimate the effects of treatment and therefore should be regarded critically.

It is important to emphasize that while results showing improvement from admission to some post-treatment follow-up point are encouraging, it is not possible to attribute those improvements to the direct effects of that treatment (See below). It is possible that these substance abuse patients would have changed significantly over this same period of time *without treatment*. Of course, random assignment designs including "no-treatment" control groups are not possible in evaluations of ongoing treatments within the real world. The interested reader is referred to studies by Moos, Finney and their colleagues on the evaluation of alcohol treatments (Moos, 1974; Moos et al., 1990). Large scale evaluations of drug abuse treatments have been performed by Simpson et al., using the DARP data (Simpson and Savage, 1980), Hubbard et al., using the TOPS data sets (Hubbard et al., 1989), DeLeon studying Therapeutic Community treatment (DeLeon, 1984) and Anglin (Anglin et al., 1989) and Ball (Ball et al., 1988) studying methadone maintenance treatments. While there are of course differences among these studies in the nature of the treatments evaluated and the evaluation paradigms, the results have typically shown significant and pervasive changes among substance dependent patients following standard treatments. In the work that follows, we review efforts designed to determine the causes of these improvements following treatment.

2) *Is Treatment More Effective Than No Treatment?* While it is ethically not possible to deny available treatment to those whose condition appears to require it, there are situations where treatments have not been applied to substance dependent persons and these situations offer some indication of what happens to substance use, personal function and the public health and safety problems of substance dependent individuals in the absence of treatment. Two recent studies provide information pertinent to this question.

Untreated Patients Metzger et al. (1992) have examined the drug use, needle sharing practices and HIV infection rates of two large samples of opiate addicted patients in the Philadelphia area. The "In-Treatment" group was comprised of 152 patients randomly selected from a large methadone maintenance program. These In-Treatment subjects were asked to refer their opiate using friends (Out-of-Treatment group—103 subjects) from the same social circles and from the same neighborhoods who had been out of all substance dependence treatments for *at least one year*. Thus, using this chain referral method, the two groups were matched on many relevant demographic, geographic, background and social factors that are associated with drug use. Despite the fact that the In-Treatment subjects were enrolled in a methadone treatment program, about 30% of patients reported continued opiate or non-opiate drug use and needle sharing. Considered alone, without indication of the prior levels of substance use and public health risk behaviors, these data might lead to a conclusion that treatment was not working. Drug use had not been reduced to zero and there was still significant public health risk in the form of needle sharing. However, the level of drug use reported by the In-Treatment sample was less than half that seen in the Out-of-Treatment group. Not surprisingly, needle sharing was also reported in a much higher proportion of the Out-of-Treatment subjects.

Perhaps the most important finding emerging from this study was the differential HIV infection rate between the two samples as seen through prospective follow-up evaluations (including serological examinations) every six months over the next six years, on over 90% of the original samples. At the initial assessment point, 13% of the In-Treatment sample and 21% of the Out-of-Treatment sample tested positive for HIV infection. Follow-up testing over the next six years showed that 51% of the Out-of-Treatment group, but only 21% of the In-Treatment group tested HIV positive. Closer examination of the role of treatment status on HIV conversion revealed that 30% of HIV-negative subjects *who remained out of treatment*, became infected with the AIDS virus over the six-year period. In comparison, only 8% of HIV-negative subjects *who remained in the treatment program*, became infected during the same time period.

It bears emphasis that nearly four times as many Out-of Treatment as In-Treatment subjects continued to engage in public health risk behaviors and thereby became infected with the AIDS virus. Though quite remarkable, it must be repeated that these data again do not prove that treatment was the causal agent responsible for these differences in infection rates. It is possible and even likely, that the "out of treatment" subjects may have lacked the motivation for treatment found among the treated subjects, and this lack of desire for personal change, rather than the effects of the treatment itself, may explain the status differences seen. For this reason, it would be important to equate level of motivation, at least at the start of treatment, in order to make any valid judgment regarding the effectiveness of treatment in reducing AIDS risk behaviors among substance dependent individuals.

Waiting List Patients An ongoing study of male veterans who applied for cocaine abuse treatment at the Philadelphia VA Medical Center helps to shed light on the relative outcomes of treated vs. untreated patients who were approximately equal in their motivation for treatment. In this 4-week study of waiting list patients by Urschel and his colleagues (See McLellan et al., 1992), 64 cocaine dependent individuals were contacted at the time of application for inpatient substance abuse treatment. Due to the unavailability of treatment beds, these individuals were put on a waiting list for the next available bed. These individuals were followed each week of their waiting period and asked questions regarding their drug use and health status, by independent evaluators. The question of interest was whether the cocaine use and the related problems would change without treatment. This is an important comparison in that these forty-two individuals had shown some motivation for change through the act of applying for treatment.

Results indicated that only 16% of this group of lower socioeconomic, male veterans received any treatment related services outside the Veterans Administration. Interestingly, those few patients who did receive some services (typically detoxification and/or temporary housing and food at a community shelter), did show some reductions in their alcohol and drug use, although essentially no improvements in their health and personal functional status. Among the remaining individuals who received no treatment services at all, there were *significant increases in the severity* of medical, psychiatric, social and drug abuse problems over the four-week waiting period. Specifically, 53% reported *increased* severity of drug problems, 57% reported increased severity of medical problems and 81% reported increased employment and support problems.

In summary, there is little evidence from these data that the drug use or the related health problems of these patients showed any improvement without treatment. In fact, there was significant worsening in the overall drug use and health status of these men who did not receive treatment, despite the fact that they were clearly motivated for change. Again, while these data are by themselves not definitive, they combine with the previous data to suggest an important role for treatment in producing behavioral change and are quite consistent with earlier studies of substance dependent patients out of treatment (Gerstein et al., 1979; Maddux and Desmond, 1986) and on waiting lists (Rua, 1989; Sosk et al., 1990).

3) *Is Treatment More Effective Than a Criminal Justice Intervention?* While the data presented thus far are quite suggestive that treatment for substance dependent individuals can produce improvements in substance use, health and personal function and in public health and safety risks, it remains possible that standard treatment approaches may actually be less effective in producing these favorable outcomes than other kinds of interventions. Perhaps the most regularly suggested alternatives to substance abuse treatment involve the criminal justice system, with incarceration, probation and parole being the major choices. In this regard, there are two important points to remember regarding the relative value of addressing substance abuse problems with incarceration. First, jail cells are expensive to build and quite expensive to operate. 1997 figures from the United States suggest that federal minimum

security prison cells cost approximately $41,000 per cell to build, a imately $29,000 to maintain per inmate, per cell, per year. Thus, im alone, even if effective in reducing alcohol and drug use, is not n cost efficient alternative as compared with treatment (Inciardi, 1988).

The second point is that in the United States alone there have been more than 100 post-incarceration evaluations of inmates who have been jailed for drug related crimes. Despite different types of crimes, different types of sentences, and different sites and years where these evaluations have taken place, the results are striking in the similarity of their outcomes. More than 70% of those who have been imprisoned for drug-related crimes—*and not treated during the course of their incarceration*—became re-addicted within the year following release. In addition, more than half of addicted inmates were re-incarcerated for drug-related offenses within a year of release. Although the public may feel protected from the effects of drug-related crime while these individuals are incarcerated, almost all will eventually get out of jail and there is little indication that prison is effective in "teaching them a lesson."

An important and policy-relevant line of research in the United States has examined the joint effects of *combining* incarceration and/or legal system interventions with treatment interventions—to determine if these two approaches are incompatible or if there are synergistic effects from the two approaches. A recent illustration is provided by a study from Cornish and colleagues evaluating the efficacy of adding the pharmacologic treatment, naltrexone to standard parole for federal offenders with opiate-related crimes (Cornish et al., 1998). Naltrexone is a widely used, orally administered, opiate antagonist that has been shown to completely block the effects of injected opiates for up to 72 hours following ingestion. In the Cornish et al., study, probationers and parolees with a history of recent and chronic opiate abuse were offered an opportunity to be randomly assigned to receive either naltrexone administered two times per week (doses of 100 mg and 150 mg) accompanied by standard health care services; or to an enhanced probation condition where they were asked to report to their probation officer two times per week. These two conditions were approximately equal with regard to the total amount of time required for participation and the total amount of contact with a counselor or probation/parole officer. All evaluations were conducted by trained technicians entirely independent from the parole process.

Though retention rates for naltrexone among many samples of opiate dependent patients have been poor (averaging fewer than 20% remaining for one month), approximately 65% of the federal parole subjects who received the medication remained on it for the entire 6 month study period. While on naltrexone, these subjects provided significantly fewer opiate positive urines than subjects in the enhanced probation control group. Although cocaine use continued to be a problem for all groups, the naltrexone subjects had lower rates of non-opiate drug use than the control subjects, as confirmed by urinalysis. Finally, 32% of naltrexone subjects were re-arrested and re-incarcerated during their first twelve months as compared with 60% of those randomly assigned to the placebo condition. Virtually all incarcerations—in both groups—were due to drug related arrests.

This study and many others not described here, illustrate three important points. First, it is possible to combine a treatment and a correctional approach to the problem of substance abuse. There are many reports of effective treatments for drug dependence designed for delivery within correctional facilities; and combined with probation and parole. Again, space considerations do not permit a complete review of this literature, but the interested reader is referred to reviews of this work (Cornish et al., 1998; Wexler et al., 1988; Anglin and Hser, 1990). A second and related point is that the addition of substance abuse treatment to a correctional intervention can result in better outcomes than with the criminal justice system intervention alone. In the above study, not only did the naltrexone treatment appear to enhance the effects of the probation/parole intervention; the external pressure applied by the criminal justice system appears to have enhanced the medication compliance and thereby the efficacy of the naltrexone. Third, while this study was focused on a pharmacological intervention used in the treatment of *opiate* addiction, this paradigm could be used to evaluate other forms of psychosocial or behavioral treatment.

4) *If Treatment Is Effective, What Makes it Effective: What are the "Active Ingredients" of Treatment*? The data presented thus far in this paper and from many prior evaluation studies indicate that substance abuse treatments *can* be effective, not just in reducing alcohol and/or drug use among those treated but also in relieving many of the important personal function and public health and safety problems so often associated with substance dependence. At the same time, there is also indication that the results of treatments are not uniform and there is typically substantial variability in the post treatment outcomes of treated patients. For example, a large national field study of drug dependent patients entering inpatient and outpatient public treatment programs (Hubbard et al., 1989) showed that at 12-month follow-up, approximately 12% of patients reported complete abstinence, employment, no crime, and no psychiatric or family problems. In contrast to these "complete successes," approximately 18% were in jail, 29% had resumed significant substance use and 13% had been readmitted to additional care since the initial treatment episode. Summarizing findings from seven large multisite studies alcohol treatment outcome, Miller and colleagues (2001) reported that on average one in four clients remained continuously, and an additional one in ten used alcohol moderately and without problems. Even controlled trials of single treatments in well-specified samples of patients have reported similar levels of variability in outcome (See for example Armor et al., 1976; Woody et al., 1984; Rounsaville et al., 1983; Edwards et al., 1977). Given substantial variability in outcome status following treatment for substance abuse, researchers have attempted to identify and study those factors that may account for this variability. Several of the most widely studied factors are discussed briefly below.

Duration and intensity of treatment. Studies of alcoholism treatment have consistently shown that patients who stay in treatment longer have greater reductions in alcohol use (Moos et al., 1990; Saxe et al., 1983; McLellan et al.,

1992; Armor et al., 1976). Similarly, studies with drug dependent patients (Gerstein and Harwood, 1990; Gerstein et al., 1979; Simpson and Savage, 1980; Hubbard et al., 1989; DeLeon, 1984) all support the finding that those patients who stay in treatment longer and who complete a standard course of care, ultimately show the best outcomes (regardless of the outcome measure). While these well-replicated findings show that a greater "dose" of treatment is associated with improved outcomes, it is quite possible that these results merely reflect the outcomes of the most motivated (thus longest-staying and most compliant) patients. In this regard, Longabaugh (Longabaugh et al., 1994) has shown that patients who are randomly assigned to longer stays in residential programs did *not* have better drinking outcomes than those randomly assigned to shorter stays. This finding suggests that merely longer lengths of time in treatment may not be adequate to produce desired outcomes. Instead, it may be that particular types of treatment "ingredients" are necessary in appropriate intensity and quality to assure patient improvement.

Treatment Process Measures While investigations of treatment processes are still relatively new, there is practical clinical value to this type of research. The identification of treatment process and management dimensions that are reliably associated with outcome might enable refinement and enhancement of the "active ingredients" of care and elimination of "inert ingredients." Recently, there have been innovations in the measurement of the treatment environment and the treatment processes that occur during substance abuse treatments (Ball and Ross, 1991; Finney et al., 1981; Allison and Hubbard, 1982; Joe et al., 1992; McLellan et al., 1992). For example, Moos and colleagues have developed and tested measures of the treatment environment in both inpatient and outpatient settings (Alterman and Cacciola, 1991; Moos, 1974; Finney et al., 1981). Similarly, Ball and his colleagues have demonstrated that it is possible to reliably and validly characterize the leadership qualities, environmental characteristics, number and types of services provided and other aspects of a drug dependence treatment program (Ball and Ross, 1991). With these additional measures it is now possible to assess potentially relevant dimensions of the treatment as it is delivered.

One clear and tangible result from the availability of these measures coupled with traditional pre-post outcome evaluation designs is the finding that treatment programs differ in the nature and amount of services provided to clients and that these differences in treatment process correlate with corresponding differences in treatment effectiveness, even after the effects of patient factors are statistically controlled. For example, early studies of alcohol treatment programs by the Rand Corporation (Armor et al., 1976), by Emrick (1975) and by Pattison (1969) found marked differences in program organization, intensity of services provided and in post-treatment outcomes among inpatient treatment programs. There have been fewer comparative studies of treatment programs for drug dependent patients but a multi-site study by Ball and Ross (Ball and Ross, 1991) examined treatment services and outcomes among methadone maintenance programs in three eastern U.S. cities. These authors found profound differences in the patterns of services provided to patients and in the outcomes from treatment despite very comparable samples of patients. Ball and Ross concluded that differences in program characteristics such as leadership, organization, staffing patterns and the amount and range of services provided during treatment, accounted for a significant proportion of the outcome differences seen among these programs.

More recently, McLellan and colleagues compared the during-treatment services and post treatment outcomes of four private substance dependence treatment programs (McLellan et al., 1993). There were substantial differences among the programs in the types and quantities of services actually provided to patients during treatment. The inpatient programs provided significantly more alcohol, drug and medical services, but services provided in the employment, family and psychiatric areas were not different between the inpatient and outpatient settings. The total group of patients in this study showed statistically significant and clinically impressive improvements by the time of the 6-month post-treatment follow-up, both in substance use and in additional measures of personal and social adjustment. At the same time, there were substantial differences in outcomes among the four programs sampled. While the results indicated that one of the four programs was particularly inferior, there was still substantial variability among the remaining three programs. Perhaps most interesting was the finding that these differential outcome results were not accounted for by differences in patient characteristics, but were related to the nature and amount of services provided.

Put simply, those programs that provided the most services, and particularly the best "fit" between the problems presented by the patients and the services directed at those problems, showed the best outcomes. Specifically, the program that provided the most services in a particular problem area showed the best outcome in that area, on nine of eleven criteria measured (McLellan et al., 1993). Thus, consistent with prior findings by Ball and Ross (Ball and Ross, 1991) and others (e.g. Brown and Miller, 1993), these data suggest that the range and fit of the treatment services provided within a program can be important in explaining the variability in effectiveness among treatment programs.

While the results of these field evaluations of multiple treatment programs provide a consistent and face valid indication that treatment services directed at the multiple problems of substance dependent patients are important "ingredients" in determining the effectiveness of those treatments, it must be clear that these results are merely associations. Without proper control groups and random patient assignment, it is impossible to infer causality. However, based upon these field studies, there have now been several controlled clinical trials comparing outcomes of treatments delivered in standard clinical settings, where the "dose" of treatment services has been systematically varied. For example, a controlled study of opiate dependent subjects extends this observation regarding the potential effectiveness of increased treatment services. McLellan and his colleagues (McLellan et al., 1993) randomly assigned opiate dependent patients to three levels of psychosocial services while in methadone maintenance: (1) Methadone only, (2) Methadone plus counseling, and

(3) Methadone plus counseling plus on-site psychiatric, employment, and family therapy services. The methadone dosage for all groups was 65 mg. At the end of six months of treatment the minimum services (methadone only) group did show some reductions in opiate use but virtually no other improvements. In addition, 69% of these patients had to be protectively terminated from the study due to unremitting drug use and/or repeated need for emergency medical care. In contrast, the standard services group showed substantial improvements in substance use as well as employment and crime reduction. The enhanced group showed the greatest number and amount of improvement, particularly in the areas of personal adjustment and public health and safety risk.

Two other studies of outpatient treatments for alcohol and for cocaine dependence also suggest that greater amounts of professional services directed at the "addiction related" problems of substance dependent individuals during treatment can produce improved outcomes. In a widely cited study of comprehensive services for alcohol dependent patients Azrin and colleagues developed the "Community Reinforcement Approach" (CRA) and tested it against other "standard" treatment interventions (Azrin, 1976). CRA includes conjoint therapy, job finding training, counseling focused on alcohol-free social and recreational activities, monitored disulfiram, and an alcohol-free social club (Azrin, 1976; Hunt and Azrin, 1973). In a study in which patients were randomly assigned to CRA or to a standard hospital treatment program, those getting CRA drank less, spent fewer days away from home, worked more days, and were institutionalized less over a 24 month follow-up (Hunt and Azrin, 1973). A second controlled study contrasted CRA, a disulfiram (Antabuse®) compliance program, and regular outpatient treatment (Azrin et al., 1982). Once again, those treated with CRA did substantially better on all outcome measures than those in the other treatment conditions.

A more recent set of studies by Higgins et al. (Higgins et al., 1991; 1994; 1993) has used the CRA approach with cocaine dependent patients. Here, cocaine dependent patients seeking outpatient treatment were randomly assigned to receive either standard drug counseling and referral to AA, or a multi-component behavioral treatment integrating contingency managed counseling, community based incentives and family therapy comparable to the CRA model (Higgins et al., 1991). The CRA model retained more patients in treatment, produced more abstinent patients and longer periods of abstinence, and produced greater improvements in personal function than the standard counseling approach. Following the overall findings, this group of investigators systematically "disassembled" the CRA model and examined the individual "ingredients" of family therapy (Higgins et al., 1994), incentives (Higgins et al., 1993), and the contingency based counseling (Higgins et al., 1991) as compared against groups who received comparable amounts of all components except the target ingredient. In each case, these systematic and controlled examinations indicated that these individual components made a significant contribution to the outcomes observed, thus proving their added value in the rehabilitation effort.

CONCLUSIONS

This examination of addiction treatment effectiveness was begun with a broad discussion of expectations placed upon substance abuse treatments. I argued that: (1) reduction in substance use; (2) improvement in health, personal and social function; and (3) reduction in public health and safety risks, represent daunting tasks given the evidence of often severe and chronic problems among substance dependent persons at the start of treatment. At the same time, the evidence presented from both "real world" field studies and from controlled clinical trials suggests that substance dependence treatments *can* meet these expectations on all three domains. For example, data from a wide range of studies indicate that treated patients show major reductions in their alcohol and drug use, lasting at least six months following completion of their treatment. These patients typically show improved medical and psychological function and often, improved earnings from employment. Finally, evaluations of drug dependent patients following treatment have shown substantial reductions in AIDS risk behaviors and in drug related crime. These outcomes have been shown in both controlled clinical trials of experimental interventions and in large-scale evaluations of standard treatments in "real world" settings.

This review has also shown that the variability in effectiveness of substance abuse treatment across different settings, modalities and programs may be related to the types and amounts of social services provided during treatment. Across several types of patients and settings of care, there was consistent and face valid evidence that patients who receive more services and particularly, more professional services targeted to the particular profile of problems presented at admission, show the best outcomes.

A final and important point implicit in the work presented is that substance abuse treatments *can be evaluated in a scientific manner* in the same way that other forms of medical, psychological, social or pharmacological interventions are evaluated. The heartening findings reported here suggest that scientific methods that have been proven in other types of intervention evaluations are equally applicable in the evaluation of multi-component treatments for addiction.

REFERENCES

Allison M. and Hubbard R.L. Drug abuse treatment process: A review of the literature. *TOPS Research Monograph*. Raleigh, N.C.: Research Triangle Press, 1982.

Alterman A.I. and Cacciola J.S. The antisocial personality disorder diagnosis in substance abusers. *Journal of Nervous and Mental Disorders*, 179:401–409, 1991.

Anglin M.D. and Hser Y. Legal Coercion and Drug Abuse Treatment. In J. Inciardi *Handbook on Drug Control in the United States*. Westport Conn., Greenwood Press, 1990.

Anglin M.D., Speckart G.R. and Booth, M.W. Consequences and Costs of Shutting off Methadone. *Addictive Behaviors*, 14(3):307–326, 1989.

Armor D.J., Polich J.M. and Stambul H.B. *Alcoholism and Treatment*. Santa Monica Ca., RAND Corp. Press, 1976.

Azrin N.H., Sisson R.W., Meyers R., and Godley M. A social-systems approach to resocializing alcoholics in the community. *Journal of Studies on Alcohol*, 43:1115–1123, 1982.

Azrin N.H. Improvements in the community reinforcement approach to alcoholism. *Behavior Research and Therapy*, 14:339–348, 1976.

Babor T., Dolinsky Z., Rounsaville B.J. and Jaffe J. Unitary versus multidimensional models of alcoholism treatment outcome: An empirical study. *J. Stud. Alc.*, 49:167–177, 1988.

Ball J.C. and Ross A. *The Effectiveness of Methadone Maintenance Treatment.* New York, Springer-Verlag, 1991.

Ball J.C., Meyers, C.P., and Friedman S.R. Reducing the Risk of AIDS Through Methadone Maintenance Treatment. *J.Health and Social Behavior.* 29(3):214–226, 1988.

Brown J.M. and Miller W.R. (1993) Impact of motivational interviewing on participation and outcome in residential alcoholism treatment. *Psychology of Addictive Behaviors*, 7:211–218.

Childrens Defense Fund Report, Washington D.C., 1994.

Clark L.T. Improving compliance and incrasing control of hypertension: Needs of special hypertensive populations. *American Heart Journal*, 121 (2 pt 2):664–669, 1991

Cornish J., Metzger D., Woody G., Wilson D., McLellan A.T., Vandergrift B. and O'Brien C.P. Naltrexone pharmacotherapy for opioid dependent federal probationers. *J. Substance Abuse Treatment*, 13:477–489, 1998.

Dekker F.W., Dieleman F.E. and Kaptein A.A. Compliance with pulmonary medication in general practice. *European Respiratory Journal*, 6(6):886–890, 1993.

DeLeon, G. The Therapeutic Community: Study of Effectiveness. *Treatment Research Monograph #84-1286*, NIDA, Rockville, Md., 1984.

Duffy DL, Martin NG, Battistutta D, Hopper JL, Mathews JD. Genetics of asthma and hay fever in Australian twins. *Am Rev Respir Dis.* 1990;142:1351–1358.

Edwards G., Orford J., Egert S., Guthrie A., Hawker C., Hensman M., Mitcheson M., Oppenheimer E. and Taylor C. Alcoholism: A controlled trial of treatment and advice, *J. Stud. Alc.*, 38:1004–1031, 1977.

Emrick C.D. A review of psychologically oriented treatments for alcoholism II. The relative effectiveness of different treatment approaches and the effectiveness of treatment versus no treatment. *J. Stud. Alc.* 36:88–108, 1975.

Fagard R, Brguljan J, Staessen J *et al.* Heritability of conventional and ambulatory blood pressures: a study in twins. *Hypertension*, 26:919–924, 1995.

Finney J.W., Moos R.H. and Chan D.A. Length of Stay and Program Component Effects in the Treatment of Alcoholism: A Comparison of Two Techniques for Process Analyses. *Journal of Consulting and Clinical Psychology*, 49:120–131, 1981.

Food and Drug Administration, *Compliance Policy Guidelines*, Associate Comm. for Regulatory Affairs, 21 CFR 310, October, 1980.

Gerstein D. and Harwood H. (Editors) *Treating Drug Problems* (Volume One). Washington D.C., National Academy Press, 1990.

Gerstein D., Judd L.L. and Rovner S.A. Career dynamics of female heroin addicts. *Am. J. Drug and Alc. Abuse*, 6(1):1–23, 1979.

Graber A.L., Davidson P., Brown A., McRae J. and Woolridge K. Dropout and relapse during diabetes care. *Diabetic Care*, 15(11):1477–1483, 1992.

Havassy B.E., Wasserman D. and Hall S.M. Social relationships and cocaine use in an American treatment sample. *Addiction*, 58:456–460, 1995.

Hesselbrock V., Meyer R and Keener J. Psychopathology in hospitalized alcoholics. *Archives of General Psychiatry*, 42:1050–1055, 1985.

Higgins S.T., Budney A.J., Bickel W.K., et al. Incentives improve treatment retention, cocaine abstinence and psychiatric symptomatology in ambulatory cocaine dependent patients. *Am. J. Psychiatry*, 151:223–225, 1994.

Higgins S.T., Budney A.J., Bickel W.K. and Badger G.J. Participation of significant others in outpatient behavioral treatment predicts greater cocaine abstinence. *Am. J. Drug and Alcohol Abuse*, 45:322–327, 1993.

Higgins S.T., Delaney D.D., Budney A.J., et al. A behavioral approach to achieving initial cocaine abstinence. *Am. J. Psychiat.*, 148:1218–1224, 1991.

Horgan C. Chartbook of Social Indicators for Substance Abuse. Princeton, N.J., Robert Wood Johnson Foundation Report., 1994.

Horowitz R.I. Treatment adherence and risk of death after a myocardial heart infarction. *Lancet*, 336(8714):542–545, 1993

Hubbard R.L., Marsden M.E., Rachal J.V., Harwood H.J., Cavanaugh E.R. and Ginzburg H.M. *Drug Abuse Treatment: A National Study of Effectiveness*. Chapel Hill: Univ. of North Carolina Press. 1989.

Hunt G.M. and Azrin N.H. A community reinforcement approach to alcoholism. *Behavior Research and Therapy*, 11:91–104, 1973.

Inciardi J.A. Some considerations on the clinical efficacy of compulsory treatment: the New York experience. In C. G. Leukefeld and F. M. Tims (Eds.) *Compulsory Treatment of Drug Abuse: Research and Clinical Practice*. NIDA Research Monograph 86: 1988.

Joe G.W., Simpson D.D. and Sells S.B. Treatment process and relapse to opioid use during methadone maintenance. *Am. J. Drug and Alcohol Abuse*, 19:124–130, 1992.

Kaprio J, Tuomilehto J, Koskenvuo M, et al. Concordance for type 1 and type 2 diabetes mellitus in a population-based cohort of twins in Finland. *Diabetologia*, 1992;35:1060–1067.

Kendler KS, Prescott C. Cannabis use, abuse and dependence in a population-based sample of female twins *Am J Psychiatry*. 1998;155:1016–1022.

Kurtz S. M. Adherence to diabetic regimes: Empirical status and clinical applications. *Diabetes Education*, 16(1):50–59, 1990.

Kyvik KO, Green A, Beck-Nielsen H. Concordance rates of insulin dependent diabetes mellitus: a population based study of young Danish twins. *BMJ*, 311:913–917, 1995.

LaPorte, D., McLellan, A.T., Erdlen, F. Alcohol and drug abuse treatment outcome as a function of follow-up difficulty. *J. Clin and Consult. Psychology*, 49(1):112–119, 1981.

Longabaugh R., Beattie M., Noel N., Stout R. and Malloy P. The effect of social investment on treatment outcome. *Journal of Studies on Alcohol*, 56:16–21, 1994.

Maddux J.F. and Desmond D.P. Relapse and recovery in substance abuse careers. In F. M. Tims and C. G. Leukefeld (Eds.) *Relapse and Recovery in Drug Abuse*, NIDA Research Monograph Series 72, DHHS Pub. No. (ADM) 86–1473, Rockville Md., 1986.

McLellan A.T., O'Brien C.P. and Kleber H.D. Drug addiction as a chronic medical illness: Implications for treatment, insurance and evaluation. *JAMA*, 284:1689–1695, 2000.

McLellan A.T. and McKay J. The treatment of addiction: What can research offer practice? In Lamb S. and McCarty D. (Eds.) *Bridging the Gap: Forging new partnerships in community-based drug abuse treatment*. 1998. Washington, DC: National Academy Press.

McLellan A.T., Arndt I.O., Woody G.E. and Metzger D. Psychosocial Services in Substance Abuse Treatment?: A dose-ranging study of psychosocial services. *J. Am. Med. Assn.*, 269(15):1953–1959, 1993.

McLellan A.T., Grissom G., Alterman A.I., Brill, P. and O'Brien C.P. Substance Abuse Treatment in the Private Setting: Are some programs more effective than others? *J. Substance Abuse Treatment*, 10:243–254, 1993.

McLellan A.T., Metzger D., Alterman A.I. et al. How effective is substance abuse treatment—Compared to what? In C.P. O'Brien and J. Jaffe (Editors) *Advances in Understanding the Addictive States*. N.Y., Raven Press, 1992.

McLellan A.T., Alterman A.I., Woody G.E. A quantitative measure of substance abuse treatments: The Treatment Services Review. *J. Nerv. Ment. Dis.*, 180:101–110, 1992.

McLellan, A.T., Luborsky, L., Woody, G.E., O'Brien, C.P., Druley, K.A. Increased effectiveness of substance abuse treatment: A prospective study of patient-treatment "matching", *J. Nerv. Ment. Dis.*, 171(10):597–605, 1983.

McLellan, A.T., Druley, K.A., O'Brien, C.P., Kron, R. Matching substance abuse patients to appropriate treatments. A conceptual and methodological approach, *Drug and Alcohol Dependence*, 5(3):189–193, 1980.

Merrill, J. *The Cost of Substance Abuse to America's Health Care System*. Center on Addiction and Substance Abuse, Columbia University, NY, NY 1993.

Metzger D., Woody G.E., DePhillipis D., et al. Risk factors for needle sharing among methadone patients. *Am. J. Psychiatry*, 121:1113–1116, 1992.

Miller W.R. and Hester, R.K. The Effectiveness of Alcoholism Treatment Methods. In Miller, W.R. and Heather, N. (Eds.) *Treating Addictive Behaviors: Process of Change*, New York: Plenum Press, 1986.

Miller W. R., Walters S. T., and Bennett M. E. How effective is alcoholism treatment? *Journal of Studies on Alcohol*, 62:211–220, 2001.

Mitchell BD, Kammerer CM, Blangero J, et al. Genetic and environmental contributions to cardiovascular risk factors in Mexican Americans. *Circulation*, 94:2159–2170, 1996.

Moos R.H., Finney J.W. and Cronkite R.C. *Alcoholism Treatment: Context, Process and Outcome.* New York, Oxford Univ. Press., 1990.

Moos, R.H. *Evaluating Treatment Environments.* New York: Wiley, 1974.

National Institute on Drug Abuse, *See How Drug Abuse Takes the Profit Out of Business*, Dept. of Health and Human Services USGPO, 1991.

Nieminen MM, Kaprio J, and Koskenvuo M. A population-based study of bronchial asthma in adult twin pairs. *Chest*, 100:70–75, 1991.

O'Brien C.P. and McLellan A.T. Myths about the treatment of addiction. *Lancet* 347:237–240, 1996.

Pattison E.M. Evaluation of alcoholism treatment: A comparison of three facilities. *Arch Gen Psychiat.* 20:478–483, 1969.

Rice D.P., Kelman S., and Miller L.S. Estimates of the economic costs of alcohol, drug abuse and mental illness, 1985 and 1988. *Public Health Reports*, 106(3):281–292, 1991.

Rounsaville B.J., Dolinsky Z.S., Babor T.F. and Meyer R.E. (1987) Psychopathology as a predictor of treatment outcome in alcoholics. *Arch. Gen Psychiat.*, 44:505–513, 1987.

Rounsaville B.J., Wilber C.H. and Kleber H. Short-term interpersonal psychotherapy in methadone maintained opiate addicts. *Arch. Gen. Psychiat.*, 40:619–626, 1983.

Rua J. *Treatment Works: The Tragic Cost of Undervaluing Treatment in the Drug War.* Paper presented at the "What Works: An International Perspective on Drug Abuse Treatment" conference. New York. New York State Division of Substance Abuse Services, 1989.

Saxe L., Dougherty D. and Fine M. *The Effectiveness and Costs of Alcoholism Treatment.* Case Study 22. Office of Technology Assessment. Washington D.C., 1983

Schuckit M.A. The clinical implications of primary diagnostic groups among alcoholics. *Arch. Gen. Psychiat.*, 42:1043–1049, 1985.

Simpson D. and Savage L. Drug abuse treatment readmissions and outcomes, *Arch. Gen. Psychiat.* 37:896–901, 1980.

Sisk J.E., Hatziandreu, E.J. and Hughes R. *The Effectiveness of Drug Abuse Treatment: Implications for Controlling AIDS/HIV Infection*, Office of Technology Assessment, Background Paper No. 6, USGPO No. 052-003-01210-3, Washington D.C., 1990.

Svetkey L.P., McKeown S.P., and Wilson A.F. Heritability of salt sensitivity in black Americans. *Hypertension*, 28:854–858, 1996.

True WR and Xian H. Common genetic vulnerability for nicotine and alcohol dependence in men. *Arch. Gen. Psychiatry.* 1999;56:655–661.

Tsuang MT, Lyons MJ, Eisen S, et al. Genetic influences on DSM-III-R drug abuse and dependence: a study of 3,372 twin pairs. *Am. J. Med. Genet.*, 1996;67:473–477.

VandenBree M., Johnson E., Neale M., Pickens R. Genetic and environmental influences on drug use and abuse/dependence in male and female twins. *Drug Alcohol Dependence*, 1998;52:231–241.

Wall Street Journal, Editorial Commentary, July 18, 1994, p. A12.

Wexler M.K., Falkin G.P. and Lipton D.S. *A Model Prison Rehabilitation Program. An Evaluation of the Stay'n Out Therapeutic Community.* New York, NDRI Press., 1988.

Williams RR, Hunt SC, Hasstedt SJ, et al. Are there interactions and relations between genetic and environmental factors predisposing to high blood pressure? *Hypertension*, 1991;18(suppl): 129–137.

Woody G.E., McLellan A.T. and Luborsky L. Psychiatric severity as a predictor of benefits from psychotherapy. *Am. J. Psychiat.*, 141(10):1171–1177, 1984.

PART B

Intervening through Health Care Systems

Alcohol/drug problems seldom occur alone. Although "dual disorders" have been described as a special subset, in fact it is the norm for people with substance abuse or dependence to have other health and social problems. Alcohol and tobacco abuse contribute to a plethora of acute and chronic illnesses of the respiratory, cardiovascular, gastrointestinal, reproductive, and central nervous systems. The devastating effects extend well beyond the individual. Unborn infants are regularly and tragically harmed by parental substance use. Those who work in family courts, domestic violence programs, rape crisis clinics, emergency and trauma departments, homeless shelters, civil and criminal courts, and child protective services see daily the suffering that surrounds substance abuse.

It is not surprising, then, that people with alcohol/drug problems are very likely to turn up in health care and social service settings. As discussed in Chapter 1, they are far more likely to be seen in medical clinics and hospitals than in addiction treatment programs. Virtually anyone who delivers health care is already treating substance abuse and its sequelae. If acute specialist treatment is not an adequate model for addressing addictions, where then should we start? To begin with, there is much that can be done to address addictive behaviors in the course of providing health care. In the chapter that opens this section, Rollnick and Boycott discuss effective ways to intervene through primary health care. Even relatively brief counseling in the context of health care can trigger a change in substance use. They also suggest that practitioners may be more willing to learn a broader counseling method that can be applied not only to addictions, but to behavior change challenges in practice more generally.

Carol Schermer, a trauma surgeon, understands her life-saving role as involving more than acute care. A large percentage of injuries seen in emergency departments and trauma centers are linked in some way to substance use. In Chapter 5 she describes how emergency and trauma care affords an opportunity not only for acute treatment, but also for preventing future injuries.

A nation's busy health care system cannot, of course, bear the full burden of treating substance use disorders. Specialized addiction treatment programs will remain an important part of the continuum of care. In Chapter 6, Robert Meyers argues that it is incumbent on programs to provide services with the greatest liklihood of efficacy. He outlines succesful evidence-based treatment methods and suggests prachcal guidelines for bridging the gap between research and practice. Pharmacies and pharmacists represent a relatively untapped resource for recognizing and addressing substance abuse. People often see pharmacists more than doctors, and therein is another opportunity for continuing care with regard to substance use. Pharmacist Ernest Dole explores in Chapter 7 how his own profession and pharmacies more generally may be an important link as health care systems address alcohol/drug problems, including the abuse of prescription medications.

Of all abused drugs, tobacco clearly is a primary contributor to disease, disability, and premature death. Yet somehow tobacco is often sequestered, and left out of discussions of substance abuse. At the same time, it is the one form of drug abuse that health care professionals are most likely to recognize as falling within their ability and responsibility to address. Effective approaches that are currently used in health care to address smoking may also be useful with alcohol and other drugs. In the closing chapter of this section, Judith Ockene considers the special case of smoking, and how it fits into the puzzle of addressing substance abuse through health care systems.

CHAPTER 4

Intervening through Primary Health Care

STEPHEN ROLLNICK AND MICHELLE BOYCOTT

This chapter[1] aims to bridge a divide in the response to substance misuse, between the addiction experts and primary health care practitioners. Both have considerable experience of substance misuse, the former for obvious reasons, the latter because the presentation of everyday health and social problems are frequently laced with the impact of alcohol and other substance misuse. The focus here will be on everyday clinical practice and how it might be improved, rather than the broader political question of whose responsibility it is to reduce the public health burden of substance misuse.

How then, can primary care practitioners make the best use of limited time to address substance misuse? What skills do they need, and how might they acquire them? Even questions like these have political implications, and the answers are likely to vary across countries, cultures and settings. With the setting of the 9th ICTAB meeting in South Africa, this chapter will be directed towards how to help practitioners working in disadvantaged communities, often ravaged by AIDS and other health problems.

[1] This is an edited and slightly enlarged version of a presentation given by Stephen Rollnick at the 9th International Congress on the Treatment of Addictive Behaviour, Cape Town, South Africa, October 6–11, 2000.

STEPHEN ROLLNICK AND MICHELLE BOYCOTT • Department of General Practice, University of Wales College of Medicine, Cardiff, CF3 7PN, Wales, United Kingdom

WHY DO IT?

In most countries there is little choice but to deal with substance misuse problems in primary care, there being few or no specialist services available (Riley & Marshall, 1999). In the United States, however, it is only relatively recently that the advantages of tackling these problems from within primary care have become apparent (Institute of Medicine, 1990): i.e. most sufferers never appear in the specialist sector anyway, but remain on the caseloads of community-based practitioners. The rationale for strengthening the primary care system in developing countries is widely acknowledged, although the reality of limited resources raises a challenge when it comes to substance misuse that cannot be ignored: intervention needs to be integrated into everyday routine and should avoid burdening practitioners unduly.

It was exactly this challenge that led the World Health Organisation to investigate the effectiveness of screening and brief intervention for alcohol problems in its still ongoing program of research. The Phase II study, conducted in 11 countries, which included Zimbabwe and Kenya, found that excessive drinkers, both men and women, responded favourably to brief advice, but not more so to more intensive intervention (WHO Brief Intervention Study Group, 1996).

This kind of program followed the lead provided by smoking researchers in developed countries, where a large body of research has strengthened the view that public health can be improved by routine advice from a respected figure like a doctor or nurse. Considerable resources have been spent on controlled trials, which confirm that "simple advice" from a doctor (Silagy & Stead, 2001) or nurse (Rice & Stead, 2001) is effective; that nicotine replacement therapy is helpful (Silagy et al., 2001); that training helps (Lancaster et al., 2001) and that more intensive interventions might also be useful (Lancaster et al., 2001). While the percentage of smokers likely to respond is relatively small, so the argument goes, if large numbers of practitioners intervened with large numbers of smokers, the impact on public health would be considerable. The mathematics clearly make sense; implementation, it will be seen in the final section of this chapter, is a little more complex.

In the alcohol field, implementation issues were put to one side in favor of following a similar strategy. Efficacy trials of brief intervention reached near identical conclusions to those in the smoking field, although not all studies were able to locate significant effects. A useful overview of this work, that includes discussion of systematic reviews of dozens of studies, can be found in Heather (2001). It is worth noting that this research was so firmly oriented towards improving public health that people with severe alcohol problems were often excluded from brief intervention studies. To the best of our knowledge, no trials of brief advice have been conducted among primary care patients who use or misuse other substances.

WHAT TO DO

There are different ways to describe the inner workings of substance misuse interventions that might be used in primary care. Research has not got to the stage where the content of different interventions have been studied in sufficient depth to provide clear, evidence-based guidelines. In truth, we are left with a range of possibilities that vary in complexity. The 3-method framework used below, involving brief advice, motivational interviewing and behaviour change counselling, is merely that which made sense to us, based on experience of working closely with health care practitioners over a number of years. Further details about the methods involved can be found in Rollnick et al. (2002) and Miller and Rollnick (2002).

Brief Advice

Advice-giving about health behavior change contains a mixture of information and a call to action, to behave differently (Rollnick et al., 1999). This activity has been conceived of as a relatively simple matter by smoking and excessive drinking researchers, and indeed, it *is* fairly straightforward to give someone clear information and some guidance about what they might do. This simplicity makes advice-giving easier to integrate into everyday practice than some of the more complex interventions described below.

Observation of practitioners reveals that this can be done with tact, sensitivity and skill. With less skill, there can be potentially damaging consequences for the morale of the patient. One seasoned practitioner told us that advice works best with the patient one knows best. The key elements here are probably an awareness of the readiness of the patient to receive the information and advice; open questions to understand the patient's views and needs; and the tailoring of content to meet the person's cultural context, language and intellectual abilities. Many years of experience can thus make a reasonably complex activity look simple, as is the case with so many sporting skills.

This view of a skilful activity might be overstated. Indeed, the promotion of routine screening and advice in the brief intervention field alludes to a quite simple procedure. One hypothesis to be discussed below in the section on implementation is that practitioners might resist such guidance because they feel that, for example, giving advice routinely to any smoker or excessive drinker ignores the complexity of the practitioner-patient relationship. There are times when it might not be appropriate to give advice, for a wide range of reasons.

To the best of our knowledge, there has been no detailed study of cultural variation in the acceptability of advice-giving in health care practice. Nevertheless, doctors and nurses we work with in the developed world say that more "traditional" patients (older, from more tightly-knit communities) often expect to be told what to do about lifestyle change, whereas other patients (whom they call "the more sophisticated ones") like to make decisions for themselves. We imagine that such variation exists between and within different cultures and groups. Indeed, one individual might like advice in one situation but prefer more autonomy in another. This suggests that while advice-giving might have considerable value in efforts to encourage changes in health behaviour, developing a wider and more flexible array of skills might be important for practitioners. Useful descriptions of the delivery of routine advice-giving can be found in accounts of the World Health Organisation Phase II alcohol study that included projects in both Zimbabwe and Kenya (WHO Brief Intervention Study Group, 1996).

More Complex Interventions

Any attempt to consider the use of more complex intervention in primary care must deal with the possibility that the burden of having to train practitioners might render it unrealistic in many settings. This issue will be addressed in the section on implementation that follows. To begin with, the clinical rationale and scientific status of interventions derived from motivational interviewing will briefly be discussed.

Motivational Interviewing

This counselling style was developed in the addictions field in response to concerns about difficult interviews in specialist clinics (Miller and Rollnick, 2002). Clients were being labelled as resistant and full of denial, somehow unwilling to listen to the messages given to them by well-intentioned counselors. Motivational interviewing is based on the rather simple notion that the way clients are spoken to about changing addictive behaviour affects their willingness to talk freely about why and how they might change. Confrontational interviewing can heighten resistance and denial; in contrast, the directive use of empathic listening can help them examine their problems with a sense of purpose, free of challenging persuasive efforts from the counselor. For this reason, motivational interviewing is defined as a counseling style, rather than a set of techniques applied to or on people. Enthusiasm for this method over the last decade is probably borne of frustration with using direct persuasion that often carries the risk of eliciting resistance. At the heart of motivational interviewing lies the idea that people are best persuaded by their own arguments for change, not by those imposed on them by a no doubt well-intentioned practitioner. Motivation to change is best elicited from the patients themselves.

Primary health care workers will recognise these challenges, not only because they have experience of talking to patients caught in the throes of addiction, but because they have daily conversations about the need to take medication and change lifestyle behaviors (Rollnick et al., 1999). However, because their setting involves time-limited consultations about a wide range of problems, it is an open question whether they have the time and resources to practice this specialist counseling style to a high standard.

Researchers also recognised the potential of motivational interviewing and set about applying "it" in various forms, using different names, in a wide variety of healthcare settings. The outcome of this effort has been mixed (Dunn et al., 2001; Burke et al., 2002), with a tendency to bypass a clear description of the content of a method under study, let alone how practitioners were trained to use it (Rollnick, 2001). Caution about this evidence base is thus warranted. It appears that the method is effective in addiction settings, while the current evidence elsewhere is more limited.

Behaviour Change Counseling

This is a name recently given by a consensus group of motivational interviewing trainers to embrace the family of derivatives of motivational interviewing used in healthcare settings (Rollnick et al., 2002) that are more suited to time-limited consultations. Many of the key skills overlap with motivational interviewing, but some of the more complex aspects of the latter method have been taken out, to be replaced by goals and skills that might be of value in more generalist settings.

Some potentially useful examples of this form of counseling are described by Rollnick et al. (2002), while others can be located in the reviews by Dunn et al. (2001) and Burke et al. (2002). Two specific strategies will be noted below, in order to illustrate that it is possible to structure a conversation about behaviour change that encourages the patient to make choices and take charge of decision-making. These are not techniques as such, but merely aids to skilful counselling.

Setting an agenda. A common problem in primary care is multiple-behavior change challenges, where the practitioner and patient might talk about a range of changes in different behaviors. For example, a man who is HIV positive, a heavy user of alcohol, and has diabetes, attends a clinic in a township, presenting with a medical problem. What behavior change does the practitioner focus on? How does he or she ensure that the patient takes charge of efforts to change?

The opening gambit of such a consultation can ensure progress or make matters difficult for both parties. Setting an agenda can help them decide what to talk about. Behavior change counseling involves a taxing maelstrom of personal and social choices. The agenda setting chart, first used in a study of behavior change in patients with diabetes, helps the two parties to select from a range of options that could be discussed: for example, eating, drinking, medication use, and so on. It also includes blank circles for the patient to add concerns not mentioned. Although the practitioner may indicate his or her preference, open questions are used to encourage the patient to make choices about where to begin the discussion. Shared decision-making is the goal. The chart itself is not an essential part of this constructive conversation. Some practitioners prefer to simply use the above guidance to structure the consultation, without visual aids (see Rollnick et al., 1999).

Assessing motivation to change. When a specific behavior is chosen, how does one encourage the patient to talk about the why and how of change? The answers to these questions will amount to an understanding of motivation or readiness to change. The assessment of importance (why change?) and confidence (how to change?) was originally designed to be done in 5–10 minutes, and can be used as the basis for encouraging the patient, often for the first time, to talk through the challenges in an accepting environment (see Rollnick et al., 1999). For example, two questions can be asked initially:

a) *How do you feel* at the moment *about* (change)? *How **important** is it to you personally to* (change)? *If 0 was "not important" and 10 was "very important", what number would you give yourself?*
b) *If you decided* right now *to* (change), *how **confident** do you feel about succeeding with this? If 0 was "not confident", and 10 was "very confident", what number would you give yourself?*

In listening to the answers to these questions the practitioner is given the opportunity, indeed the privilege, of stepping inside the patient's beliefs and expectations about change. The practitioner maintains an attitude of curiosity while gently steering the discussion towards a shared understanding of why and how change might occur.

How do I raise the subject? This is a common call from the consulting room, independent of the method being used. Judging by the reports of practitioners, concern about how to raise the subject might well account for a substantial number of missed opportunities to deal with substance misuse. Our supervision and training experiences have led us to the rather obvious conclusion that raising the issue is not a problem, but what happens afterwards is. Most patients will go along with a polite request to talk about a particular subject. What they might resist or resent is insensitive questioning thereafter.

If this hypothesis is correct, then anything that makes patients feel at ease will help. Among the possibilities we have explored are avoiding premature action talk, using open questions to give patients center stage to say how they feel, regular summarising by the practitioner, asking the patient to talk about a typical day (see Rollnick et al., 1999) and using the importance and confidence assessment described above.

HOW TO DO IT: IMPLEMENTATION

It has been difficult to implement in practice the findings of brief intervention research on smoking and drinking. Practitioners seem to resist even an apparently simple recommendation like delivering brief advice to all smokers. With excessive drinkers, the challenge is greater because practitioners often have ambivalent attitudes towards drinking, and they fail to identify most potential cases, many of whom do not present with the medical consequences of their drinking in the first place. When one talks to practitioners about other kinds of drug misuse, military metaphors are often used to describe bruising encounters with apparently unreasonable patients.

In trying to bridge the divide between substance misuse experts and primary health care practitioners, our hunch is not to view resistance in the latter group as entirely their problem. Rather, we hope that an understanding of their concerns might lead to more constructive programmes and recommendations for addressing the widespread problem of substance abuse.

The Concerns of Primary Care Practitioners

A number of studies of the experiences, attitudes and behavior of practitioners towards substance misuse intervention in primary care have been carried out in the alcohol field (see for example, Aalto, Seppä, K and Mattila, P. et al., 2001; Aalto et al., 2001; Angove & McBride, 2001; Andreasson et al., 2001; Kaner et al., 1999; Deehan et al., 1998) and in the smoking field (see for example, McEwan et al., 2001; Keller et al., 2000). The findings are broadly congruent with our own discussions with practitioners about why they don't spend more time on substance misuse: they often feel over-burdened with acute medicine, making it difficult to give priority to preventive work; most are primarily concerned with the needs of the individual and are less committed to public health promotion than are specialists in the substance abuse field. They also indicate that they are concerned to maintain good relationships with their patients, and sometimes fear that raising the subject of behavior change might put this relationship in jeopardy. It is not uncommon to hear accounts of feeling unskilled to deal with the consequences of raising the subject, particularly with a short consultation time of 5–15 minutes, and that they would like more training. Some talk about the relatively low success rate with brief advice, whatever the public health benefits might be. Finally, they sometimes fear outright abuse from patients who might demand particular medications (e.g. tranquilizers).

A Flexible Approach to Implementation

No single idea, method or program is likely to address these concerns and ensure that routine intervention with substance misuse takes place. We identify below a number of possibilities that might encourage practitioners to become more involved.

1. Bottom-up initiatives

Implementation is effectively an attempt to change the behavior of practitioners. Among the most pressing recent examples in developing countries is the over-prescribing of antibiotics for acute respiratory problems in primary care. Strongly-worded guidelines, thoroughly disseminated and backed up by evidence that these drugs are not appropriate for most acute respiratory problems, have apparently had little impact on practice. It seems that inside the consultation, a number of forces promote prescribing, for example, limited time and the doctor's belief that patients want this kind of medication. Doctors are aware of the pressure from above to change, but this is not enough for implementation to succeed. They need success experiences that leave them and their patients comfortable about managing the problem without antibiotics. Learning new ways of handling the consultation might be central to this effort. Implementation without clinically relevant training might not get very far.

The lessons from this account are borne out by the reviews of the literature on the implementation of guidelines. Where valid guidelines have been developed and disseminated, the final hurdle of implementation is best overcome by an overtly educational strategy in which guidelines are adapted by the individuals who will use them, with a focus on consultations with individual patients rather than general performance (Grimshaw and Russell, 1993). Such an approach is suited to helping primary care practitioners in the field of substance abuse, whether in industrialized or developing countries. It calls for a bottom-up approach in which research findings and externally developed guidelines are used to encourage practitioners themselves take charge of developing a response to the problem that is sensitive to their needs and the cultural context in which they work.

2. Loosening the guideline to screen all patients

It is not uncommon to encounter screening and brief intervention viewed as part of the same activity. In the alcohol field, for example, both the World Health Organization and other leading researchers (Babor & Higgens-Biddle, 2000) even use the letters "SBI" (screeing and brief intervention) to describe the heart of their proposal for primary care. The idea is to screen all patients who enter the system using one of the validated questionnaires developed for this purpose. Practitioners might resist the use of routine screening for a number of reasons. Not only does this involve much more work, but the administration of patient care requires adjustment for this to take place. Screening might be the answer in some settings and circumstances, but not in others. Some practitioners might be concerned about the rationale for this work. Indeed, it has been pointed out from within the alcohol field (Rollnick et al., 1997) that screening for *young* heavy drinkers might violate the usual rationale for screening, since epidemiological research shows that most of these excessive drinkers spontaneously reduce their drinking in later life. Leaving this as an explicitly optional element might reduce resistance among practitioners.

3. Opportunistic screening inside the consultation

If practitioners do not screen all patients systematically, how else might they identify those who misuse different substances? Guidelines for doing this in primary care were provided by Stott (1983), who suggested that practitioners might take advantage of the unique circumstances of each consultation to consider opportunities for promoting good health, at a time that seems right to the practitioner and patient. His use of the term *opportunistic* thus referred not to taking advantage of all patients entering a clinic setting, but to well-timed decisions to raise the subject with selected individuals. Taking this approach might relieve practitioners of the expectation that they should be delivering systematic screening to all patients in a busy clinical setting.

4. Raising the subject with all levels of problem severity

In the alcohol field, brief intervention research has focussed only upon at-risk excessive drinkers, because public health experts would like to see consumption reduced in this group. Practitioners we meet talk about having more concerns about the severe end of the problem drinking spectrum. It might make better sense to develop programs that include intervention for all kinds of drinkers, thus encouraging practitioners to acquire skills to raise the subject with any patient who might have a problem with alcohol.

5. Core skills for behaviour change problems

While specialists understandably work on the challenges of their chosen topic (e.g. heavy drinking or smoking), primary care practitioners experience health behavior problems as integrated with social, economic, medical and other behavioral problems. Asking them to intervene with a particular behavior in isolation from other related problems might thus prove troublesome. For example, if a young man presents with a medical problem associated with smoking, drinking and abuse of some other illegal drug, how does the practitioner decide where to focus health promotion efforts? What consulting skills are needed? Is brief advice adequate? It is this kind of dilemma that led to the development of the methods described above, that can be used with any behavior change scenario. Physicians may have more interest in receiving training in these methods, which is what we turn to now.

6. Broad content of training

There is probably no escape from some investment in training if practitioners are to realistically tackle the behavioral problems associated with AIDS, substance abuse and other problems. Simply encouraging them to *do more*, for example, "give more advice about drinking" might be insufficient. For training to be successful, we assume that there must be something of value to them in it, something that will make their lives easier rather than more demanding.

What, then, could substance abuse training consist of? One obvious component is information about the manifestations of substance abuse and its relation to other problems like AIDS, family problems, and so on. Another is information about the cost-effectiveness of brief advice. This is the kind of material that could easily be integrated into both pre- and post-qualification training curricula.

For the qualified practitioner, what is likely to make everyday practice easier? However tempting it might be for specialists from different sectors of the substance abuse field to champion their chosen subject and associated intervention method, use of a single broad model of behavior change intervention skills carries clear advantages. At its heart, such a method involves good communication about the consultation in which a patient's very personal values and preferences frequently rub up against the aspirations of the practitioner. Much like the common consultation about breaking bad news, some particular skills and sensitivities are required, by no means beyond the reach of the primary care practitioner. To ignore the common elements across different problem areas in favor of topic-specific education might not only be more expensive, but might bypass the generic skills most needed by practitioners.

The suggestion here is not that substance abuse training should be replaced by generic behavior change training, but that the emphasis might be on the latter, which could provide the platform upon which more substance-specific educational material is placed. Thus, for example, of 100 training units, 50 units could be assigned to generic behaviour change consulting skills, with the remaining 50 units given to information about specific topics like alcohol problems, smoking, AIDS, and so on.

The field of AIDS provides a good example. With so many developing countries ravaged by double digit prevalence rates of HIV infection, there will be undoubted pressure to use international aid and local resources in the fight against this disease. Training primary care practitioners might well be one result of this effort. The temptation to run HIV-specific training will be great. However, it might be worth considering the broader behavior change challenges that arise in consultations about HIV, and run training courses that provide practitioners with the basic framework and consulting skills for dealing with any behavior change challenge.

7. Context-bound training methods

It is one thing to speculate about what training might consist of, quite another to consider how this might be delivered. This is a poorly researched area, weighed down in developed countries by decades of traditional, standard practice, often called continuing medical education (CME): practitioners are offered doses of education delivered off-site by different experts in various fields. There seems little reason for those in developing countries to follow suit, because the effectiveness of CME of this kind has been questioned in favor of more personally tailored and context-bound learning (Davies et al., 1995). The implication is that practitioners need to grapple with everyday medical and social problems *in context* in order to define their learning needs and work on solutions to clinical challenges.

Sensitivity to local cultural attitudes could be critical in substance misuse training. For example, if a young female nurse is talking to an older man whose culture defines a status gap between them, an intervention about sexual behavior change and substance misuse will demand skilful negotiation. Trainers need to structure learning opportunities that match the context. Strengthening the educational base *within* primary care might be preferable, for example, to constructing centers of excellence outside of it. The developing world has many good examples of locally-directed learning and practice, and the substance abuse field offers a good opportunity to strengthen the skill base on the front line of care.

One area of recent development has been the construction of an alternative to the commonly used off-site training workshop, which tends to rely on relatively artificial role-play learning techniques. We have used the term *context-bound training* (Rollnick et al., in press a) to describe a different way of thinking and training, some elements of which should be applicable in settings where resources are limited. Practitioners are trained on-site, and the approach of the trainer is not to teach them new methods, but to become immersed in everyday consulting challenges they face. Typical scenarios are constructed by practitioners, and an actor is used to consult with them in the clinic setting before and after each brief seminar. These seminars are used to share experiences and consider how to handle the same actor immediately afterwards. The trainer's ideas are merely used in the meeting to bolster this attempt to develop more flexible consulting skills. In its most sophisticated form, we have used tape recordings, and asked practitioners to examine in private their transcript before and after attending the seminar. Some evidence that practitioners actually change their consulting patterns has been collected (Rollnick et al., in press b).

CONCLUSION: TOWARDS STRONGER GENERALISTS

Substance abuse problems appear in primary care in large numbers and often cannot be avoided. The potential for preventive work and public health gain has been well argued and researched. In most developing countries this is the only realistic way forward. Specialist services have a role, but are limited by the sheer numbers of people involved. Whatever the intervention methods may be called, it does seem reasonable to conclude that the opportunity is there for practitioners to improve their repertoire of consulting skills for tackling problems like substance abuse.

It is one thing to have evidence from efficacy trials of different interventions, quite another to encourage realistic implementation in demanding circumstances. We have raised a number of implementation topics for debate in a field in which easy solutions are not evident, and in which practitioners on the ground will need considerable support to become more skilled at taking a deep breath and tackling the ravages of substance misuse. An obvious bias in this discussion has been our view of the need to enhance the *generalist* skills of practitioners; this is where we believe the strength of primary care lies, particularly in the developing world. It might be better to work with this strength than to risk overwhelming practitioners with specialist expertise that might well be beyond their ability to take on board.

REFERENCES

Aalto M., Seppä K., Mattila P., Mustonen., Ruuth K., Hyvärinen H., Pulkkinen H., Alho H. & Sillanaukee P. (2001). Brief intervention for male heavy drinkers in routine general practice: a three-year randomized controlled study. *Alcohol & Alcoholism*, 36: 224–230.

Aalto, M., Pekuri P. & Seppä K. (2001). Primary health care nurses' and physicians' attitudes, knowledge and beliefs regarding brief intervention for heavy drinkers. *Addiction*, 96: 305–311.

Andréasson S., Hjalmarsson K. & Rehnman C. (2001). Implementation and dissemination of methods for prevention of alcohol problems in primary health care: a feasibility study. *Alcohol & Alcoholism*, 35: 525–530.

Angove R. and McBride A.J. (2001). Swimming upstream: how and why an alcohol misuse screening and intervention service using the AUDIT can have limited impact in primary care. *Journal of Substance Misuse*, 6: 70–79.

Babor T. & Higgens-Biddle J. (2000). Alcohol screening and brief intervention: dissemination strategies for medical practice and public health. *Addiction*, 95: 677–686.

Burke B., Arkowitz H. & Dunn C. (2002). The efficacy of motivational interviewing and its adaptations: what we know so far. In: Miller W.R. & Rollnick S. *Motivational Interviewing: Preparing People for Change*. New York: Guilford Press.

Butler C,. Rollnick S., Cohen D., Russell I., Bachmann M. & Stott N. (1999). Motivational consulting versus brief advice for smokers in general practice: A randomized trial. *British Journal of General Practice*, 49: 611–616.

Davies D., Thomson M, Oxman A. & Haynes B. (1995). Changing physician performance: A systematic review of the effect of continuing medical education strategies. *Journal of the American Medical Association*, 274: 700–705.

Deehan A., Templeton,L., Taylor, C., Drummond D.C., & Strang J. (1998). Low detection rates, negative attitudes and the failure to meet "Health of the Nation" targets: findings from a national survey of GPs in England and Wales. *Drug and Alcohol Review*, 17(3): 249–258.

Dunn C., Deroo L. & Rivara (2001). The use of brief interventions adapted from motivational interviewing across behavioural domains: a systematic review. *Addiction*, 96: 1725–1742.

Grimshaw J. & Russell I. (1993). Achieving health gain through clinical guidelines, I: Developing scientifically valid guidelines. *Quality in Health Care*, 2: 243–248.

Heather N, Peters T. & Stockwell T. (2001). *International Handbook of Alcohol Dependence and Problems.* Chichester: John Wiley & Sons.

Institute of Medicine (IOM) (1990). *Broadening the Base of Treatment for Alcohol Problems.* Washington, DC: National Academy Press.

Kaner E., Heather N., Gilvarry E., McAvoy B. & Lock C. (1999). Intervention for excessive alcohol consumption in primary health care: attitudes and practices of English general practitioners. *Alcohol & Alcoholism*, 34: 559–566.

Keller S., Donner-Banzhoff N., Kaluza G., Baum E. & Basler H-D. (2000). Improving Physician-delivered Counseling in a Primary Care Setting: Lessons from a Failed Attempt. *Education for Health: Change in Learning & Practice*, 13: 387–397.

Lancaster T, Silagy C. & Fowler G. (2001). *Training Health Professionals In Smoking Cessation (Cochrane Review).* The Cochrane Library, 4. Oxford: Update Software.

McEwen A., Akotia N. & West R. (2001). General Practitioners' views on the English national smoking cessation guidelines. *Addiction*, 96: 997–1000.

Miller W. R. & Rollnick S. (2002). *Motivational Interviewing: Preparing People for Change* (2nd edition). New York: Guilford Press.

Rice V.H. & Stead L.F. (2001). *Nursing interventions for smoking cessation (Cochrane Review).* The Cochrane Library, 4. Oxford: Update Software.

Riley L. & Marshall M. (Eds) (1999). *Alcohol and Public Health in 8 Developing Countries.* Geneva: World Health Organisation (WHO/HSC/SAB/99.9).

Rollnick S, Butler C. & Hodgson R. (1997). Brief alcohol intervention in medical settings: Concerns from the consulting room. *Addiction Research*, 5: 331–342.

Rollnick S., Mason, P. & Butler C. (1999). *Behavior Change: A Guide for Practitioners.* Edinburgh: Churchill Livingstone.

Rollnick, S. (2001). Enthusiasm, quick fixes and premature controlled trials. *Addiction*, 96: 1769–1770.

Rollnick S., Allison J., Ballasiotes S., Barth T., Butler C., Rose G. & Rosengren D. (2002). Variations on a theme: motivational interviewing and its adaptations. In: Miller, W.R. & Rollnick, S. *Motivational Interviewing: Preparing People for Change.* New York: Guilford Press.

Rollnick S., Kinnersley P. & Butler C.C. (in press a). Context-bound communication skills training: Development of the SPICE training method. *Medical Education.*

Rollnick S., Kinnersley P., Rees M., Butler C.C., Hood K. & Anderson L. (in press b). "Developing a new line of patter": can doctors change their consultations for sore throat? *Medical Education.*

Silagy C. & Stead L.F. (2001). *Physician advice for smoking cessation (Cochrane Review).* The Cochrane Library, 4. Oxford: Update Software.

Silagy C., Lancaster T., Stead L., Mant D., Fowler G. (2001). *Nicotine replacement therapy for smoking cessation (Cochrane Review).* The Cochrane Library, 4. Oxford: Update Software.

Stewart M, Belle Brown J, Wayne Weston W, McWhinney IR, McWilliam C.L. & Freeman T.R., (1995). eds. *Patient-Centered Medicine. Transforming the Clinical Method.* Thousand Oaks: Sage Publications.

Stott N.C.H. (1983). Primary Care: Closing the Gap between Theory and Practice. London: Wiley.

WHO Brief Intervention Study GROUP (1996) A randomized cross-national clinical trial of brief interventions with heavy drinkers. *American Journal of Public Health*, 86: 948–955.

CHAPTER 5

Intervening through the Emergency Department and Trauma Center

CAROL R. SCHERMER

INTRODUCTION

Alcohol is the leading risk factor for injury, with a high prevalence of alcohol-related injuries reported by emergency departments and trauma centers worldwide. Problem drinkers use healthcare resources more than the general population and are at increased risk for recurrent injury and death. This chapter will discuss the magnitude of the problem of alcohol and injury, screening tests that have been evaluated in the injured population, and the status of interventions.

Nearly half of all trauma deaths occur at the trauma scene and are not responsive to improvements in care but would respond to injury prevention (Cales 1984, West 1979). Although nearly one-half of US trauma beds are occupied by patients who were injured while under the influence of alcohol, alcohol abuse and dependence typically are not addressed during the period of trauma care for the patient (Soderstrom 1987, 1992, Gentilello 1988, Colquitt 1987, Reyna 1985).

The appeal of intervening in the Emergency Department (ED) or trauma center is that treatment can come to the patient, rather than waiting for the patient to seek treatment. Appropriate screening identifies patients that otherwise may not have been recognized as problematic drinkers. Additionally, patients may be more motivated to change and receptive to treatment in a moment of crisis (Longabaugh 1995, Bombardier 1997). Two advantages of intervening in the emergency room or trauma center setting are that the proportion of heavy drinkers is

---

CAROL R. SCHERMER • Department of Surgery, University of New Mexico Health Sciences Center, Albuquerque, New Mexico 87131

high and most injured patients are young and thus may be detected at an early stage of problem drinking. Treatment of the drinking problem can naturally evolve from treatment of the injury.

MAGNITUDE OF THE PROBLEM

Injuries are the leading cause of death among persons under 44 years old and the leading cause of years of life lost due to premature death (NCIPC 1991) Injury is more costly than any health condition. When lost goods and services are accounted for costs exceed $110 billion US dollars per year (Rice et al. 1989). Numerous studies report that alcohol is the leading risk factor for injury. In 40 to 50% of fatal motor vehicle crashes (MVCs) and 30–40% of nonfatal MVCs at least one occupant is legally intoxicated. Alcohol plays a role in a large proportion of falls, drownings, hypothermia, burns, and intentional injuries. (Reyna 1985, Lowenfels 1984) The mean blood alcohol concentration in patients admitted to trauma centers is routinely reported as over 150 mg/dl (Rivara 1993a, McLellan 1990, Schermer 2001a).

Cherpitel has extensively reviewed alcohol and injuries. The ED population in general, whether urban or suburban, injured or non-injured has more alcohol-related problems than the general population. The international prevalence of alcohol problems in patients evaluated in the ED ranges from 5% to 31% (Cherpitel 1993, Rund 1981, Teplin 1989). Approximately one-third of all patients presenting to the ED are legally intoxicated at the time of visit or are deemed to have alcohol problems by screening questionnaires. (Bernstein 1997, Jurkovich 1992) The highest group of patients having a positive blood alcohol concentration (BAC) tend to be those presenting with psychiatric problems, the second highest are those involved in accidents. ED studies the world over have consistently suggested that patients seeking treatment for injury are more likely to be positive for alcohol than those seeking treatment for medical reasons. Alcohol use is more common in injured than non-injured patients, and heavy drinkers have more severe injuries. Moreover, intoxicated injured patients are more likely to report previous alcohol related injuries (Cherpitel 1988, Borges 1998). In an ED study of vehicular crash victims, Maio et al. found a 15% prevalence of abuse or dependence in patients treated and released and 30% abuse or dependence for patients admitted to a trauma center (Maio 1997). Similar results have been found in various studies in the UK and Thailand (Thom 1999, Dowey 1993, Lapham 1998).

US and Canadian studies have shown that alcohol and drug abusers are twice as likely as the general population to be hospitalized for injury (Miller 2001) and that 20% to 86% of hospitalized trauma patients test positive for alcohol or other drugs (Gentilello 1988, Sloan 1989, Soderstrom 1992, Rivara 1993a,b, McLellan 1990). Soderstrom (1992) and Rivara (1993a) have found 25% to 45% of patients admitted for trauma met criteria for abuse or dependence. Treno and colleagues found a 14.9% rate of alcohol related diagnoses including withdrawal, abuse, dependence and cirrhosis among more than 22,000 patients in the California Trauma Registry (Treno 1996).

The risk of death due to injury in those with alcohol problems is 2.5 to eight times that of the general population (Popham 1984, Welte 1987, Weiczorek 1990, Evans 1990). Rivara et al. (1993b) and Schermer et al. (2001a) examined recurrent injury rates in trauma patients. Patients who were intoxicated at the time of admission were 2.5 times more likely to sustain a second injury or recurrent hospitalization in the 2 years following admission to be readmitted for injury. Those with chronic alcohol disorders were 3.5 times more likely. A similar study by Sims (1989) in Detroit showed that 44% of trauma patients sustained 2 or more recurrent injuries within 5 years of the initial admission. Alcohol abuse was identified in 67% of those requiring recurrent admission and in 60% of those with a single admission. Kaufman has shown that recidivists are more likely to be BAC positive (Kaufman 1998).

Blose and Holder have shown that problem drinkers utilize injury related medical care at a rate of 1.6 times that of a comparison group (Blose and Holder 1991), and Anda (1988) and colleagues estimate that those who consume 5 to 9 or more drinks per occasion have 1.9- to 3.3-fold greater chances of dying from injury compared to those who do not. Li and colleagues found that a larger proportion of people who die from injury drink alcohol than those who die from disease (Li 1994).

Costs related to injury are higher than for cancer or heart disease, but only a small portion of the healthcare dollar is spent on prevention of recurrent injury. In general when people are admitted to a hospital, the underlying causes of their diseases are examined, such as smoking, exercise and diet for heart disease. But for injury, the underlying causes are rarely examined. In the U.S., Soderstrom and Cowley assessed clinical practices in trauma centers involving alcohol in 1987 (Soderstrom 1987). They showed that BACs were routinely obtained in 55% of centers responding to their survey but fewer than 1/3 of centers employed an alcoholism counselor and less than 5% of patients received a treatment referral. Colquitt (1987) examined referral patterns in a community hospital with an inpatient detoxification unit and alcohol and drug counselors. None of the motor vehicle crash victims with high BACs were referred for treatment. Lowenstein (1990) has also shown that injured intoxicated patients are three times less likely than non-injured intoxicated patients to be referred for counseling.

Injury should be viewed as a public health problem rather than as accidental since it often results from the interaction of many factors including substance use. The US preventive services task force (1996) recommends that "all persons who use alcohol should be informed of the health and injury risks associated with consumption." The American Medical Association (AMA) believes that trauma centers are ideal sites for implementation of brief interventions and encourages hospitals to promote alcohol and drug testing of injured patients and to implement appropriate substance abuse evaluation and treatment.

SCREENING IN THE ED OR TRAUMA SETTING

EDs now recognize they can function in a prevention capacity for patients who do not have other health services. The Society of Academic Emergency Medicine (SAEM) has created a preventive services task force that identifies alcohol and drug screening as the primary intervention that could readily be performed in the ED (Irvin 2000). Screening may be performed by any member of the health care team: the social worker, the nurse or the physician. Screens, such as the CAGE need to be administered verbally in an empathic manner or results may be suspect. The AUDIT, generally a self-administered instrument, may also be given verbally in situations where patients with multiple injuries cannot fill out the form. Screening instruments have been well tested in the ED in the US, Mexico, Spain and the United Kingdom (Cherpitel 1998, 2000, Becker 1995, Peters 1998).

In addition to screening tests identifying those with problematic alcohol use, other benefits include better medical management, safer and more effective pain management, improvements in aftercare planning and treatment, enhanced patient compliance, and possible prevention of future alcohol related injuries. Universal screening keeps the process from being biased against certain cultural, ethnic, gender and age groups.

Clinical suspicion of acute alcohol intoxication and of chronic alcohol problems is inaccurate and fraught with bias (Gentilello 1999a, Becker 1995). In one study, physicians and Emergency Department nurses failed to identify 23% of acutely intoxicated injured patients with the miss rate increasing as severity of injury increased. Young, disheveled, uninsured males with low socioeconomic status were likely to be falsely suspected of acute intoxication. Also staff identified fewer than 50% of patients screening positive for chronic alcohol problems (Gentilello 1999a). Becker found that only 52% of emergency physicians and ED nurses correctly identified alcohol positive patients (Becker 1995).

Some have argued for using the blood alcohol concentration to screen for alcohol problems (CSAT TIP series). However, BAC alone should not be used to screen for alcohol problems since many patients with alcohol problems will be negative at the time of admission (Yates 1987, Rivara 1993b, Maio 1997, Soderstrom 1996). The sensitivity of BAC to check for alcohol problems is at best 75%. In one study, 45% of patients who had alcohol abuse or dependence had no measurable BAC in the ED (Maio 1997). Traditional laboratory tests of GGT, AST, MCV even when combined with BAC are not predictive of alcohol dependence in the trauma setting (Ryb 1999). Breath alcohol analysis also has poor sensitivity of 20%, but high specificity 94% (Cherpitel 1989).

The need for brevity cannot be overemphasized in the busy ED setting. In London, Smith and colleagues evaluated a simple 3 item Paddington Alcohol Test which contains a quantity question, a frequency question and an item relating alcohol to the patients' attendance in the ED. The screen alone increased referral rates by ten-fold over a prior study done in the same ED (Smith 1996, Gentilello 1999a). Cherpitel found that the TWEAK had a sensitivity of 87% and specificity of 86% when detecting harmful and dependent drinkers in the ED when compared to other commonly available instruments. The AUDIT was comparable (Cherpitel 1998). The CAGE, Brief MAST, and AUDIT have been evaluated by Soderstrom and colleagues in trauma inpatients and when compared to the structured clinical interview from the DSM-III-R, lifetime alcohol dependence is diagnosed in 35.5%, abuse in 8.1% (Soderstrom 1997). Screening tests such as the short MAST are positive for alcohol problems in as many as 75% of trauma patients and are even positive in 26% of patients with no detectable BAC on admission (Rivara 1993a). Self-report data seems to be reliable in the US, Mexico and Spain where studies report low rates of patients reporting not drinking, who then measure positive by BAC or breathalyzer (Cherpitel 1992). Soderstrom found the CAGE questions to be the best predictor of lifetime dependence in injured patients (Soderstrom 1997) and found the sensitivity and specificity of the AUDIT to detect current alcohol dependence were 95% and 82% (Soderstrom 1998).

Cherpitel developed a brief screening instrument, the RAPS (Rapid Alcohol Screen), for problem drinking specifically tested for use in the ED (Cherpitel 2000) since routine questionnaires had previously not performed well in identifying female problem drinkers or those of some ethnic groups (Cherpitel 1998). The RAPS developed from an ED study outperformed other screening instruments with 98% sensitivity and 78% specificity across all subgroups. Salivary alcohol testing (SAT) has been evaluated in Scotland where 22% of accident victims consenting to study were SAT positive (Simpson 2001). In the US, in subcritically injured patients, SAT was compared to AUDIT scores to examine it as a screen for hazardous or harmful drinking. A SAT result of 4 mmol/L (20 mg/dl) or greater identified patients with an AUDIT score of 8 or more (Tu 1992, Becker 1995).

Although a number of screening instruments have been evaluated, the AUDIT appears to have the most international appeal; norms have been developed based on its evaluation in a number of countries. (Saunders, 1993). Research centers in Australia, Bulgaria, Kenya, Mexico, Norway and the US all participated in the evaluation of the AUDIT. Unlike the CAGE, it has good operating characteristics for different gender and ethnicity (Cherpitel 1995, Volk 1997). It is designed to detect early or mild problem drinking rather than detecting alcohol dependence. It therefore may be a more appropriate screening test for the trauma population that tends to be younger and have fewer problems than treatment seeking populations or patients hospitalized for complications of alcohol dependence.

Interventions

There are only a handful of intervention studies and reports of referral patterns reported from EDs and Trauma Centers. In a retrospective series of intoxicated patients seen in an ED, only 12.5% were asked about depression, suicide or other dangerous behaviors or referred for alcohol treatment and only 15% were advised to stop drinking whereas nearly half of the intoxicated patients were referred for outpatient medical or surgical follow-up. Injured patients were even less likely to receive treatment or referral for alcohol problems than non-injured patients (Lowenstein 1990).

Bernstein and colleagues developed project ASSERT to facilitate access to the substance abuse treatment system and to primary care and preventive services for ED patients with drug and alcohol related health problems via the use of health promotion advocates (Bernstein 1997). They had previously shown that only 50% of emergency department patients kept treatment appointments after an active referral process (Bernstein 1996). The health promotion advocates screened, administered a brief negotiated interview and used an active referral process. In the ASSERT study many referrals were made, but only a small proportion (25%) of enrolled patients kept follow-up appointments. Those who kept follow-up appointments demonstrated a reduction in severity of drug problems, and a reduction in alcohol consumption and in binge drinking frequency. Patient satisfaction, an outcome measure, was high: 91% of patients reported they were satisfied with their referrals, thought things were explained well, and 99% thought the health promotion advocates respected them as individuals. Case management initiated in the ED for patients who have repeated visits has also been shown to decrease alcohol and drug consumption, homelessness and recurrent ED and hospital visits (Okin 2000).

Monti and colleagues evaluated the efficacy of a brief motivational interview (MI) in the ED in 18 and 19 year olds after an alcohol related event (Monti 1999). Patients receiving MI had a significantly lower incidence of drinking and driving, traffic violations, alcohol related injuries and problems than those who received standard therapy. In summary, studies on brief intervention in the ED (Peters 1998, Bernstein 1997, Monti 1999) show that 1/3 to 2/3 of patients drank less and 8–61% got further help for their alcohol problems after the intervention. In an urban ED, of 1034 patients approached, 78% agreed to participate in screening and brief on-site intervention and referral as needed. Although follow-up interviews only reached 28%, one-half of those re-contacted at 3-months reported decreased drinking, harm and dependence symptoms. Readiness to change also improved for 43% of the patients. Screening and brief intervention was reported as helpful by 15 of 23 patients (Hungerford 2000). Screening staff and location were independent determinants of consent to participate. Consent to participate varied from 65 to 94% by which personnel interviewed the patient and by where the patient was interviewed. Patients across severity levels accepted equally.

In London, alcohol health workers (AHW) have been evaluated in the ED setting to perform an initial brief intervention and to act as a catalyst for patients to seek treatment (Wright 1998). The introduction of the AHW to the ED resulted in a 3-fold increase in referral to counseling services. For the patients in which follow up data were obtained, almost half followed up with their referral for further counseling. Only 6% of patients declined further help. Of questionnaires returned, 65% were drinking less at 6 months.

Screening and intervention in the inpatient trauma population has the advantage of time to allow the patient to sober up. It is also a more select population that has suffered a greater adverse impact and patients are fewer in number than the ED population. Trauma centers have more time to perform screening and to adequately address the results with hospitalized patients.

In 1988 Chang reported that in 346 patients who tested positive for alcohol with a mean BAC of 200 mg/dl, not a single patient was referred for alcohol evaluation and treatment (Chang 1988). In a small study of 19 trauma patients, 17 accepted referral and completed therapy (Gentilello 1988). Fuller and colleagues describe a substance abuse consultation team's role in a trauma center. In a retrospective review of 100 consecutive trauma admissions who were considered to be at high risk and referred to the substance abuse consultation team, all 100 patients were diagnosed with psychoactive substance use disorders and 78 were referred for rehabilitation. Of those referred, 62% accepted a treatment referral (Fuller 1995).

In Finland, Antti-Poika (1988) and colleagues studied 120 injured male drinkers randomized to control versus intervention. The control group was given the results of the lab tests (GGT). Intervention involved a discussion with an assistant nurse and a booklet on how to control drinking. The intervention patients also received additional counseling by the surgeon, during their returns as outpatients. Intervention patients had decreases in alcohol consumption by more than 1/3 versus controls.

Surgical units were included in a Health Care Intervention Service quasi-experimental study (Welte 1998). Patients were initially screened with the CAGE questions and those with evidence of tolerance or negative consequences received a full intervention and referral to treatment. The intervention took the form of persuading the patient to accept formal treatment, to "overcome denial" by reviewing the harmful effects of drinking, to clarify the difference between the patient's current and preferred conditions and to set improvement goals. The full intervention group sought more help than the control group.

The same research group (Welte 1998) evaluated an education-based, risk-reduction intervention. It was given to patients who did not meet criteria of abuse or dependence but were still perceived to be drinking too much. It included the provision of factual information, expression of concern over the patient's drinking, and agreement on a plan to counter the risks from alcohol. The risk-reduction intervention decreased the number of drinking days versus controls that received no intervention.

Gentilello (1999b) and colleagues evaluated a randomized controlled trial of brief intervention versus standard of care in an inpatient trauma population. A single brief motivational interview decreased alcohol consumption and perhaps more importantly, reduced recurrent injury by 47%. That same study showed that 66% of screen positive patients readily consented to the study, however, the consent did not tell patients that alcohol use and problems were being measured. Roughly 15% of patients in both treatment and controls arms went to self-help groups afterwards, nearly 5% in each arm sought more formal alcohol treatment. Prior alcohol treatment was associated with a lack of response.

Forsberg et al. looked at brief intervention versus an extensive counseling session in patients admitted to a Swedish emergency surgical ward. Six and

12 month follow-ups found that patients drank as frequently as before, but they were drinking fewer drinks per occasion. There was no difference between groups. Patients in both groups had also moved to a stage of increased readiness to change (Forsberg 2000).

The Society of Academic Emergency Medicine (SAEM) has stated that "no other specialist sees more of the negative consequences of disease than the emergency physician" (D'Onofrio 1998a). A task force was developed to introduce brief screening tools applicable to the ED to detect at risk drinkers and to show that they could be realistically performed in the busy ED setting (D'Onofrio 1998a). They recommend assessment and intervention techniques once the at-risk individuals had been identified (D'Onofrio 1998b). One-half of Emergency Medicine directors teach their residents methods of screening for alcohol and substance abuse. (Krishel 1999), only 24.7% provide education on specific screening questionnaires. The SAEM task force has provided a curriculum for training residents in screening and brief intervention.

The Center for Substance Abuse Treatment (CSAT) as part of its Treatment Improvement Protocol series (CSAT 1995) published recommendations for screening hospitalized trauma patients for alcohol and other drug problems in 1995. From Gentilello's study, Dunn et al. also developed guidelines for performing alcohol interventions in trauma centers (Dunn 1997). However, despite a significant amount of alcohol research in trauma centers, there is no clear evidence that screening and interventions in trauma centers are more frequent than five or ten years ago.

UNIQUE CONCERNS IN THE HOSPITAL SETTING AND BARRIERS TO IMPLEMENTATION

Patients presenting to the ED and Trauma centers for injury are not often actively seeking alcohol or drug treatment. Ethically, caregivers need to have a clear understanding of when it is necessary and appropriate to obtain alcohol use information and share it with others. Untreated substance use can lead to recurrent injury or death. If the physician suspects that the patient has a treatable disorder the question arises if it is ethical to not refer the patient to treatment. Caregivers need to be careful to not invade a patient's privacy in the name of society's greater good since it will cause patients to lose trust in their caregivers. If confidentiality is breached, patients may lose employment or family access.

Many patients have committed crimes, particularly driving under the influence, prior to their admission to the hospital. The phenomenon of drunk drivers escaping detection through the emergency department and trauma center has been well described (Cydulka 1998, Barillo 1993, Evett 1994, Krause 1998, Schermer 2001b). Patients may legitimately fear the criminal justice system or that the insurance companies won't pay their bills. Another issue in the trauma setting is that some patients may not be able to communicate due to head injury, tracheostomy, or medications. Where to assess and intervene can also be a problem since the patients may not have a private room and thus it may be difficult to have a confidential conversation with a patient.

In general, trauma center staff have negative attitudes regarding alcohol treatment since they often repeatedly see the same patient (Silver 1990). It is difficult for physicians to realize who cuts down on their drinking, since they only see the failures time and time again and do not get follow up on who does well. Providers have attitudes of disinterest, avoidance, pessimism, and disdain especially when confronted with a hostile, manipulative or combative patient (Lowenstein 1990).

One barrier expressed by the emergency medicine community is that screening of all patients may not be feasible. A study in the UK demonstrated that researchers were able to screen only 28% of adult patients in a busy Accident and Emergency department (Peters 1998). Barriers to implementation of screening and intervention programs expressed by the trauma community are lack of knowledge of effective treatments, lack of confidence in performing interventions, concerns that patients will view an intervention as a violation of privacy, and the cost of implementing alcohol screening and counseling. Additional concerns include whether it is the trauma surgeon's responsibility to screen and intervene and whether screening will alter reimbursement for care (Danielsen 1999, Rivara 2000). Conclusions of Soderstrom's survey of current practice was "trauma centers still do not view alcohol problems as relevant to their mission" (Soderstrom 1994).

CONCLUSION

Trauma and emergency physicians are not specifically trained to address alcohol issues nor are alcohol issues thought to be a critical part of their practice. ED physicians and Trauma surgeons are clearly aware of the problem of alcohol and trauma but many still perceive treatment as ineffective and believe that costs and time constraints may prohibit screening and intervening. In essence, tertiary care physicians are being asked to perform a primary care service. In fact, Ryb and colleagues studied laboratory markers to try to identify patients with alcohol problems because "it is difficult to get nurses and doctors to always question patients, and in fact not all patients can be questioned at the time of arrival, so adding a laboratory marker would help identify at-risk patients" (Ryb 1999).

Despite a large number of published articles over the last quarter century describing the problem and magnitude of substance abuse and its relationship to injury and ED visits, there is a relative paucity of studies on intervention. Most recommendations for screening and interventions rely on extant literature based on treatment seeking and primary care populations. However, the few intervention studies performed in the ED and Trauma setting appear to have promising results and thus give hope for effectiveness. More studies in the ED and inpatient trauma setting should be performed. In the meantime, at least some effort should be focused on screening and treatment if subsequent decreased use of healthcare resources and secondary injury prevention are to occur.

Trauma patients tend to be younger than many study treatment populations with most studies reporting mean ages in the low 30's. Also many trauma patients abuse alcohol and have suffered adverse consequences, but are neither dependent nor have physical impairment from alcohol. The argument to intervene should be self-evident but somehow it has not captured the attention of trauma centers. Since brief interventions are inexpensive, short, and can be performed by a healthcare provider, they seem to make the most sense in the ED and trauma center. Emergency physicians and trauma team members need to acquire the knowledge and skills necessary to provide care to the patient with alcohol problems. Tools need to be specific to the environments of the ED and Trauma center to deal with the hectic environment and the high turnover of patients. Policy decisions on what physicians and hospitals can and cannot do in terms of legal consequences should be decided prior to the development of a screening program.

Traumatic injury should be viewed as a disease like heart disease with its attendant risk factors. Screening and brief intervention needs to be customized to meet the needs of organizations, professional groups and risky drinkers in specific settings (Babor 2000). Particularly in the US, hospitals need specific guidelines for dealing with patient confidentiality and privacy of records containing alcohol and other drug information otherwise the reluctance to screen will continue. Alcohol treatment interventions with patients at risk for multiple injury episodes hold promise for the prevention of a significant portion of traumatic injuries. Changes in substance abuse treatment may improve nursing morale, patient and family satisfaction and patient management and follow-up. Implementation of hospital based screening and treatment programs needs to be an organizational approach that focuses on optimal patient care while protecting reimbursement for services, privacy rights and confidentiality. Trauma patients may represent a uniquely motivated group of patients since they may be able to reflect on the consequences of alcohol use. The opportunity for intervention should not be overlooked.

REFERENCES

American Medical Association. Screening for alcohol and other drug use in trauma patients (House of Delegates, Resolution A91). *Chicago: American Medical Association* 1991.

Anda RF, Williamson DF, Remington PL. Alcohol and fatal injuries among U.S. adults: Findings from the NHANES I. *JAMA* 1988;260(17):2529–2532.

Antti-Poika I, Karaharju E, Roine R, Salaspuro M. Intervention of heavy drinking—a prospective and controlled study of 438 consecutive injured mail patients. *Alcohol & Alcoholism* 1988;23(2):115–121.

Babor TF, Higgins-Biddle JC. Alcohol screening and brief intervention: dissemination strategies for medical practice and public health. *Addiction* 2000;95(5):677–686.

Barillo DJ. Arrest and conviction of injured intoxicated drivers in eastern Pennsylvania. *Acid Anal Prev* 1993;25:635–639.

Becker B, Woolard R, Nirenberg TD, Minugh PA, Longabaugh R, Clifford PR. Alcohol use among subcritically injured emergency department patients. *Acad Emerg Med* 1995;2(9):784–790.

Bernstein E, Tracey A, Bernstein J, Williams C. Emergency department detection and referral rates for patients with problem drinking. *Subst Abuse* 1996;17:69–76.

Bernstein E, Bernstein J, Levenson S. Project ASSERT: an ED based intervention to increase access to primary care, preventive services, and the substance abuse treatment system. *Acad Emerg Med* 1997;30:181–189.

Blose JO, Holder HD. Injury related medical care utilization in a problem drinking population. *Am J Public Health* 1991;81:1571–1575.

Bombardier CH, Ehde D, Kilmer J. Readiness to change alcohol drinking habits after traumatic brain injury. *Arch Phys Med Rehabil* 1997;78:592–596.

Borges G, Cherpitel CJ, Medina-Mora ME, Mondragon L. Alcohol consumption in emergency room patient general population: a population-based study. *ACER* 1998;22(9):1986–1991.

Cales RH. Trauma Mortality in Orange County: The effect of implementation of a regional trauma system. *AEM* 1984;13:1–10.

Chang G, Astrachan BM. The emergency department surveillance of alcohol intoxication after motor vehicle accidents. *JAMA* 1988;260:2533–2536.

Cherpitel CJ. Drinking patterns and problems associated with injury status in emergency room admissions. *ACER* 1988;12(1):105–110.

Cherpitel CJ. Breath analysis and self-reports as measures of alcohol-related emergency room admissions. *JSA* 1989;50(2):155–161.

Cherpitel CJ, Pares A, Rodes J, Rosovsky H. Validity of self-reported alcohol consumption in the Emergency room: data in the United States, Mexico and Spain. *J Stud Alcohol* 1992;53(3): 203–207.

Cherpitel C. Alcohol and injuries: a review of international emergency room studies. *Addiction* 1993;88:923–937.

Cherpitel CJ. Differences in performance of screening instruments for problem drinking among blacks, whites and Hispanics in an emergency room population. *J Stud Alcohol* 1998;59: 420–426.

Cherpitel CJ. A brief screening instrument for problem drinking in the emergency room: the RAPS4. *J Stud Alcohol* 2000;May 447–449.

Colquitt M, Fielding LP, Cronan JF. Drunk drivers and medical and social injury. *NEJM* 1987; 371:1262–1266.

CSAT TIP series: #16 Alcohol and other drug screening of hospitalized trauma patients. Substance Abuse and Mental Health Services Administration. Rostenberg, PO MD chair USDHHS Rockville MD 1995.

Cydulka RK, Harmody MR, Barnoski A, et al. Injured intoxicated drivers: citation, conviction, referral, and recidivism. *Ann Emergency Medicine* 1998;22:349–352.

Danielssen PE, Rivara FP, Gentilello LM, Maier RV. Reasons why trauma surgeons fail to screen for alcohol problems. *Archives of Surgery* 1999;134:564–568.

D'Onofrio G, Bernstein E, Bernstein J, Woolard RH, Brewer PA, Craig SA, Zink BJ. Patients with alcohol problems in the emergency department, Part 1: Intervention and referral. *Academic Emergency Medicine* 1998a;5(12):1210–1217.

D'Onofrio G, Bernstein E, Bernstein J, Woolard RH, Brewer PA, Craig SA, Zink BJ. Patients with alcohol problems in the emergency department, Part 2: Intervention and referral. *Academic Emergency Medicine* 1998b;5(12):1210–1217.

Dowey KE. Alcohol-related attendances at an accident and emergency department. *Ulster Med Journal* 1993;62(1):53–62.

Dunn C, Donovan D, Gentilello LM. Practical guidelines for performing alcohol interventions in trauma centers. *J Trauma* 1997;42:299–304.2

Evans L. The fraction of traffic fatalities attributable to alcohol. *Accident Analysis Prevention* 1990;22:587.

Evett JK, Finley CJ, Armida N, et al. Judicial outcome for the intoxicated driver admitted to a regional trauma center. *Acad Emerg Med* 1994;1:254–257.

Forsberg L, Ekman S, Halldin J, Ronnberg S. Brief interventions for risk consumption of alcohol at an emergency surgical ward. *Addict Behav* 2000;25(3):471–475.

Fuller MG, Diamond DL, Jordan ML, Walters MC. The role of a substance abuse consultation team in a trauma center. *J Studies Alcohol* 1995;56:267–271.

Gentilello LM, Duggan P, Drummond D, Tonnesen A, Degner EE, Fischer RP, Reed RL II. Major injury as a unique opportunity to initiate treatment in the alcoholic. *Am J Surgery* 1988; 156:558–560.

Gentilello LM, Kobean R, Walker A, Moore E, et al. Acute ethanol intoxication increases the risk of infection following penetrating abdominal trauma. *J Trauma* 1993;34:669–675.

Gentilello LM, Villaveces A, Ries RR, et al. Detection of acute alcohol intoxication and chronic alcohol dependence by trauma center staff. *J Trauma* 1999a;47:1131–1139.

Gentilello LM, Rivara FP, Donovan DM, Jurkovich GJ, Daranciang E, Dunn CW, Villaveces A, Copass M, Ries R. Alcohol interventions in a trauma center as a means of reducing the risk of injury recurrence. *Ann Surgery* 1999b;230(4):473–483.

Hungerford DW, Pollock DA, Todd KH. Acceptability of Emergency Department based screening and brief intervention for alcohol problems. *Acad Emerg Med* Dec 2000;7(12):1383–1392.

Institute of Medicine, National Academy of Sciences. Broadening the base of treatment for alcohol problems. *Washington, DC: National Academy Press*; 1990.

Irvin CB, Wyer PC, Gerson LW. Preventive care in the emergency department, Part II: Clinical preventive services—an emergency medicine evidence-based review. *Acad Emerg Med* 2000;7: 1042–1054.

Jurkovich GJ, Rivara FP, Gurney JG, Seguin D, et al. Effects of alcohol intoxication on the initial assessment of trauma patients. *Ann of Emerg Med* 1992;21:704–708.

Kaufman CR, Branas CC, Brawley ML. A population-based study of trauma recidivism. *J Trauma* 1998;45:325–332.

Krause KR, Howells GA, Bair HA, et al. Prosecution and Conviction of the Injured Intoxicated Driver. *J Trauma* 1998 45(6):1069–1073.

Krishel S, Richards CF. Alcohol and substance abuse training for emergency medicine residents: a survey of U.S. programs. *Acad Emerg Med* 1999;6(9):964–6.

Kristenson H, Ohlin H, Hulten-Nosslin MB, Trell E, et al. Identification and intervention of heavy drinking in middle-aged men: results and follow-up of 24–60 months of long-term study with randomized controls. *ACER* 1983;7:203–209.

Lapham SC, Skipper BJ, Brown P, Chadbunchachai W, Suriyawongpai Paisarnsilp S. Prevalence of alcohol problems among emergency room patients in Thailand. *Addiction* 1998;93(8): 1231–1239.

Li G, Smith GS, Baker SP. Drinking behavior in relation to cause of death among US adults. *Am J Pub Health* 1994;84:1402–1406.

Longabaugh R, Minugh A, Nirenberg T, Clifford P, Becker B, Woolard R. Injury as a motivator to reduce drinking. *Acad Emerg Med.* 1995;2:817–825.

Lowenfels AV Miller TT. Alcohol and trauma. *Annals of Emerg Med* 1984; 13:1056–1060.

Lowenstein SR, Weissberg MP, Terry D. Alcohol intoxication, injuries, and dangerous behaviors—and the revolving emergency department door. *J Trauma* 1990;30:1252–1258.

Maio RF, Waller PF, Blow FC, Hill EM, Singer KM. Alcohol abuse/dependence in motor vehicle crash victims presenting to the emergency department. *Acad Emerg Med* 1997;4:256–262.

McLellan BA, Vingilis E, Liban CB, Stoduto G, et al. Blood alcohol testing of motor vehicle crash admissions at a regional trauma unit. *J Trauma* 1990 30:418–421.

Miller TR, Lestina DC, Smith GS. Injury risk among medically identified alcohol and drug abusers. *ACER* 2001;25(1):54–59.

Monti PM, Colby SM, Barnett NP, et al. Brief intervention for harm reduction with alcohol-positive older adolescents in a hospital emergency room. *JCCP* 1999;67(6):989–994.

National Center for Injury Prevention and Control. Ten leading causes of injury death in the united states. *Atlanta: Centers for Disease Control and Prevention* 1991.

Okin RL, Boccellari A, Azocar F, Shumway M, O'Brien K, Gelb A, Kohn M, Harding P, Wachsmuth C. the effects of clinical case management on hospital service use among ed frequent users. *Am J Emerg Med* 2000;18(5);603–608.

Peters J, Brooker C, McCabe C, Short N. Problems encountered with opportunistic screening for alcohol-related problems in patients attending an accident and emergency department. *Addiction* 1998;93(4):589–94.

Popham RE, Schmidt W, Israelstram S. Heavy alcohol consumption and physical health problems: A review of the epidemiologic evidence. *Research Advances In Alcohol And Drug Problems*, vo18 New York, Plenum Press. 1984 pp. 149–182.

Reyna TM, Hollis HW, Hulsebus RC. Alcohol-related trauma: the surgeon's responsibility. *Annals of Surgery* 1985;201:194–197.

Rice DP, MacKenzie EJ, et al. Cost of injury in the United States: A report to congress. *San Francisco: Institute for Health and Aging, University of California, and Injury Prevention Center, Johns Hopkins University* 1989.

Rivara FP, Jurkovich GJ, Gurney JG, Seguin D, et al. The magnitude of acute and chronic alcohol abuse in trauma patients. *Archives of Surgery* 1993a;128:907–913.

Rivara FP, Koespsell TD, Jurkovich GJ, Gurney JG, et al. The effects of alcohol abuse on readmission for trauma. *JAMA* 1993b;270(16):1962–1964.

Rivara FP, Tollefson S, Tes E, Gentilello LM. Screening trauma patients for alcohol problems: Are insurance companies barriers? *J Trauma* 2000;48(1):115–118.

Rund DA, Summers WK, Levin M. Alcohol use and psychiatric illness in emergency patients. *JAMA* 1981;245(12):1240–1241.

Ryb GE, Soderstrom CA, Kufera JA, Dischinger PC, Ho SM. Use of blood alcohol concentration and laboratory tests to detect current alcohol dependence in trauma center patients. *J Trauma* 1999;47(5):874–880.

Saunders JB, Aasland OG, Babor TF de la Fuente JR Grant M. Development of the Alcohol Use Disorders Identification Test (AUDIT): WHO collaborative Project on Early Detection of Persons with Harmful Alcohol Consumption II. *Addiction* 1993;88(6):791–804.

Schermer CR, Qualls CR, Brown CL, Apodaca TR. Intoxicated motor vehicle passengers: An overlooked at-risk population *Archives of Surgery* 2001a;136:1244–1248.

Schermer CR, Apodaca TR, Albrecht RM, Lu SW, Demarest GB. Intoxicated motor vehicle passengers warrant screening and treatment similar to intoxicated drivers. *J Trauma* 2001b;51:1083–1086.

Selzer ML, Vinokur A, Van Rooijen L. A self-administered short Michigan Alcoholism Screening Test (SMAST). *J Alcohol* 1975;36:117–126.

Silver BA, Sporty LD. Behavioral correlates and staff recognition of alcohol use in a university hospital trauma service. *Psychomatics* 1990;31:420–425.

Simpson T, Murphy N, Peck DF. Saliva alcohol concentrations in accident and emergency attendances. *Emerg Med J* 2001;18(4):250–254.

Sims DW, Bivins BA, Obeid FN, Horst HM, et al. Urban trauma: a chronic recurrent disease. *J Trauma* 1989;29:942–957.

Sloan EP, Zalenski RJ, smith RF, Sheaff CM, et al. Toxicology screening in urban trauma patients: drug prevalence and its relationship to trauma severity and management. *J Trauma* 1989;29: 1647–1653.

Smith SG, Touquet R, Wright S, Das Gupta N. Detection of alcohol misusing patients in accident and emergency departments: the Paddington alcohol test (PAT). *J Accid Emerg Med* 1996; 13(5):308–312.

Soderstrom CA, Cowley RA. A national alcohol and trauma center survey. *Archives of Surgery* 1987;122:1067–71.

Soderstrom Ca, Dischinger PC, Smith GS, McDuff DR, et al. Psychoactive substance dependence among trauma center patients. *JAMA* 1992;267:2756–2759.

Soderstrom CA, Dailey JT, Kerns TJ. Alcohol and other drugs. *J Trauma* 1994;36:68–73.

Soderstrom CA, Kerns TJ, Ho SM, Dischinger PC, Read KM, Smith GS. Assessment of current alcoholism rates among vehicular and non-vehicular patients admitted to a level I trauma center. 40th Annual Proceedings. *Assoc Adv Auto Med* 1996;40:247–261.

Soderstrom CA, Smith GS, Kufera JA, Dischinger PC, Hebel JR, McDuff DR, Gorelick DA, Ho SM, Kerns TJ, Read KM. The accuracy of the CAGE, the brief Michigan Alcoholism Screening test, and the alcohol use disorders identification test in screening trauma center patients for alcoholism. *JAMA* 1997;43(6):962–969.

Soderstrom CA, Dischinger PC, Kerns TJ, et al. Screening trauma patients for alcoholism according to NIAAA Guidelines with Alcohol Use Disorders Identification Test Questions. *ACER* 1998;22:1470–1475.

Teplin LA, Abram KM, Michaels SK. Blood alcohol level among emergency room patients: a multivariate analysis. *J Stud Alcohol* 1989;50(5):441–447.
Thom B, Herring R, Judd A. Identifying alcohol-related harm in young drinkers: the role of accident and emergency departments. *Alcohol Alcohol* 1999;34(6):910–915.
Treno AJ, Gruenewald PJ, Ponicki WR. Use of ICD-9-CM codes in the estimation of alcohol-involved injury: Search for a surrogate II. *ACER* 1996;20:320–326.
Tu GC, Kapur B, Isreal Y. characteristics of a new urine, serum, and saliva alcohol reagent strip. *Alcoholism* 1992;16:222–227.
US Preventive Services Task Force. Guide to clinical preventive services. 2nd Ed. Baltimore: Williams & Wilkins, 1996.
Volk RJ, Steinbauer JR, Cantor SB, Holzer CE 3rd. The Alcohol Use Disorders Identification Test (AUDIT) as a screen for at-risk drinking in primary care patients of different racial/ethnic backgrounds. *Addiction* 1997;92(2):197–206.
Weiczorek WF, Miller BA, Nochajski TH. Alcohol diagnoses among DUI offenders. In: Problem drinker-driver project research note. *Buffalo, NY: Research Institute on Alcoholism* 1990: 90–96.
Welte JW, Miler BA. Alcohol use by violent and property offenders. *Drug and Alcohol Dependence* 1987;19:313–324.
Welte JW, Perry P, Longabaugh R, Clifford PR. An outcome evaluation of a hospital-based early intervention program. *Addiction* 1998;93(4):573–581.
West JG, Trunkey DD, Lim RC. Systems of trauma care. *Archives of Surgery* 1979;114:455–460.
Whitfield RA, Zador P, ife D. Projected mortality from injuries. *Accid Anal Prev* 1985;17:367–371.
Wright S, Moran L, Meyrick M, O'Connor R, Touquet R. Intervention by an alcohol health worker in an accident and emergency department. *Alcohol Alcohol* 1998;33(6):651–656.
Yates D, Hadfield J, Peters K. The detection of problem drinkers in the accident and emergency departments. *British Journal of Addiction* 1987;82:163–167.

CHAPTER 6

Establishing and Maintaining Evidence-Based Treatment in Community Programs

ROBERT J. MEYERS AND NATASHA SLESNICK

Over the past 40 years, an abundance of research has focused on which alcohol treatment approaches are most effective. Adult alcoholism treatment research clearly indicates that even brief treatment is generally better than no treatment at all, that certain treatments are more consistently effective than other methods, and also that there is no single treatment that is superior to all others. However, a handful of treatments seem to rise to the top in all meta-analytic reviews of the alcohol treatment literature. Even though most of these well-supported treatments have been available for some time, the gap between science and practice remains vast.

EVIDENCE FOR THE EFFICACY OF ALCOHOL TREATMENT METHODS

There now is an abundance of research evidence to guide clinicians and funding agencies toward effective treatment methods for alcohol use disorders, at least for adults. While few clinicians have the time to read and analyze hundreds of outcome studies, there have been several recent meta-analytic reviews of this literature. Two reviews focused on the relative effectiveness of treatment methods (Miller et al., 1995; Miller, Wilbourne, & Hettema, 2001) and two others focused on cost-effectiveness (Holder et al., 1991; Finney & Monahan, 1996). Miller et al. (1995) evaluated 211 studies that encompassed 43 treatment modalities, taking into account the methodological strength of each study's

ROBERT J. MEYERS AND NATASHA SLESNICK • Center on Alcoholism, Substance Abuse, and Addictions, University of New Mexico, Albuquerque, New Mexico 87106

design and its support or non-support for specific treatment modalities. The five modalities that emerged as most effective were: (1) brief interventions, (2) social skills training, (3) motivational enhancement, (4) the community reinforcement approach, and (5) behavioral contracting. The most recent version of this review (Miller, Wilbourne & Hettema, in press) included 383 controlled trials, and again included these five approaches among the top ten empirically-supported methods. For the first time, two medications also appeared among the methods most strongly supported: naltrexone and acamprosate. The top ten list was rounded out by behavioral self-control training, behavioral marital therapy, and self-help manuals (bibliotherapy).

Attending to cost-effectiveness, Holder and colleagues (1991) reviewed 224 published results from controlled clinical alcohol treatment trials. Using a system for counting positive and negative trials, they reported their top five treatments as: (1) social skills training, (2) self-control training, (3) brief motivational counseling, (4) behavioral marital therapy, and (5) the community reinforcement approach. All five of these also fell into the low-cost category, whereas more expensive approaches showed less evidence of efficacy. Finally, Finney and Monahan (1996) extended the work of Holder et al. (1991) by re-examining the same studies with different and more stringent criteria. Taking into account the strength of the design and additional outcome measures, their top five treatment modalities were: (1) the community reinforcement approach, (2) social skills training, (3) behavioral marital therapy, (4) disulfiram implants, and (5) other marital therapy. Once again, these top treatments all fell into the low to medium-low cost category.

Clearly, there is a cluster of alcohol treatment methods that seem to have "the right stuff". In the above meta-analyses there are two treatments that appear in the "supported" list for all four (social skills training and community reinforcement approach) and five more that are common to two or three of the reviews (brief counseling, motivational enhancement, behavior contracting, behavioral self-control training, and behavioral marital therapy). It should be noted, of course, that most of these treatment outcome studies have been conducted in North America.

Far fewer studies have evaluated substance abuse treatments for adolescents. Multiple psychosocial intervention approaches have been developed during the past two decades to address adolescent alcohol and other drug abuse, but the vast majority of available interventions have not been adequately evaluated as to their effectiveness. In the early 1990's Catalano, Hawkins, Wells, Miller and Brewer (1990/1991) found only 16 treatment outcome studies. A recent review by Williams and Chang (2000) identified 53 adolescent treatment outcome studies. Comparatively, there have been well over 1000 studies on alcohol treatment for adults (Miller et al., 1995). Conclusions regarding adolescents are that treatment is superior to no treatment, but there is insufficient evidence to designate treatment methods that are more effective than others. The exception to this is that outpatient family therapy appears to be consistently more effective than other forms of outpatient treatment with which it has been compared (Williams & Chang, 2000).

BRINGING SCIENCE INTO PRACTICE

Although most alcohol treatment program directors and staff want to have successful outcomes for their clients, relatively few focus their treatment on methods with the best evidence of efficacy. Without clear incentives to adopt and maintain optimal practice methods, it is clear that practitioners and programs tend to continue with or drift back to familiar and often outmoded treatment approaches. The central objective of this chapter is to suggest ways of bringing evidence-based treatment methods into practice.

Getting Started

A first step is for the program or practitioner to make a commitment to the use of evidence-based treatment methods. Some programs, for example, have adopted a policy that they will use only treatment methods with adequate scientific evidence of efficacy. When scarce public funds are used to treat citizens of a community, is it not incumbent on programs to provide services with the greatest likelihood of efficacy? This commitment can also come from the funding agency, by requiring that programs receiving public support shall use only evidence-based treatment methods.

While this may sound like a common-sense approach, addiction treatment in many nations has historically relied upon methods with little or no empirical support, using treatment methods until or even long after they have been found to be ineffective. Such traditional methods, developed without the benefit of modern clinical trial methodology, have often been used for decades, and become entrenched in practice. They become familiar and comfortable methods, with little incentive for practitioners to adopt newer, empirically sound intervention. Thus emerges the gap between science-based treatments and clinical practice.

Bridging this gap is a challenge for both researchers and practitioners. Reliable information about what works usually appears first in scientific publications written and read by researchers, in journal articles and conference presentations. Distilling this information is no simple matter. As noted above, even carefully-done meta-analyses of outcome research can come to different conclusions. By the time this information is disseminated into publications read by practitioners, it is difficult to separate reliable, data-based evidence from the writer's own unsubstantiated opinion.

When an evidence-based treatment method is identified and adopted, there is still the challenge of ensuring that therapists are competently delivering it. This, too, is challenging. If supervision occurs at all, it typically occurs by the counselor describing to the supervisor what has transpired behind closed doors. Clinicians may inaccurately perceive, recall, or describe what they did. The audiotaping or videotaping of counseling sessions permits a supervisor to observe directly what is being done in treatment. Even in highly-controlled clinical trials, counselors often drift from delivering the intended method and require redirection (Miller & Meyers, 1995). The basics in getting started, then, are to make a commitment to the use of evidence-based methods, and have a means of directly monitoring what is happening in treatment delivery.

Hiring New Staff

The largest influence on changing the culture of a treatment program is held by the person who does the selection and hiring of new staff. One way to disseminate new methods into programmatic practice is to hire staff who have already been trained in them. Again, counselor self-description of competence is insufficient. Hiring decisions are among the most important, and we recommend directly observing the applicant's skills as part of the hiring process, as through a work sample or role play. Know what skills, style, and treatment approaches you want, and then ask candidates to demonstrate them. Experience and training do not guarantee competence. There is evidence, for example, that counselors who are highly empathic, skillful in client-centered reflective listening (Truax & Carkhuff, 1967), tend to have better outcomes in substance abuse treatment. A hiring interview might therefore include a role-play demonstration of the counselor's skill in empathic listening. Evidence-based treatment methods (such as CRA, behavioral marital therapy, or social skills training) also often require the counselor to take quite an active role in the treatment process.

People already competent in the desired evidence-based treatment methods will not always be available for hire. Therefore, consider the willingness and eagerness of potential staff to learn new methods through training and direct supervision. If there is a probationary period for new hires, this period can be used to determine that the counselor can learn and apply in practice the desired methods.

Training Staff

Implementing new, evidence-based treatment methods often requires significant changes in practice behavior, which usually happens in a gradual, fashion. Reading and talking *about* a new approach is not enough. Usually a training workshop is not enough. Practice with feedback is how new skills are learned. Ordinary clinical practice resembles learning how to play golf in a dense fog Ziskin (1970). One hits the ball and has some feeling for immediate effect, but there is no reliable feedback to help correct one's drive. Indeed, one could labor for years on a fog-bound driving range without improving much at the game. Even in a fog, however, systematic feedback about the length and trajectory of drives could improve one's swing in a matter of hours, especially with a golf pro at hand to offer specific coaching and positive feedback. Good clinical supervisors act a bit like a golf pro, observing practice, giving ongoing feedback, and reinforcing the desired skills.

To be sure, specific guidelines can be helpful. Many therapist manuals and videotapes are now available to aid in learning evidence-based methods. These can be supplemented by discussions with a knowledgeable supervisor or trainer. Yet reading and discussing a book about golf or watching others play it can only take you so far. It is just preparation for the next level of training.

Feedback on practice and positive reinforcement for steps in the right direction are two basic elements for the acquisition of a new skill. These two common-sense and empirically-grounded learning aids—systematic feedback and positive reinforcement—are sensible strategies to be included in any efforts to teach new practice behavior. One way of shaping practice is through role playing in the presence of a knowledgeable supervisor. Role-play has the advantage of flexibility. Various clinical scenarios can be constructed without waiting for them to occur in actual practice. A role-play can be tried over, using different approaches, or "fast forwarded" to a later point in treatment.

Another commonly used strategy in training therapists is pairing them with a more experienced clinician. The trainee participates in co-therapy in order to observe and practice new skills in an actual session. The experienced therapist also debriefs with the trainee at the end of the session to provide further direction, for example, through explaining the reasoning behind utilizing certain strategies in the session. As skills increase, the experienced therapist may be phased out of the therapy process as the trainee assumes greater responsibility. As an alternative to co-therapy, an experienced therapist or clinical supervisor may sit in on the session, or observe live via a one-way mirror or video link to ensure clinical integrity. Sessions may also, of course, be videotaped or audiotaped for later review. If an experienced clinician or supervisor for the new treatment approach is not available on-site, arrangements may be made with a suitably qualified professional from another agency or city to offer training.

Ongoing Supervision

Training is not a one-time event, as skill acquisition is a continuous process. Therapists' level of skill and experience in providing the intervention will vary, requiring different levels and frequency of supervision.

One point to remember here is that therapists' self-reports of what occurred in treatment sessions are at best incomplete. When learning a new approach, inexperienced therapists often do not recognize or may not report mistakes. There is thus no substitute for direct observation of sessions, usually via audio or videotaping, to monitor exactly what the therapist is doing. This allows the supervisor to point out and shape behaviors of which the therapist may be unaware. This can also work well in a group format, allowing several therapists to learn from the review of specific session takes, and permitting group discussion of problems that they are likely to encounter. It has been our experience that clients rarely object to confidential taping for research or supervision purposes, if it is presented un-apologetically as an important and routine procedure.

The supervisor's role can also include working with therapists' own issues that may arise from or affect their treatment sessions. Supervisors can help therapists to be aware of their own reactions or biases, which may influence the direction of the treatment they provide. Supervisors can also monitor therapists' frustrations with client outcomes, therapy processes, and other job related issues that may interfere with learning new clinical methods. Good monitoring and positive feedback within a supportive supervisory relationship is key in putting new evidence-based methods into practice.

A certain degree of therapist self-monitoring can be aided by providing checklists or concise reminder guidelines to be used when delivering new treatment procedures. Because of the critical nature of their work, even highly experienced airline pilots continue to use checklists to ensure that they have followed correct procedures. Such checklists can help therapists keep from drifting back to old habits, and can be used by the supervisor in assessing the accuracy of self-appraisal.

PROGRAM EVALUATION

When trying out new treatment procedures in a practice setting, it is sensible to implement program evaluation procedures to study the relative impact of the new approach in this real-life setting. Getting outcome data can be useful for many reasons including program development, agency documentation, personal reinforcement and development of staff. Funding sources often request information as to how well the program is meeting the client needs and program goals. Furthermore, having consistent evaluation procedures underlines a program's commitment to evidence-based practice.

Useful program evaluation need not be complicated. Often it can be accomplished via relatively modest adjustments in routine procedures. To discover the impact of a new procedure, however, one does need three essential elements: (1) client assessment at intake, (2) consistency of treatment, and (3) follow-up evaluation.

Client Assessment

A first step in a reliable program evaluation is to implement a consistent assessment of clients at intake. Depending upon the purposes it will serve, this assessment need not be extensive, and surely it is important not to overburden clients and staff or to delay treatment with needless paperwork and questions. A stable intake assessment system provides consistent baseline information for all clients, against which outcomes can be compared. It can also be useful in determining treatment needs. Reliable assessment information is helpful to the clinician, by supplying early important information about the client (about motivation, problem severity, etc.). The assessment process can also constitute a type of triage, screening for special or acute problems that need to be addressed. Finally, research has shown that clients themselves highly value assessment and that programs with formal assessment batteries are more likely to retain clients in treatment (Institute of Medicine, 1990; Sobell, 1993). Initial engagement and retention, in turn, are important to the process and outcomes of therapy (Slesnick, Meyers, Meade & Segelken, 2000).

Clinically, however, it is important that bombardment with questions is not the client's first experience in treatment. Without a context of care, prolonged impersonal assessment can be invasive or stressful to clients who are seeking help, and could discourage a client from returning. One strategy that we have found useful is for the first person that a client sees to be one of the program's more experienced clinical staff. Even half an hour of attentive listening, allowing clients to tell their story and feel heard, can establish a positive relationship with the program that then offers a context for completing assessment. It may also increase the accuracy of assessment. Attrition and drop-out rates with clients in the addiction field is usually high. Anything a program can do to reduce these rates of drop-out can improve overall client outcome results. Length of time in active treatment is one variable that has been associated with a positive treatment outcome (Moos & Moos, 1995).

Some assessment can be administered via computer, not requiring interviewer time. Many assessment questionnaires can be completed by the client with little assistance, again reducing actual time a staff member needs to be present (Allen & Columbus 1995; Miller, Westerberg & Waldron, in press).

Consistent Treatment

A second quality assurance element is to ensure that the treatment being evaluated is, in fact, being delivered with fidelity. It's hard to evaluate the value of a treatment if therapeutic procedures are unreliable or changing. The training, supervision and monitoring methods described above help to ensure that treatment is being delivered properly and consistently.

This is not to say that treatment has to be done with cookie-cutter sameness. Clients can be offered a menu of evidence-based treatment methods, and involved actively in the choice of their own treatment plan. Such active involvement can enhance clients' commitment to, involvement in, and outcomes from their treatment. Keeping track of which clients chose and received which treatment components can provide clues to what seems to be working best. Total amount of treatment (e.g., number of sessions) is also useful to document, both because it is an index of service delivery and because it tends to be associated with client outcomes.

No matter how consistent you try to be, however, it is likely that therapists will differ in their competence with and outcomes from treatment. It appears, in fact, that one of the strongest determinants of clients' outcome is the therapist to whom they happen to be assigned (Najavits & Weiss, 1994). Another useful component of program evaluation, then, is to track client outcomes in relation to the primary therapist who treated them.

Follow-up Assessment

If you have consistent information about where clients started and what treatment they received, then the remaining piece is to find out what happened to them. How did they fare?

A rudimentary level of program evaluation is to assess client satisfaction with treatment, via a questionnaire routinely administered during or at the completion of their treatment. The Working Alliance Inventory (Horvath & Greenberg, 1986), for example, is a widely-used instrument for this purpose, and clients' reports on this scale as early as the second session often predict treatment retention and outcome. Satisfaction ratings do not, of course, indicate whether therapists were using the intended treatment procedures or document their outcomes.

Outcome data are collected directly from at least a representative sample of clients, usually via questionnaires or follow-up interviews. Perhaps the simplest way to do this is to routinely contact all clients (or a representative subset) at an anniversary date of their intake or treatment completion. A good interval is 3–6 months, because it allows enough time to study initial impact of treatment, but it is also soon enough that contact is less likely to be lost. Mailed questionnaires can be used, but the problem is usually a poor return rate. Interviews provide direct contact, and may also be useful (even billable) continuing care. While there are some advantages in having outcome data collected by an interviewer other than the client's therapist, it appears that therapists themselves can collect reasonably accurate outcome data (Breslin, Sobell, Sobell, Buchan & Kwan, 1996).

SUMMARY

In the alcohol field, and in substance abuse treatment more generally, we now have access to a range of treatment methods with strong evidence of efficacy. Such methods do little good, however, unless and until they are put into practice. Although it may be more comfortable to continue offering treatment in the same, familiar ways, we owe it to our clients to offer them the most effective treatments we can find. This involves making a personal and programmatic commitment to offering only evidence-based treatment methods, then hiring, training, and supervising staff to ensure their competence to provide those treatments. Program evaluation represents a further commitment to the use of evidence in guiding treatment, and involves a systematic intake assessment, clarity and consistency of treatment delivery, and follow-up monitoring to evaluate clients' outcomes.

REFERENCES

Allen, J. P., & Columbus, M. (1995). *Assessing alcohol problems: A guide for clinicians and researchers.* Bethesda, MD: National Institute on Alcohol Abuse and Alcoholism.

Breslin, C., Sobell, L. C., Sobell, M. B., Buchan, G., & Kwan, E. (1996). Aftercare telephone contacts with problem drinkers can serve a clinical and research function. *Addiction, 91*, 1359–1364.

Budney, A. J., & Higgins, S. T. (1998). *National Institute on Drug Abuse therapy manuals for drug addiction: Manual 2. A Community Reinforcement Approach: treating cocaine addiction.* (NIH Publication No. 98 4309). Rockville, MD: U.S. Department of Health and Human Services.

Catalano, R. F., Hawkins, J. D., Wells, E. A., Miller, J. L., & Brewer (1990–1991). Evaluation of the effectiveness of adolescent drug abuse treatment, assessment of risk for relapse, and promising approaches for relapse prevention. *International Journal of Addictions Special Issue: Relapse prevention in substance misuse, 25(9A–10A)*, 1085–1140.

Finney, J. W., & Monahan, S. C. (1996). The cost-effectiveness of treatment for alcoholism: A second approximation. *Journal of Studies on Alcohol, 57(3)*, 229–243.

Godley, S. H., Meyers, R. J., Smith, J. E., Karvinen, T., Titus, J. C., Godley, M. D., Dent, G., Passetti, L., & Kelberg, P. (in press). Adolescent Community Reinforcement Approach (ACRA) for Adolescent Cannabis Users. Volume 4 of the Cannabis Youth Treatment Manual series. Center for Substance Abuse Treatment (CSAT), *U.S. Department of Health and Human services (DHHS).*

Holder, H., Longabaugh, R., Miller, W. R., & Rubonis, A. (1991). The cost effectiveness of treatment for alcoholism: A first approximation. *Journal of Studies on Alcohol, 52*, 517–540.

Horvath, A. O., & Greenberg, L. (1986). The development of the working alliance inventory. In L. S. Greenberg & W. M. Pinsof (Eds.), The psychotherapeutic process: A research handbook (p. 529–556). New York: Guilford Press.

Institute of Medicine, (1990). *Broadening the Base of Treatment Problems.* Washington, DC: National Academy of Press.

Kadden, R., Carroll, K. M., Donovan, D., Cooney, N., Monti, P., Abrams, D., Litt, M., & Hester, R. (1992). *Cognitive-behavioral coping skills therapy manual: A clinical research guide for therapists treating individuals with alcohol abuse and dependence* (NIAAA Project MATCH Monograph, Vol. 3, DHHS Publication No. ADM 92-1895. Washington DC: US Government Printing Office.

Meyers, R. J., & Smith, J. E. (1995). *Clinical guide to alcohol treatment: The Community Reinforcement Approach.* New York: Guildford Press.

Miller, W. R., Brown, J. M., Simpson, T. L., Handmaker, N. S., Bien, T. H., Luckie, L. F., Montgomery, H. A., Hester, R. K., & Tonigan, J. S. (1995). What works? A methodological analysis of the alcohol treatment outcome literature. In R. K. Hester & W. R. Miller (Eds.), *Handbook of alcoholism treatment approaches: Effective alternatives* (2nd ed., pp. 12–44). Boston: Allyn and Bacon.

Miller, W. R., & Hester, R. K. (1995). *Handbook of Alcoholism Treatment Approaches: Effective Alternatives* Needham Heights, MA, US: Allyn & Bacon, Inc.

Miller, W. R., & Meyers, R. J. (1995). Beyond generic criteria: Reflections on life after clinical science wins. *Clinical Science, Spring*, 4–6.

Miller, W. R., & Rollnick, S. (2002). *Motivational Interviewing: Preparing people for change* (2nd ed.) New York: Guilford Press.

Miller, W. R., Westerberg, V. S., & Waldron, H. B. (in press). Evaluating alcohol problems in adults and adolescents. In: R. K. Hester & W. R. Miller (Eds.), *Handbook of Alcoholism Treatment Approaches: Effective alternatives.* (3rd Ed). Boston: Allyn and Bacon.

Miller, W.R., Zweben, A., DiClemente, C.C., Rychtarik, R.G., (1992). Motivational enhancement therapy manual: A clinical research guide for therapist treating individuals with alcohol abuse and dependence (NIAAA Project MATCH Monograph Vol 2, DHHS Publication No. ADM 94-3723). Washington DC: US printing office.

Moos, R. H., & Moos, B. S. (1995). Stay in residential facilities and mental health care as predictors of readmission for patients with substance use disorders. *Psychiatric Services, 46*, 66–72.

Monti, P. M., Abrams, D. B., Kadden, R. M., & Cooney, N. L. (1989). *Treating Alcohol Dependence: A coping skills training guide.* New York: Guilford Press.

Najavits, L. M., & Weiss, R. D. (1994). Variations in therapist effectiveness in the treatment of patients with substance use disorders: An empirical review. *Addiction, 89*, 679–688.

National Institute on Alcohol Abuse and Alcoholism (1995). *The Physicians' Guide to Helping Patients with Alcohol Problems.* NIH Pub No. 95-3769. Bethesda, MD: the Institute.

National Institute on Drug Abuse Research Monograph No. 156. Rockville, MD: National Institutes of Health.

Newcomb, M. D. (1995). Identifying high-risk youth: prevalence and patterns of adolescent drug abuse. In. E. Rahdert and D. Czechowicz (Eds.), *Adolescent drug abuse: Clinical assessment and therapeutic interventions* (pp. 7–38).

O'Farrell, T. J. (1993). *Treating alcohol problems: Marital and family interventions.* New York: Guilford Press.

Sobell, L.C., (1993) *Motivational Interventions with problem drinkers.* Presented at the sixth meeting of the international conference on treatment of addictive behaviors, Santa Fe, New Mexico.

Williams, R. J., & Chang, S. Y. (2000). A comprehensive and comparative review of adolescent substance abuse treatment outcomes. *Clinical Psychology: Science and Practice, 7(2)*, 138–166.

Ziskin, J. (1970). *Coping with psychiatric and psychological testimony.* Beverly Hills, CA: Law and Psychology Press.

CHAPTER 7

Intervening through Pharmacy Services

ERNEST J. DOLE

PATIENT CARE AND THE PHARMACY PROFESSION

The public, at least in the United States, has long held the pharmaceutical profession in high esteem and pharmacists are among the most accessible health-care providers (Gallup News Service, 1997). Often the community utilizes the pharmacist as a reliable and available source of medical and pharmaceutical information. The profession of pharmacy has a covenant with society regarding safe and appropriate medication use. Pharmacists possess a unique knowledge base that brings together the pharmacology, pharmacokinetics, pharmacodynamics, toxicology, mechanism of action, adverse effects and interaction potential of pharmaceutical agents. Pharmacists then integrate this knowledge with an in-depth understanding of pathophysiology to improve patient care.

In addition to possessing specialized knowledge, pharmacy has tried to evolve from a profession of medication dispensing to one that encompasses direct patient care and patient empowerment (Dole, 1994; Berger, Anderson-Harper, Kavookjian, 1997; Berger & Suchanek-Hudmon, 1997; Berger, 1997; Berger, 1999). This move was facilitated by a new mission statement of pharmacy defined as "pharmaceutical care" (Heplar & Strand, 1990; Heplar, 1985). Pharmaceutical care is: "the direct, responsible provision of medication-related care for the purpose of achieving definite outcomes that improve a patient's quality of life. The principal elements of pharmaceutical care are that care is directly provided to the patient, it is provided to produce definite outcomes, these outcomes are intended to improve the patient's quality of life and the provider [pharmacist] accepts personal responsibility for the outcomes" (American Society of Health-System Pharmacists, 1993).

ERNEST J. DOLE • Department of Pharmaceutical Care, Lovelace Health Systems, Albuquerque, New Mexico 87108

Pharmaceutical care, as proposed by Hepler and Strand, would increase the involvement of pharmacists in the areas of patient data gathering, evaluation, and developing strategies in collaboration with physicians and other members of the health care team to improve medical care, resolve drug-related problems, and assume responsibility for outcomes. Numerous studies have demonstrated the benefits of pharmacist participation on a multidisciplinary team to improve control of chronic conditions such as heart failure (Gattis, Hasselblad, Whellan, 1999), hyperlipidemia (Bozovich, Rubino, Edmunds, 2000), diabetes mellitus (Coast-Senior, Kroner, Kelley, 1998), asthma (Rupp, McCallian, Sheth, 1997), hypertension (Carter, Barnette, Chrischilles, 1997), coronary artery disease (Carson, 1999), and anticoagulation (Foss, Schoch, Sintek, 1999). Additionally, pharmacist-managed refill clinics have been shown to be time efficient while continuing to preserve quality of care (Cassidy, Keith, Coffey, 1996; Smith, Barnette, Maffeo, 2000). Finally, improved medication adherence has been documented in patients who received pharmacist consultation in conjunction with routine medical care (Lipton & Bird, 1994).

According to a recent report, pharmacists are essential in providing a safe medication delivery system to patients (Kohn, 2000). Pharmacist interventions to reduce inappropriate drug prescribing in the elderly in ambulatory care settings have resulted in improved outcomes (Hanlon, Weinberger, Samsa, 1996; Wilcox, Himmelstein, Woolhandler, 1994; Hanlon, Fillenbaum, Schmader, 2000). In a 1-year randomized trial, Hanlon et al., evaluated the effect of clinical pharmacist interventions involving elderly outpatients (≥65 years) with polypharmacy (≥5 chronic medications) and their primary physicians (Hanlon, Weinberger, Samsa, 1996). Patients in the control group ($n = 103$) received usual care (clinic nurse reviewing patients' current medications before and after their visit and the physician visit), whereas patients randomized to the intervention group ($n = 105$) received usual plus clinical pharmacist care. The clinical pharmacist reviewed each patient's medical record, determined current medication use, identified drug-related problems by meeting with patients and caregivers, and evaluated patients' medications for appropriateness by using a medication appropriateness index criteria and relative weights. The outcomes of the study were prescribing appropriateness, health-related quality of life (HRQOL), adverse drug reactions (ADRs), medication compliance and knowledge, number of medications, patient satisfaction and physician receptivity. At three months, there was a 24% improvement in inappropriate prescribing in the intervention group, compared with a 6% improvement in the control group ($p = 0.0006$). This improvement was sustained at 12 months, with a 28% improvement in the intervention group versus a 5% improvement in the control group ($p = 0.0002$). Fewer patients in the intervention group had adverse events when compared with the control group. The two groups were comparable when HRQOL was evaluated, and there were no significant differences between groups with regard to medication compliance or knowledge, number of medications, or patient health care satisfaction. Physicians who had contact with the clinical pharmacist indicated that they were highly satisfied with their interactions. In fact, approximately 55% of written recommendations made for the intervention group were acted upon, as compared with 20% of those made for the control group ($p < 0.001$). The authors concluded that a clinical pharmacist providing care for elderly primary care patients could reduce inappropriate prescribing and ADRs without affecting quality of life.

The economic impact of pharmacist interventions has been documented in several studies (Bond, Raehl, Franke, 1999; Bond, Raehl, Franke, 2000; Bond, Raehl, Franke, 2001; Blakely and Hixson-Wallace, 2000; Jameson, VanNoord, Vanderwoud, 1995; Cowper, Weinberger, Hanlon, 1998; Sorrento, Bonanza, Salisbury, 1996). For every dollar invested in clinical pharmacy practice there has been an associated reduction in drug costs (Bond, Raehl, Franke, 1999). Blakey et al. determined the effectiveness of a pharmacist in recognizing and resolving drug therapy problems, decreasing drug therapy costs, and maintaining positive clinical outcomes in a geriatric ambulatory clinic in a VAMC (Blakey & Hixson-Wallace, 2000). In this non-randomized study, pharmacists reviewed upcoming patients' computerized drug lists and available electronic medical records. Patients targeted were those with polypharmacy (≥5 chronic medications/day). All other patients received traditional medical care alone (controls). The clinical effect of each intervention was rated as positive (patient achieved therapeutic goal), negative (patient's disease state worsened or patient had ADR after the intervention), or neutral. During the 8-month study, the team saw 178 patients over 250 visits. Of these, traditional medical care was provided at 144 visits and traditional medical care plus pharmacist evaluation was provided at 106. A total of 220 actual and potential drug-related problems were identified in the intervention group. Of these, 217 of the pharmacist-recommended changes in drug therapy were accepted. Most of the interventions involved identifying agents being used without indications. Discontinuation of unnecessary agents resulted in a significant reduction in number of medications in both groups, from 7.4 to 7.0 ($p = 0.0007$) in the control group and from 10.6 to 7.2 ($p < 0.0001$) in the intervention group. At six months, 85% of the discontinued medications remained inactive. Positive effects of changes in therapy were seen in 47.5%, neutral in 52%, and negative in 0.5% of interventions. When drug cost avoidance was compared with pharmacy costs associated with team services, the net savings to the VAMC was $7788/year.

Jameson et al. conducted a randomized clinical trial in a primary care practice to measure the following outcomes: number of chronic prescription medications, number of individual doses/day, monthly cost of prescription drugs, patient self-reports of compliance and of drug regimen convenience, and adverse effects (Jameson, VanNoord, Vanderwoud, 1995). Patients were randomized to intervention ($n = 27$) and control groups ($n = 29$) and outcomes were measured at baseline and at six months. A clinical pharmacist gave patients (average age 60.5 years) in the intervention group a 45- to 60-minute pharmacotherapy consultation, performed medication reviews for drug-related problems, collaborated with a physician in the development of a new drug regimen and educated the patient on the new medication changes. One month after the intervention, the pharmacist contacted the patient by phone (5–10 minutes) to review and reinforce the treatment plan. Outcomes were again measured six months later. At baseline, the average number of medications was six/day, with almost 10 doses/day. Annual drug costs averaged $1800 per person. At six months, the number of drugs, doses, and the 6-month cost decreased in the intervention group and increased in the control; the net difference was 1.1 drugs ($p = 0.004$), 2.15 doses ($p = 0.007$), and $293 per six months ($p = 0.008$). Patients in the intervention group experienced a reduction in adverse effects and an improvement in understanding and compliance, although the reductions were not statistically significant.

Evidence that the pharmacist role is changing from a dispensing role to a patient-focused role is shown by the growth of collaborative practice agreements between the provider and the pharmacist. There is ample evidence to show that pharmacists can have a positive impact on patient outcomes and may also lower costs of treatment; thus, it is important to grant pharmacists a means by which they can become full partners in the health care team. Collaborative practice involves agreements between a qualified pharmacist and a physician to allow the pharmacist to initiate, adjust (prescribe), or continue pharmacotherapy in accordance with pre-approved, written protocols (Mitrany & Elder, 1999; Koch, 2000; Carmichael, O'Connell, Devine, 1997; Hammond & Dole, 1996). The team approach inherent in collaborative practice can help to address and attempt to resolve escalating costs, insufficient access to medical care, and inconsistent quality of care in today's managed health care environment. As patients with chronic diseases account for a high percentage of health care costs, management and prevention of complications and comorbidities places emphasis, and increases reliance upon pharmacotherapy (Maddux, Dong, Miller, 2000). Additionally, with managed formularies, the complexities of pharmaceutical care increase as physicians are inundated with calls from pharmacists for permission for drug interchange. Collaborative practice can improve both the quality and availability of patient care as pharmacists are easily accessible and have the ability to counsel patients on disease management. Also, qualified pharmacists can improve the cost-effectiveness of physicians' time by overseeing routine laboratory testing, prescribing, patient counseling, and follow-up tasks. Importantly, the written treatment protocols may increase consistency of treatment and will not reduce the quality of care as periodic review and revisions of the protocols will allow for continued provision of quality care (Mitrany & Elder, 1999; Koch, 2000; Carmichael, O'Connell, Devine, 1997).

PHARMACISTS AND SUBSTANCE ABUSE

Given their expanding role in patient care and their extensive knowledge of drugs and their effects, pharmacists represent a potentially valuable and relatively untapped resource for substance abuse intervention. This is particularly so for pharmacotherapies. Pharmacists provide the essential role of dispensing medication to patients and managing the inventory control aspects of pharmacotherapy. They are often the health care providers with the best knowledge and insight into the regulatory aspects of substance abuse pharmacotherapy, e.g., in regards to the use of methadone and other agents in the treatment of patients with opioid dependence. Pharmacists are particularly well prepared and in a unique position to assess and manage the pharmacotherapy of persons with substance use disorders and co-morbid issues such as pain management. They are optimal health care providers to consider the implications of medication interactions both in terms of prescribed medication (e.g. pharmacotherapy of addictions with concomitant illnesses such as diabetes mellitus, hypertension, asthma) and interactions with non-prescribed or illicit medications. Pharmacists have the knowledge and ability to extrapolate empirical data on drug interactions from prescribed to illicit substances. They are trained to obtain a detailed medication history from patients and to help them with medication adherence. As more pharmacotherapies are developed to treat substance use disorders, pharmacists, are well positioned to bring these new approaches to the front line safely and effectively (Dole & Tommasello, in Press).

Pharmacists create and deliver educational programs for health professionals and patients about the pharmacology, pharmacodynamics, pharmacokinetics, toxicology, adverse drug reactions (ADRs), and drug interactions between prescribed medications and substances of abuse. As part of an interdisciplinary team treating individuals with substance abuse disorders, pharmacists have a unique perspective utilizing their specialized knowledge base to improve the pharmaceutical care of hospice, palliative care or chronic pain patients (Dole & Tommasello, in press). Although pharmacists have a specialized knowledge base, however, the majority in practice today do not interact routinely to provide information to an interdisciplinary healthcare team, nor are they universally integrated into an interdisciplinary system of care (Dole & Tommasello, in press).

Pharmacists, by virtue of their trust and frequent contact with patients, may also be well positioned for detection, early intervention, and referral of substance use disorders. This is a pharmacist role already developed with regard to tobacco, an example to which we now turn.

How Pharmacy is Currently Involved in Addressing Addictions

Intervening through Pharmacy and Smoking Cessation

The majority of the literature of pharmacy interventions in substance abuse and chemical dependency is in the area of smoking cessation (Suchanek-Hudmon & Berger, 1995; Suchanek-Hudmon, Corelli, Berger, 2001; Suchanek-Hudmon, Corelli, Kroon, 2001; Berger, Braxton-Lloyd, Suchanek-Hudmon, 2001; Sinclair, Bond, Lennox, 1998; Smith, McGhan, Lauger, 1995; McGhan & Smith, 1996). Pharmacists are logical persons to provide smoking cessation assistance to patients who are nicotine dependent (Suchanek-Hudmon & Berger, 1995; Suchanek-Hudmon, Corelli, Berger, 2001; Suchanek-Hudmon, Corelli, Kroon,

2001; Berger, Braxton-Lloyd, Suchanek-Hudmon, 2001). Recent research indicates that pharmacists can increase the cessation rate of patients whom they counsel regarding medications for smoking cessation (Sinclair, Bond, Lennox, 1998; Smith, McGhan, Lauger, 1995; McGhan & Smith, 1996). Additionally, in an analysis of the pharmacoeconomics of smoking cessation, pharmacy consultation was determined to be an important and cost-beneficial component of the overall therapy plan (McGhan & Smith, 1996).

Despite their extensive knowledge and skills, pharmacists' role in helping patients in smoking cessation has not been fully realized. Only about 8% of licensed U.S. pharmacists have received formal training in smoking cessation, although 70% believe that training will increase the number of patients they counsel, and 94% believe that advanced training for smoking cessation will increase the quality of the assistance that they provide patients (Suchanek-Hudmon & Berger, 1995; Suchanek-Hudmon, Corelli, Kroon, 2001; Hudmon, Prokhorov, Corelli, 2000). If the profession of pharmacy is to realize its full potential in promoting smoking cessation, it is important for practicing pharmacists and pharmacy students to receive training for counseling their patients (Suchanek-Hudmon & Berger, 1995; Suchanek-Hudmon, Corelli, Kroon, 2001; McElnay, Maquire, Drummond, 2000). As described by Rollnick and Boycott in Chapter 4, such training can be in general behavior change counseling skills that are applicable to a broad range of patient concerns.

Pharmacy Intervention in Alcohol and Other Substances of Abuse

As readily accessible healthcare providers, pharmacists should be actively involved in reducing substance abuse. Pharmacists are **already** involved in methadone and detoxification clinics and in the dispensing and monitoring of patients receiving medications such as acamprosate, disulfiram and naltrexone. Pharmacists make significant contributions in resolving drug-related practice and workplace problems. Some participate in organizations to help impaired pharmacists and other health professionals. Pharmacists have a unique perspective from which to counsel patients and other healthcare colleagues about medications.

Given this unique position, pharmacists should develop the skills needed to fulfill a significant role in substance abuse prevention, education, and treatment, both in healthcare settings and in the community (Dole & Tommasello, in press). Thus far, pharmacy involvement in substance abuse intervention has mostly been limited to the dispensing of medications. Less progress has been made in a clinical involvement of pharmacists in interventions. One study has investigated brief motivational intervention by pharmacists in an outpatient medical setting (Gettman, Swanson, Miller, 1999), but clinical intervention by pharmacists remains largely undeveloped in this field.

In part, this lack of progress exists because there has been little formal training in addiction medicine for pharmacists, despite their expertise in drug effects (Dole & Tommasello, in press; Erickson, 2001). Of the 460 residency programs accredited by the American Society of Health-System Pharmacists, only nine focus on psychiatry. Yet there are no U.S. pharmacy residencies or fellowships dedicated to post-graduate training in substance abuse, despite calls for such training from leading professional associations. The American Association of Colleges of Pharmacy (AACP) has published curricular guidelines for pharmacy in substance abuse education (Baldwin, Light, Stock, 1991), although implementation has been less than desired (Baldwin, Dole, Levine, 1994). Both the American Society of Health-System Pharmacists (1998) and the American Pharmaceutical Association (1982) have issued position statements regarding pharmacy's role and responsibility in the education, prevention and assistance of those with substance use. The American Association of Colleges of Pharmacy (AACP) has also recently published revised guidelines for policies and procedures for students and faculty of colleges and schools of pharmacy with substance use disorders (Dole, Baldwin, Murawski, 1999). In certain practice settings (e.g., with geriatric patients), screening for and intervention with alcohol and other substance use disorders may be more particularly challenging and warrant special training (Dole & Gupchup, 1999). Pharmacy students themselves feel a need for training in substance abuse. In one recent survey, more than 60% of students said they would need a working knowledge of substance use disorders in their professional practice (Murawski & Juergens, 2001.)

OPPORTUNITIES FOR PHARMACISTS IN INTERVENTION IN ADDICTIONS

As discussed above, pharmacists have opportunities for intervening in addictions, and could be uniquely positioned to help patients. With their unique knowledge of pharmacology, pharmacokinetics, pharmacodynamics and pathophysiology, they should be able to identify possible medication abuse situations while counseling patents about their prescriptions. Impeding pharmacists' involvement is a lack of consistent education, not only within residencies but in the training curricula of schools of pharmacy (Gettman, Sosa, Dole, 2000). While some pharmacy programs do address substance abuse, their effort is not reflected at the national level. Some programs offer advanced training; others may have an elective substance abuse course or none at all. Some programs require minimum competencies in the area of substance abuse; others do not. As described above, postgraduate training opportunities in substance abuse for pharmacists are virtually nonexistent (Dole & Tommasello, in press). Funding mechanisms have not been developed to address this gap in substance abuse education for pharmacy faculty and their students.

Challenges for Pharmacy Training

Complexity. A number of challenges face the pharmacy profession in expanding training opportunities in substance abuse educations. The pathophysiology of substance abuse is complex and incompletely understood. In order to understand the proper place of a medication in a disease state, the pathophysiology of that disease must be known. The medications used to treat substance use disorders are complex, and are incompletely addressed in the training of pharmacists.

Over-crowded Curricula. Schools and colleges face the more general dilemma of teaching more complex material in a more integrated, multidisciplinary fashion and in a shorter amount of time. In this context, teaching about many specific therapeutic areas is condensed. Given an already-overloaded curriculum, further specialist training in substance abuse may be met with resistance by pharmacy faculty.

Stigma. Few diseases carry the stigma, prejudice, and misinformation that substance use disorders do. Such stigma can dissuade professionals from seriously addressing this widespread health problem, and education is the key to overcoming such barriers. Implementation of substance abuse education in the pharmacy curriculum is a place to begin.

Lack of Faculty Interest and Expertise. Given the history of ignoring substance abuse, few pharmacy faculty have adequate expertise to teach in this area. Few members of the pharmacy profession are engaged in substance abuse research. This creates a self-perpetuating cycle at colleges and schools of pharmacy.

Patient Expectations. Patients themselves may not expect to be counseled by their pharmacist. Although required to counsel patients before providing medication, pharmacists have long been perceived as professionals who simply dispense medication. Few patients expect their pharmacists to educate or counsel them regarding personal issues such as substance use.

Need for Postgraduate Training Opportunities. An infrastructure to support the initial training and further development of pharmacy practitioners and researchers in substance use disorders needs to be created.

Pharmacist Confidence. Pharmacists are accustomed to counseling patients on their medication when it is dispensed. Many pharmacists, however, do not feel confident discussing substance use disorders with their patients, in part because they lack not only the specific knowledge but also the communication tools to do so.

Funding. Whether in for-profit or public systems, pharmacies are funded primarily to dispense medications. In the U.S., pharmacists have only recently been recognized in some states as primary providers who are authorized to be reimbursed for the provision of counseling or educational services. Such counseling may be seen as time-consuming and distracting pharmacy staff from their primary mission.

CORE COMPETENCIES FOR PHARMACISTS

Too little is known about the pharmacy profession's training in substance use disorders, attitudes towards substance use disorders, and pharmacists' skill level in providing services to patients with substance use disorders. A framework needs to be developed to begin to identify and teach core competencies in substance abuse education for the profession of pharmacy. We suggest the following as optimal competencies to be targeted in the education of pharmacists (Dole & Tommasello, in press).

Knowledge

- Pharmacology, pharmacokinetics, pharmacodynamics, toxicology, mechanism of drug action, drug–drug interactions, and the adverse reactions between alcohol, tobacco, and common drugs of abuse and agents used in the pharmacotherapy of substance use disorders; and
- Knowledge of the pathophysiology of chemical dependence and the theories of addiction, including the biological basis of addiction and the social, environmental, and genetic risk factors that contribute to its expression.

Clinical Skills

Pharmacists should have the ability to:

- Assist in the early identification of individuals with substance use disorders by using standard screening instruments;
- Develop and deploy culturally sensitive assessments for individuals with substance use disorders;
- Intervene effectively with these patients by using motivational interviewing (BMI) and other effective counseling methods;
- Create a list of substance abuse treatment resources in their communities, including the responsible contact person for each program or provider;
- Refer individuals affected by substance use disorders for appropriate evaluation; and
- Participate in multidisciplinary efforts to intervene and care for clients and colleagues recovering from substance use disorders.

Attitudes

Pharmacists should be able to:

- Approach and treat substance abuse and addiction as any other chronic disease; and
- Approach and treat substance abuse and addiction without personal bias and judgment of the patient.

Treatment

Pharmacists should be able to:

- Provide recommendations for the appropriate use of mood-altering substances in individuals recovering from substance use disorders to health care providers and the public;

- Instruct drug abuse counselors and other health professionals working in drug treatment programs on the pharmacology, pharmacodynamics, pharmacokinetics, toxicology, adverse drug reactions, drug–drug interactions, and mechanisms of action of abused substances and of medications used for to treat substance use disorders;
- Provide information about support group meetings (e.g., Alcoholics Anonymous, Narcotics Anonymous) appropriate to the needs of individuals whose lives are affected by substance use disorders;
- Provide pharmaceutical care to patients treated for substance use disorders;
- Assist in the development of pharmacotherapy options for drug detoxification protocols used by health care providers; and
- Be aware of the different types of treatment modalities, their expected outcomes, and their cost-effectiveness;

Public Health Awareness

Pharmacists should be able to:

- Participate effectively in public discourse on the implications of policies related to illicit drugs, substance abuse prevention, and the treatment of chemical dependence; and
- Describe the potential ramifications of changes in the illicit drug market on the clinical manifestations and nature of substance abuse and chemical dependence in the community.

SUPPORT FOR TRAINING

If public resources are devoted to increasing pharmacists' involvement in addressing substance abuse as a public health issue, the following initiatives could be considered (Dole & Tommasello, in press):

- Assess substance abuse education in the schools and colleges of pharmacy to determine the need for curriculum reform in this area;
- Create a process for developing a consensus on the core competencies in substance abuse education for the pharmacy profession;
- Train at least two faculty at every school or college of pharmacy in substance abuse education. These faculty can then be responsible for integrating the core competencies in substance abuse education into the standard curriculum at each school;
- Develop and maintain an infrastructure that will ensure continued faculty development in substance abuse education;
- Develop continuing education (CE) programs in substance use disorders for practicing pharmacists;
- Inform accrediting, certifying, and licensing bodies for the profession of pharmacy of the need for curricular improvement in substance abuse education; and

- Assist pharmacists and pharmacy students who are themselves impaired by substance abuse.

SUMMARY

Substance use disorders permeate almost any health care system. As readily accessible health care providers, pharmacists could play an active role in addressing substance abuse among their patients. Pharmacists have a unique perspective and expertise from which to counsel patients and other health care providers about medications. Pharmacists are in a unique position to intervene and counsel patients with smoking, alcohol and other substance abuse problems. This role is only beginning to be recognized. Pharmacists are an untapped resource among the health professionals available to address and study addictions. To assume a greater role in substance abuse prevention, education, and treatment in organized health care settings and in the community, pharmacists need more specific training in substance abuse knowledge and skills.

REFERENCES

American Pharmaceutical Association. Official Policy of the American Pharmaceutical Association. Subject: Impaired Pharmacists. 1982.

ASHP position statement on pharmaceutical care. Am J Hosp Pharm 1993;50:1720–1723 Kohn LT.

Baldwin JN, Alexander JW, Dole EJ et al. American Society of Health-System Pharmacists. ASHP Statement on the Pharmacist's Role in Substance Abuse Prevention, Education and Assistance. *Am J Health-Syst Pharm.* 1998;55:1721–1724.

Baldwin JN, Dole EJ, Levine PJ et al. Survey of pharmacy substance abuse course content. *Am J Pharm Ed.* 1994;58:47S–52S.

Baldwin JN, Light KE, Stock C et al. Curricular guidelines for pharmacy education: substance abuse and addictive disease. *Am J Pharm Ed.* 1991;55:311–316.

Berger BA. Readiness for change: improving treatment adherence. Glaxo-Wellcome Continuing Education. 1997;8.

Berger BA. Motivational interviewing helps patients confront change. US Pharmacist 1999;24:88–95.

Berger BA, Anderson-Harper HM, Kavookjian J. Patient empowerment. US Pharmacist 1997;12

Berger BA, Braxton-Lloyd K, Suchanek-Hudmon K. The pharmacist's role in smoking cessation. US Pharmacist 2001;26:57–64.

Berger BA, Suchanek-Hudmon K. Readiness for change: implications for patient care. *J Am Pharm Asso.* 1997;may/june:321–8.

Blakey SA, Hixson-Wallace JA. Clinical and economic effects of pharmacy services in a geriatric ambulatory clinic. *Pharmacotherapy.* 2000;20:1198–1203.

Bond CA, Raehl CL, Franke T. Clinical pharmacy services, pharmacist staffing, and drug costs in United States hospitals. *Pharmacotherapy.* 1999;19:1354–62.

Bond CA, Raehl CL, Franke T. Clinical pharmacy services, pharmacy staffing, and the total cost of care in United States hospitals. *Pharmacotherapy.* 2000;20:609–21.

Bond CA, Raehl CL, Franke T. Interrelationships among mortality rates, drug costs, total cost of care, and length of stay in United States hospitals: Summary and recommendations for clinical pharmacy services and staffing. *Pharmacotherapy.* 2001;21:129–41.

Bozovich M, Rubino C, Edmunds J. Effect of a clinical pharmacist-managed lipid clinic on achieving national cholesterol education program low density lipoprotein goals. *Pharmacotherapy.* 2000;20:1375–83.

Carmichael JM, O'Connell MB, Devine B, et al. Collaborative drug therapy management by pharmacists. *Pharmacotherapy.* 1997;17:1050–61.

Carson JJ. Pharmacist-coordinated program to improve use of pharmacotherapies for reducing risk of coronary artery disease in low-income adults. *Am J Health-Syst Pharm.* 1999;56:2319–24.

Carter BL, Barnette DJ, Chrischilles E, et al. Evaluation of hypertensive patients after care provided by community pharmacists in a rural setting. *Pharmacotherapy.* 1997;17:1274–85.

Cassidy IB, Keith MR, Coffey EL, et al. Impact of pharmacist-operated general medicine chronic care refill clinics on practitioner time and quality of care. *Ann Pharmacother.* 1996;30:745–51.

Coast-Senior EA, Kroner BA, Kelley CL, et al. Management of patients with type 2 diabetes by pharmacists in primary care clinics. *Ann Pharmacother.* 1998;32:636–41.

Cowper PA, Weinberger M, Hanlon JT, et al. The cost-effectiveness of a clinical pharmacist intervention among elderly outpatients. *Pharmacotherapy.* 1998;18:327–32.

Dole EJ. Beyond pharmaceutical care. *Am J Hosp Pharm.* 1994;51:2183–4.

Dole EJ, Baldwin JN, Murawski MM et al. American Association of Colleges of Pharmacy Guidelines for the Development of Psychoactive Substance Use Disorder Policies for Colleges of Pharmacy. *Am J Pharm Ed.* 1999;63:28S–34S

Dole EJ, Gupchup GV. A review of the problems associated with screening instruments used for alcohol use disorders in the elderly. *Consult Pharm.* 1999;14:294–9.

Dole EJ, Tommasello AC. Recommendations for implementing effective substance abuse education in pharmacy practice. HRSA/AMERSA/SAMHSA/CSAT Federal Number: 222 978 919. 2001. In Press.

Erickson CT. Pharmacists can now play a bigger role in reducing drug problems. Texas State Board of Pharmacy Newsletter. 2001;3:1–3.

Foss MT, Schoch PH, Sintek CD. Efficient operation of a high-volume anticoagulation clinic. *Am J Health-Syst Pharm.* 1999;56:443–9.

Gallup News Service. 1997. Honesty and ethics poll: Pharmacists strengthen their position as the most highly rated occupation. Gallup Organization Poll Releases; December 13, 1997. Princeton, NJ.

Gattis WA, Hasselblad V, Whellan DJ, et al. Reduction in heart failure events by the addition of a clinical pharmacist to the heart failure management team. *Arch Intern Med.* 1999;159:1939–45.

Gettman DA, Swanson KM, Miller WR. Brief interventions by pharmacists to understand and motivate change among veteran outpatients misusing alcohol. *J Am Pharm Asso.* 1999;39:265. abstract

Gettman DA Sosa PC, Dole EJ. Barriers and strategies for educating pharmacy students about detecting and managing substance abuse. Am J Pharm Ed 2000;64 (winter supplement):108S.

Hammond RW, Dole EJ. The pharmacist clinician: prescriptive authority in New Mexico. *JMCP.* 1996;2:594–6.

Hanlon JT, Weinberger M, Samsa GP, et al. A randomized, controlled trial of a clinical pharmacist intervention to improve inappropriate prescribing in elderly outpatients with polypharmacy. *Am J Med.* 1996;100:428–37.

Hanlon JT, Fillenbaum GG, Schmader KE, et al. Inappropriate drug use among community-dwelling elderly. *Pharmacotherapy.* 2000;20:575–82.

Heplar CD. Pharmacy as a clinical profession. *Am J Hosp Pharm.* 1985;42:1298–1306.

Heplar CD, Strand LM. Opportunities and responsibilities in pharmaceutical care. *Am J Hosp Pharm.* 1999;47:533–543.

Hudmon KS, Prokhorov AV, Corelli RL, et al. Helping tobacco users to quit: Pharmacists' counseling role. Presented at: American Society for Preventive Oncology 24th Annual Meeting, March 5–7, 2000, Bethesda, MD. abstract.

Jameson J, VanNoord G, Vanderwoud K. The impact of a pharmacotherapy consultation on the cost and outcome of medical therapy. *J Fam Pract.* 1995;41:469–72.

Koch KE. Trends in collaborative drug therapy management. *Drug Benefit Trends.* 2000;12:45–54.

Lipton HL, Bird JA. The impact of clinical pharmacists' consultations on geriatric patients' compliance and medical care use: a randomized controlled trial. *The Gerontologist.* 1994;34:307–15.

Maddux MS, Dong BJ, Miller WA, et al. A vision of pharmacy's future roles, responsibilities, and manpower needs in the United States. *Pharmacotherapy.* 2000;20:991–1020.

McElnay JC, Maquire RA, Drummond A, Hughes CM. Smoking cessation: the contribution of community pharmacy. *Dis Manage Health Outcomes.* 2000;8(3):147–158.

McGhan WF, Smith MD. Pharmacoeconomic analysis of smoking-cessation interventions. *Am J Health-Syst Pharm.* 1996;53:45–52.

Mitrany D, Elder R. Collaborative pharmacy practice: an idea whose time has come. *JMCP.* 1999;5:487–91.

Murawski MM, Juergens JP. Analysis of longitudinal pharmacy student alcohol and drug use survey data. *Am J Pharm Educ.* 2001;65:20–29.

Rupp MT, McCallian DJ, Sheth KK. Developing and marketing a community pharmacy-based asthma management program. *JAPhA.* 1997;NS37:694–9.

Sinclair HZ, Bond CM, Lennox AS, et al. Training pharmacists and pharmacy assistants in the stage-of-change model of smoking cessation: A randomized controlled trial in Scotland. *Tob Control.* 1998;7:253–261.

Smith ML, Barnette DJ, Maffeo C. Refill program using pharmacy student interns in a primary care clinic. *Am J Health-Syst Pharm.* 2000;57:756–9.

Smith MD, McGhan WF, Lauger G. Pharmacist counseling and outcomes of smoking cessation. *Am Pharm.* 1995;NS35(8):20–9.

Sorrento TA, Bonanza KC, Salisbury DW. Pharmaceutical services in a capitated geriatric care program. *Am J Health-Syst Pharm.* 1996;53:2848–52.

Suchanek-Hudmon K, Berger BA. Pharmacy applications of the Transtheoretical model in smoking cessation. *Am J Health-Syst Pharm.* 1995;52:282–7.

Suchanek-Hudmon K, Corelli RL, Berger BA. Treating tobacco use and dependence. RX consultant. 2001. In press

Suchanek-Hudmon K, Corelli RL, Kroon LA et al. Reducing pulmonary disease: the pharmacist's role in smoking cessation. *J Pharm Prac.* 2001;14:143–59.

To Err is Human: Building a Safer Health System. Washington, D.C., National Academy Press. 2000.

Willcox SM, Himmelstein DU, Woolhandler S. Inappropriate drug prescribing for the community-dwelling elderly. *JAMA.* 1994;272:292–96.

CHAPTER 8

The Case of Tobacco

JUDITH K. OCKENE AND LORI PBERT

INTRODUCTION

Tobacco treatment provides an excellent case for the importance of treating substance use and other health-related problem behaviors within healthcare settings and systems as well as through other community settings. The incontrovertible evidence linking cigarette smoking with serious illness and premature death has placed increasing demands on the medical and mental health community to intervene with smokers. However, despite the known health risks, tobacco use remains high worldwide. In the United States, roughly 25% of adults smoke (Centers for Disease Control and Prevention, 1999), with current prevalence estimates indicating that 28% of adult males and 22% of adult females smoke (Corrao, Guindon, Sharma & Shokoohi, 2000). Individuals with a current or past history of significant psychiatric problems including depression, schizophrenia, and alcoholism, have much higher rates of smoking and are less likely to stop smoking than those in the general population (Glassman, 1993). For instance, among individuals identified as alcoholic, the incidence of smoking is 80–90%, with alcoholic persons also more likely to smoke heavily (Bien & Burge, 1990; Bobo, 1989).

Internationally, the smoking prevalence among adults (aged 15 or older) ranges from 20% (South Asia) to 59% (East Asia and Pacific, and Eastern Europe and Central Asia) for men, and from 1% (South Asia) to 26% (Eastern Europe and Central Asia) for women (World Health Organization, 1997). Recognizing the global pandemic of tobacco use which kills 4 million people a year, the World Health Organization has initiated a Framework Convention on Tobacco Control (FCTC) (World Health Organization, 2000). This international body is set up to focus attention, financial and technical resources and action on the tobacco problem, especially in non-industrialized countries.

JUDITH K. OCKENE AND LORI PBERT • Division of Preventive and Behavioral Medicine, University of Massachusetts, Worcester, Massachusetts 01655

Viewed as an addictive behavior, tobacco use can be treated from psychosocial, behavioral, and pharmacological perspectives. There is clear and strong evidence that tobacco use interventions, both brief and intensive, in ambulatory settings and inpatient services within hospitals are effective and make a difference. Preliminary evidence suggests the potential for interventions in pharmacy services. Each setting and system presents its own challenges which need attention if routine and effective treatment is to take place. This chapter will cover: opportunities and needs for tobacco treatment in each healthcare setting and system; the evidence for the effectiveness of tobacco treatment in each setting; the prevalence of tobacco treatment in different settings; suggestions for methods for screening and intervening; and the application of the treatment methods discussed to non-industrialized countries. We also will provide principles for integrated tobacco treatment programs and present an effective statewide program as a model.

OPPORTUNITIES AND NEEDS FOR TOBACCO TREATMENT IN HEALTHCARE SETTINGS

Opportunities for tobacco treatment are available in multiple healthcare settings. In the outpatient setting opportunities include acute care, chronic care, and well care visits both within primary care and specialty ambulatory settings such as cardiac and pulmonary clinics. Healthcare organizations and settings, and the providers who work in them, have tremendous opportunities to affect the health of a large percentage of the population. For example, 83% of adults in the United States saw or spoke to a health professional in 1998 (78% of smokers and 85% of non-smokers) (Ockene, Zapka, Pbert, Brodney & Lemon, in press). Although we don't have those figures for non-industrialized countries, in general individuals who provide some level of healthcare to people, whether it be providing medications or free clinics generally have contact with a large proportion of the population. The health assessment visit is an obvious time to implement tobacco treatment. In the United States 56.3% of smokers (compared to 65% of non-smokers) have had a physical examination or routine check-up in 1998 (unpublished data, Dr. Maria Hewitt, Institute of Medicine). The acute and chronic care visit, when the presenting problem is related to the behavior of interest such as smoking, also is an excellent time for intervention (Stange, Flocke & Goodwin, 1998). For instance, the primary care clinician or the cardiologist and pulmonologist have valuable opportunities to provide brief treatment to a smoker seen for chest pain, vascular problems and other cardiac concerns or for a cough or chronic bronchitis and greatly affect the individual's risk of mortality. Additionally, other acute care visits for problems not directly related to smoking present an opportunity, but are less likely to be used for this purpose (Sesney, Kreher, Hickner & Webb, 1997).

Opportunities for intervention also exist in the inpatient setting among medical and surgical patients. For example, in the United States at least 1 in 4 of the over 33 million patients hospitalized annually is a smoker (Smith, Kraemer, Miller, DeBusk & Taylor, 1999), with smokers hospitalized more often than non-smokers (Haapanen-Niemi, Miilunpalo, Vuori, Pasanen & Oja, 1999; Penttinen, 1997). Smokers often are receptive to discussion about smoking and perceive themselves to be more vulnerable when they are sick (Ockene, Kristeller, Goldberg, Ockene, Merriam, Barrett, Pekow, Hosmer & Gianelly, 1992). Long-term quit rates after hospitalization, both for patients hospitalized with smoking-related disease (e.g. 30–50% post-myocardial infarction) (Frid, Ockene, Ockene, Merriam, Goldberg, Kristeller & Barrett, 1991) as well as non-smoking-related problems or non-cardiac surgery (15% for general hospitalization and 24% for non-cardiac surgery (Glasgow, Stevens, Vogt, Mullooly & Lichtenstein, 1991; Simon, Browner & Mangano, 1992), are higher than the annual quit rates of 3–5% in the general population. Hospital-based treatments could enhance the likelihood of cessation at such "teachable moments". Establishing a policy to make hospitals in non-industrialized countries smoke-free would further support abstinence during the inpatient stay.

The availability of over-the-counter nicotine replacement products in pharmacies in the United States and European countries such as England has increased the opportunity for intervention in the pharmacy setting. Given the extensive use of pharmacists for medical advice in non-industrialized countries (Kamat & Nichter, 1998), pharmacists have the potential to serve an important role in providing advice and assistance to tobacco users in these countries. In addition, pharmacists are often members of inpatient hospital teams and, given their knowledge of pharmacotherapies and their counseling training, they could play a valuable role as part of a tobacco treatment protocol.

All types of clinicians—physicians, nurses, nurse practitioners, respiratory therapists, dentists, psychologists, pharmacists, health educators, dietitians and others—can effectively deliver smoking cessation messages and counseling, and the use of multiple providers increases cessation (Fiore, Bailey, Cohen, Dorfman, Goldstein, Gritz, Heyman, Holbrook, Jaen, Kottke, Lando, Mecklenburg, Mullen, Nett, Robinson, Stitzer, Tommasello, Villejo & Wewers, 1996; Fiore, Bailey, Cohen, Dorfman, Goldstein, Gritz, Heyman, Holbrook, Jaen, Kottke, Lando, Mecklenburg, Mullen, Nett, Robinson, Stitzer, Tommasello, Villejo & Wewers, 2000; Raw, McNeill & West, 1998). This finding has implications for non-industrialized countries, where a cadre of healthcare workers other than physicians may be more accessible to smokers and can be instructed on how to incorporate tobacco treatment into the care they routinely deliver. The different levels of intensity of treatment needed by different smokers can be met by providers who do brief interventions, such as physicians, pharmacists, or other health professionals more readily accessible to individuals in non-industrialized countries, and by specialists who can implement more intensive treatment in the healthcare setting or through other venues such as telephone counseling or computer-assisted interventions.

EVIDENCE FOR THE EFFECTIVENESS OF TOBACCO TREATMENT IN EACH SETTING

Ambulatory Settings

Implementing a tobacco use status identification system within the health-care setting significantly increases the rate at which clinicians intervene with their patients who smoke, and results in higher rates of smoking cessation. Brief tobacco interventions (generally 3 minutes or less) following the 5A model described later in this chapter are one of the most cost-effective routinely-performed medical procedures in the United States (Meenan, Stevens, Hornbrook, LaChance, Glasgow, Hollis, Lichtenstein & Vogt, 1998). However, no studies have been found that evaluate the effectiveness or cost-effectiveness of brief smoking cessation advice by healthcare providers in non-industrialized countries (Novotny, Cohen, Yurekli, Sweanor & de Beyer, 2000).

To guide the clinician in delivering brief tobacco dependence treatment, the United States Public Health Service (PHS) developed the *Treating Tobacco Use and Dependence Clinical Practice Guideline* for primary care clinicians (Fiore et al., 2000), and the Health Education Authority in England (Raw et al., 1998) developed *Smoking Cessation Guidelines for Health Professionals: A guide to effective smoking cessation interventions for the health care system.* They provide assessment and intervention models for the treatment of nicotine dependence, as well as evidence-based strategies. In the USPHS document the model is summarized as the 5 As: Ask, Advise, Assess, Assist and Arrange followup (Figure 1). It is recommended that smoking status be assessed and

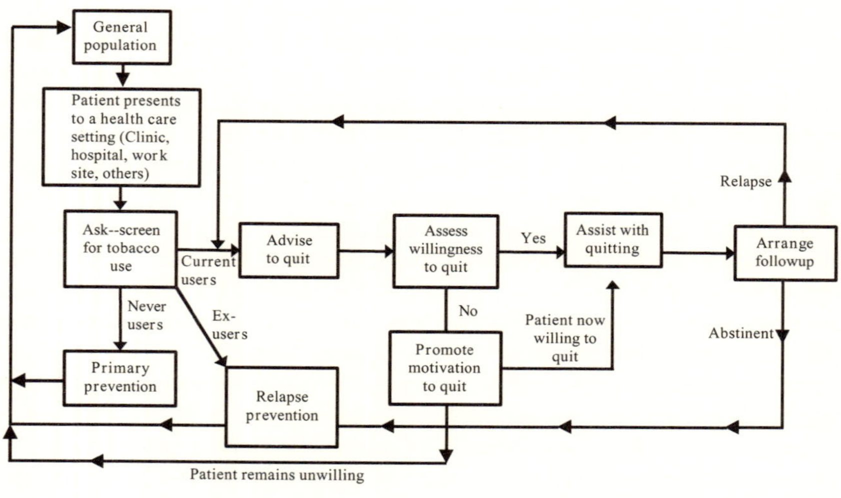

Figure 1 Model for nicotine dependence assessment and treatment

Source: Fiore MC, Bailey WC, Cohen SJ, et al: *Treating Tobacco Use and Dependence.* Clinical Practice Guideline. Rockville, MD: U.S. Department of Health and Human Service. June 2000.

documented at every clinical contact (Ask). Systems must be put in place within any healthcare setting to ensure that screening and treatment occur on a regular basis. All current smokers should be provided clear, strong and personalized advice to stop smoking (Advise) and assessed for their willingness to make a quit attempt at each contact (Assess).

For smokers unwilling to quit, a brief motivational intervention involving the 5 Rs—relevance, risks, rewards, roadblocks, and repetition—delivered by the clinician in a manner that expresses empathy, supports the individual's self-efficacy, promotes choice and avoids arguments has been found to be helpful in encouraging the consideration of smoking cessation (Miller & Rollnick, 1991; Prochaska & Goldstein, 1991). For smokers ready to quit, brief intervention with followup should be provided (Assist and Arrange). When appropriate, referral may be made for more intensive treatment. Higher intensity counseling and more frequent contacts result in higher abstinence rates. In developing an individual treatment plan, the physiological, psychological and social aspects of the patient's dependence need to be taken into consideration, and both behavioral and pharmacological treatment provided.

Because smoking and cessation patterns can be expected to differ in different countries, brief provider-delivered interventions may well need to be adapted to fit the needs of different cultures and countries. The 5A model found to be effective in the United States can serve as a model, but will need to be tailored and evaluated in non-industrialized countries to maximize applicability and effectiveness.

Inpatient Settings (Hospitals)

High-intensity behavioral interventions that include at least one month of followup contact are the most effective in promoting smoking cessation in hospitalized patients beyond usual care (Ockene et al., 1992). In one effectiveness study where very brief interventions were delivered by regular but relatively in-experienced hospital personnel (respiratory therapists) who had other hospital duties, no difference was found for the intervention compared to usual care (Stevens, Glasgow, Hollis & Mount, 2000). Based on this study and three other negative studies of brief hospital treatment, Stevens and colleagues recommend that smoking treatment programs for hospitalized smokers should use experienced accountable professional counselors for whom treatment is a primary responsibility. This person also could implement other addictions-related and lifestyle counseling involving patient behavior change. Given the strong evidence that inpatient tobacco treatment programs for patients with smoking-related disease are efficacious, such programs should be a standard component of hospital treatment (Orleans & Ockene, 1993).

Important elements of a treatment program for smokers in the hospital include smoke-free hospitals, assessing and documenting tobacco status of every patient admitted to the hospital, initiating treatment in the hospital, including physician advice as well as counseling from other healthcare providers, and providing the smoker with coping and relapse-prevention skills. The same basic 5A counseling approach and pharmacologic therapies used in outpatient settings can be used in the hospital.

Telephone followup is an effective and acceptable method of relapse prevention for smokers after hospital discharge, as in other types of smoking treatment (Lichtenstein, Glasgow, Lando, Ossip-Klein & Boles, 1996; Ockene et al., 1992). Use of nurse managers (Houston-Miller, Smith, DeBusk, Sobel & Taylor, 1997) and health educators (Kristeller, Merriam, Ockene, Ockene & Goldberg, 1993; Ockene et al., 1992) are effective in managing the treatment of smokers in programs initiated in the hospital and continued through telephone counseling.

Pharmacies

There are only two studies (Maguire, McElnay & Drummond, 2001; Sinclair, Bond, Lennox, Silcock, Winfield & Donnan, 1998) which we could find that have investigated the efficacy of pharmacists conducting tobacco treatment. Sinclair and colleagues (Sinclair et al., 1998) in the U.K. found in a randomized clinical trial that patients in the intervention condition were significantly more likely to discuss smoking with pharmacy personnel who were trained in tobacco cessation counseling and rated their discussion more highly than did usual care patients. The former also reported higher rates of abstinence at up to 9 months followup. Although the rates between intervention and usual care patients were not significant, trends were evident. Another study conducted in the U.K. (Maguire et al., 2001) also demonstrated that community-based services in pharmacies in which pharmacists were taught counseling and given a package, the Pharmacists Action on Smoking (PAS) method, which includes identification, health education materials and counseling by the pharmacists, was effective in assisting smokers to stop and to remain abstinent. Each of the noted studies suggest that community pharmacists have the potential to help smokers stop smoking. This is encouraging as pharmacists are used extensively for medical advice in less-industrialized countries (Kamat & Nichter, 1998).

Although more research is clearly needed in this area, the American Society of Health-System Pharmacists (ASHP) Therapeutic Position Statement on smoking cessation (American Society of Health-System Pharmacists, 1999; Gauen, 1999) highlights opportunities for pharmacists to become involved in tobacco treatment and to actively promote tobacco abstinence. Since pharmacists provide direct patient care and have high interest in providing health education to patients (Bond, Sinclair, Winfield et al., 1993) they can use opportunities for advising patients about smoking cessation. Computerized or manual systems can prompt pharmacists to initiate smoking cessation efforts and distribution of tobacco products can be discouraged (American Society of Health-System Pharmacists, 1999; Gauen, 1999). Printed self-help materials can be available in pharmacies and strategically placed at point-of-purchase locations. British community pharmacists are required to provide health education, at least through the display of education material (Sinclair, Bond, Lennox, Taylor & Winfield, 1995).

PREVALENCE OF PROVIDER-DELIVERED TOBACCO TREATMENT

Given the strong evidence on the effectiveness of clinician-delivered tobacco treatment, the national *Healthy People 2010* objectives issued in the United States set a goal of increasing to at least 85% the proportion of primary care providers who routinely identify their patients' smoking status and offer smoking cessation advice, assistance and followup for all their patients who smoke (U.S. Department of Health and Human Services & Office of Disease Prevention and Health Promotion, 2000). However, according to surveys and interviews with patients, physicians in the United States are far from meeting the recommended rates for delivering tobacco treatment in the outpatient setting. Only about half of U.S. smokers report receiving advice (e.g. Centers for Disease Control and Prevention 1993; Doescher & Saver, 2000; Thorndike, Rigotti, Stafford & Singer, 1998) and far fewer report receiving assistance or followup as recommended by the Public Health Service clinical practice guideline (Fiore et al., 2000) and the *Healthy People 2010* goal. The rates are even lower when patients are asked about specific steps taken by the physician (Goldstein, Niaura, Willey-Lessne, DePue, Eaton, Rakowski & Dube 1997; Rogers, Johnson, Young & Graney, 1997). Rates of physician or other healthcare provider-delivered smoking treatments in non-industrialized countries were not found.

There is evidence that physicians are more likely to provide smoking cessation advice during wellness visits versus acute visits and for patients who have smoking-related diseases versus those with conditions not related to smoking, and that physicians are less likely to offer advice to smokers not considering quitting compared to those thinking or ready to quit, (e.g., Jaen, 1997; Sesney et al., 1997; Thorndike et al., 1998). Clinicians should intervene with all smokers at all visits regardless of whether or not the visit is for illnesses caused or complicated by tobacco use, or the addiction level of the smoker. Also, specialist physicians need to make better use of the opportunities afforded by their visits, as specialist physicians are less likely to screen and treat smokers than are primary care physicians.

While there are no national U.S. or international data describing the prevalence of hospital-based tobacco treatment programs (France, Glasgow & Marcus, 2001), several studies have investigated the prevalence of smoking cessation efforts in the inpatient setting. Findings document that hospitalized smokers in a CVD unit tend to receive more information from their healthcare providers than patients in a general medical or surgical unit (Halpern, Schmier, Ward & Klesges, 2000; Orleans & Ockene, 1993).

We found only one study (Williams, Newsom & Brock, 2000) that addresses the prevalence of pharmacist-delivered tobacco treatment. The findings suggest that although pharmacists believe they are qualified to perform smoking cessation interventions, they do not routinely identify smokers. This is an area that is very open for important exploration and research.

MODELS OF INTEGRATED TOBACCO TREATMENT PROGRAMS IN INDUSTRIALIZED AND NON-INDUSTRIALIZED COUNTRIES

Primary care clinicians have considerable opportunities to deliver tobacco treatment services in industrialized and non-industrialized countries and subsequently prevent millions of cases of disability, illness and death. The optimal approach is to use comprehensive programs which use multiple clinician types and opportunities. However, what can be considered a model comprehensive program in one setting or country may not be so for another setting or country, or indeed for the same setting or country at another time. Barriers and facilitators to maximize screening and counseling vary by time, technology, target group and setting.

The WHO Framework Convention on Tobacco Control has discussed the importance of including treatment of tobacco dependence in the framework which member states would be held to if it were ratified. As part of the discussion it was noted that treatment should be viewed as part of a comprehensive cessation strategy integrated in primary healthcare and should include advice, and behavioral and pharmacologic treatment tailored to countries' circumstances (World Health Organization, 2001). Although many of the WHO member states believe in the importance of the recommendation, several countries note that technical and financial assistance would be essential to implement the treatment of tobacco dependence in their countries.

The rest of this section reviews characteristics or model principles (Ockene et al., in press) of optimal tobacco treatment programs and presents an effective statewide or nationwide program which can be used as a model for other countries.

Model Principles

1. Consider multiple target groups, e.g. include strategies aimed at provider, patient and community. Include tobacco treatment interventions that move towards a public health model which could be delivered in a less-intensive format to a large proportion of the population. Such interventions include self-help booklets, outreach telephone counseling and group sessions.
2. Consider factors outside of the individual clinician's control, e.g. reimbursement, availability and accessibility of services.
3. Ensure that intervention strategies and expectations about performance standards reflect the state of science, professional consensus, and professional norms.
4. Use strategies which may be differentially needed by population sub-groups (i.e. promote equity).

5. Establish systems to screen, track and monitor patients' smoking and providers' delivery of treatment.
6. Be prepared to modify program components over time to maximize the delivery of and access to tobacco treatment as patient needs and environmental factors change.

An Example of a U.S. Statewide Program to Provide Tobacco Treatment

Statewide or country-wide programs which include tobacco treatment in clinical settings are important and challenging to implement. In 1992, a voter approved referendum in Massachusetts, U.S., established the Health Protection Fund, with revenue generated from a 25 cent increase in the excise tax on cigarettes and smokeless tobacco (Koh, 1997; Massachusetts General Law, 1992). A portion of this revenue funds the Massachusetts Tobacco Control Program (MTCP), whose aims are to reduce tobacco-related health risk by: (1) motivating and helping smokers stop smoking; (2) preventing young people from initiating tobacco use, interrupt habituated use, and reduce youth access to tobacco products; and (3) reducing non-smokers' exposure to environmental tobacco smoke (Robbins & Krakow, 2000). The MTCP funds a comprehensive media campaign, community-based programs, tobacco-related research and evaluation, and statewide capacity-building projects including a quitline that provides tobacco treatment counseling, self-help materials, referrals and crisis intervention for smokers who want to quit; a clearinghouse that develops, distributes and maintains a database of educational materials; and programs that provide training and technical assistance to primary healthcare sites and community-based programs. The tobacco control program is integrated into the existing public health system, including a public/private partnership system of hospitals, health centers, community-based agencies, local boards of health and city health departments, and schools.

Local programs are at the center of MTCP's tobacco control activities. Boards of health/health departments and local tobacco control community coalitions are funded to raise public awareness and enact and enforce local ordinances and regulations designed to reduce youth access and environmental tobacco smoke. Innovative outreach and intervention programs respond to the particular need of a target population at home, at public events and in other public settings. Innovative intervention for risk-taking youth programs foster youth leadership in tobacco control and provide smoking cessation interventions for youth participants. Tobacco treatment programs located within a variety of community healthcare settings provide free or low-cost, evidence-based tobacco treatment services (e.g. 5A intervention, individual and group counseling) and pharmacologic interventions, and are reimbursed by the MTCP for delivery of each unit of service, with the intent of providing a coordinated system of care at the community level. The MTCP requires tobacco treatment providers within funded programs to both complete the competency-based training and achieve certification through the University of Massachusetts Medical School (Pbert, Ockene, Ewy, Leicher & Warner, 2000).

The Massachusetts Tobacco Control Program uses the model principles noted above by targeting strategies at smokers, providers and the community through availability of one-on-one intervention, community-based media and other strategies and training of specialists and primary care providers. It uses multiple types of providers in a comprehensive model and provides systems for tracking and monitoring. Many of these model principles can be applied in non-industrial countries with necessary adaptations to the environment and culture in which the program exists. Unfortunately, there has been little or no research to document the applicability of these model principles in non-industrialized countries. An important research agenda would be to evaluate this transferability. As an encouraging sign, The U.S. National Institutes of Health (NIH) already has begun to offer funds for research in this important area.

REFERENCES

American Society of Health-System Pharmacists. (1999). ASHP Therapeutic Position Statement on Smoking Cessation. *Am J Health-Syst Pharm* 56(5): 460–464.

Bien, T. & Burge, R. (1990). Smoking and drinking: A review of the literature. *Int J Addict* 25: 1429–1454.

Bobo, J. (1989). Nicotine dependence and alcoholism epidemiology and treatment. *J Psychoactive Drugs* 21(3): 323–329.

Bond, C., Sinclair, H., Winfield, A. & et al. (1993). Community pharmacists' attitudes to their advice giving role and the deregulation of medicines. *Int J Pharm Pract* 2: 26–30.

Centers for Disease Control and Prevention. (1993). Physician and other health-care professional counseling of smokers to quit: United States 1991. *MMWR* 42: 854–857.

Centers for Disease Control and Prevention. (1999). Cigarette smoking among adults—United States, 1995. *Morb Mortal Wkly Rep* 46: 1217–1220.

Corrao, M., Guindon, G., Sharma, N. & Shokoohi, D., Eds. (2000). Tobacco Control Country Profiles. Atlanta, GA, American Cancer Society.

Doescher, M.P. & Saver, B.G. (2000). Physicians' advice to quit smoking. The glass remains half empty. *J Fam Pract* 49(6): 543–7.

Fiore, M., Bailey, W., Cohen, S., Dorfman, S., Goldstein, M., Gritz, E., Heyman, R., Holbrook, J., Jaen, C., Kottke, T., Lando, H., Mecklenburg, R., Mullen, P., Nett, L., Robinson, L., Stitzer, M., Tommasello, A., Villejo, L. & Wewers, M. (1996). Smoking Cessation: Clinical Practice Guideline No. 18. Rockville, MD, U.S. Department of Public Health and Human Services, Public Health Service, Agency for Health Care Policy and Research.

Fiore, M., Bailey, W., Cohen, S., Dorfman, S., Goldstein, M., Gritz, E., Heyman, R., Holbrook, J., Jaen, C., Kottke, T., Lando, H., Mecklenburg, R., Mullen, P., Nett, L., Robinson, L., Stitzer, M., Tommasello, A., Villejo, L. & Wewers, M. (2000). Treating Tobacco Use and Dependence. Clinical Practice Guideline. Rockville, MD, US Department of Health and Human Services, Public Health Services.

France, E., Glasgow, R. & Marcus, A. (2001). Smoking cessation interventions among hospitalized patients: What have we learned? *Prev Med* 32: 376–388.

Frid, D., Ockene, I., Ockene, J., Merriam, P., Goldberg, R., Kristeller, J. & Barrett, S. (1991). Severity of angiographically proven coronary artery disease predicts smoking cessation. *Am J Prev Med* 7(3): 131–135.

Gauen, S. (1999). Ways to help patients quit smoking (editorial). *AM J Health Syst Pharm* 56: 425.

Glasgow, R., Stevens, V., Vogt, T., Mullooly, J. & Lichtenstein, E. (1991). Changes in smoking associated with hospitalization: quit rates, predictive variables, and intervention implications. *Am J Health Promot* 6(1): 24–29.

Glassman, A. (1993). Cigarette smoking: Implications for psychiatric illness. *Am J Psychiatry* 150: 546–553.

Goldstein, M.G., Niaura, R., Willey-Lessne, C., DePue, J., Eaton, C., Rakowski, W. & Dube, C. (1997). Physicians counseling smokers. A population-based survey of patients' perceptions of health care provider-delivered smoking cessation interventions. *Arch Intern Med* 157(12): 1313–1319.

Haapanen-Niemi, N., Miilunpalo, S., Vuori, I., Pasanen, M. & Oja, P. (1999). The impact of smoking, alcohol consumption, and physical activity on the use of hospital services. *Am J Public Health* 89(5): 691–698.

Halpern, M., Schmier, J., Ward, K. & Klesges, R. (2000). Smoking cessation in hospitalized patients. *Respir Care* 45(3): 330–336.

Houston-Miller, N., Smith, P., DeBusk, R., Sobel, D. & Taylor, C. (1997). Smoking cessation in hospitalized patients. Results of a randomized trial. *Arch Intern Med* 157(4): 409–415.

Jaen, C.R. (1997). Primary-care physicians. *Tob Control* 6(Suppl 1): S34–36.

Kamat, V. & Nichter, M. (1998). Pharmacies, self-medication and pharmaceutical marketing in Bombay, India. *Soc Sci Med* 47: 779–794.

Koh, H. (1997). An analysis of the successful 1992 Massachusetts Tobacco Tax Initiative. *Tobacco Control* 6: 213–218.

Kristeller, J., Merriam, P., Ockene, J., Ockene, I. & Goldberg, R. (1993). Smoking Intervention for Cardiac Patients: In Search of More Effective Strategies. *Cardiology* 82: 317–324.

Lichtenstein, E., Glasgow, R., Lando, H., Ossip-Klein, D. & Boles, S. (1996). Telephone counseling for smoking cessation. *Health Educ Res* 11: 243–257.

Maguire, T., McElnay, J. & Drummond, A. (2001). A randomized controlled trial of a smoking cessation intervention based in community pharmacies. *Addiction* 96: 325–331.

Massachusetts General Law (1992). Chapter 254, Section 2T, Acts of 1992.

Meenan, R., Stevens, V., Hornbrook, M., LaChance, P., Glasgow, R., Hollis, J., Lichtenstein, E. & Vogt, T. (1998). Cost effectiveness of a hospital-based smoking cessation intervention. *Med Care* 36: 670–678.

Miller, W. & Rollnick, S. (1991). Motivational interviewing: Preparing people to change addictive behavior. New York, Guilford Press.

Novotny, T., Cohen, J., Yurekli, A., Sweanor, D. & de Beyer, J. (2000). Smoking cessation and nicotine-replacement therapies. In: *Tobacco control in developing countries.* Jha, P. & Chaloupka, F., Eds. New York, Oxford University Press: 287–307.

Ockene, J., Kristeller, J., Goldberg, R., Ockene, I., Merriam, P., Barrett, S., Pekow, P., Hosmer, D. & Gianelly, R. (1992). Smoking cessation and severity of disease: The Coronary Artery Smoking Intervention Study. *Health Psychol* 11(2): 119–126.

Ockene, J., Zapka, J., Pbert, L., Brodney, S. & Lemon, S. (in press). Provider, System and Policy Strategies to Enhance the Delivery of Cancer Prevention and Control Activities in Primary Care.In: *The Institute of Medicine Report, Fulfilling the Promise of Cancer Prevention and Early Detection* Washington, DC, National Academy Press.

Orleans, C. & Ockene, J. (1993). Routine hospital-based quit-smoking treatment for the postmyocardial infarction patient: An idea whose time has come (editorial). *J Am Coll Cardiol* 22(6): 1703–1705.

Pbert, L., Ockene, J., Ewy, B., Leicher, E. & Warner, D. (2000). Development of a state wide tobacco treatment specialist training and certification programme for Massachusetts. *Tobacco Control* 9(4): 372–381.

Penttinen, J. (1997). Smoking and risk of hospitalization [letter]. *Epidemiol* 8(2): 220–221.

Prochaska, J. & Goldstein, M. (1991). Process of smoking cessation: Implications for clinicians. *Clin Chest Med* 12(4): 727–735.

Raw, M., McNeill, A. & West, R. (1998). Smoking cessation guidelines for health professionals: A guide to effective smoking cessation interventions for the healthcare system. *Thorax* 53(Suppl 5): S1–S19.

Robbins, H. & Krakow, M. (2000). Evolution of a comprehensive tobacco control programme: building system capacity and strategic partnerships—lessons from Massachusetts. *Tobacco Control* 9: 423–430.

Rogers, L.Q., Johnson, K.C., Young, Z.M. & Graney, M. (1997). Demographic bias in physician smoking cessation counseling. *Am J Med Sci* 313(3): 153–158.

Sesney, J.W., Kreher, N.E., Hickner, J.M. & Webb, S. (1997). Smoking cessation interventions in rural family practices: an UPRNet study. *J Fam Pract* 44(6): 578–585.

Simon, J., Browner, W. & Mangano, D. (1992). Predictors of smoking relapse after noncardiac surgery. Study of Perioperative Ischemia (SPI) Research Group. *Am J Public Health* 82(9): 1235–1237.

Sinclair, H., Bond, C., Lennox, A., Silcock, J., Winfield, A. & Donnan, P. (1998). Training pharmacists and pharmacy assistants in the stage-of-change model of smoking cessation: A randomised controlled trial in Scotland. *Tobacco Control* 7: 253–261.

Sinclair, H., Bond, C., Lennox, A., Taylor, R. & Winfield, A. (1995). Nicotine replacement therapies: smoking cessation outcomes in a pharmacy setting in Scotland. *Tobacco Control* 4:338–343.

Smith, P., Kraemer, H., Miller, N., DeBusk, R. & Taylor, C. (1999). In-hospital smoking cessation programs: Who responds, who doesn't? *J Consult Clin Psychol* 67(1): 19–27.

Stange, K.C., Flocke, S.A. & Goodwin, M.A. (1998). Opportunistic preventive services delivery. Are time limitations and patient satisfaction barriers? *J Fam Pract* 46(5): 419–24.

Stevens, V., Glasgow, R., Hollis, J. & Mount, K. (2000). Implementation and effectiveness of a brief smoking-cessation intervention for hospital patients. *Med Care* 38: 451–459.

Thorndike, A.N., Rigotti, N.A., Stafford, R.S. & Singer, D.E. (1998). National patterns in the treatment of smokers by physicians. *Jama* 279(8): 604–608.

U.S. Department of Health and Human Services & Office of Disease Prevention and Health Promotion (2000). Healthy People 2010: Understanding and Improving Health *and* Objectives for Improving Health. Washington, D.C., U.S. Department of Health and Human Services.

Williams, D., Newsom, J. & Brock, T. (2000). An evaluation of smoking cessation-related activities by pharmacists. *J Am Pharm Assoc* 40(3): 366–370.

World Health Organization (1997). Tobacco or Health: A Global Status Report. Geneva, Switzerland.

World Health Organization. (2000). Second Meeting of the Working Group on the WHO Framework Convention on Tobacco Control. http://www.who.int/gb/fctc/wg2/fEwg2.htm, December 28, 2001.

World Health Organization. (2001). Intergovernmental Negotiating Body on the WHO Framework Convention on Tobacco Control—Third Session. http://www.who.int/gb/fctc/inb3/Einb3.htm, December 28, 2001.

PART C

Intervening through Mental Health Services

As clinicians are well aware, it is quite common for people with substance use disorders to present with a variety of mental health problems as well. Similarly, among those treated in mental health systems the prevalence of concomitant substance use disorders is high.

People with such "dual disorders" present special challenges in treatment. One important issue is whether their problems should be understood as separate disorders to be addressed through different specialist treatment systems, or as intertwined problems to be addressed in an integrated fashion. The extent of integration versus segregation of substance abuse and mental health care varies across nations.

The two chapters of this section examine the special issues involved in treating concomitant mental and substance use disorders. In Chapter 9, Melanie Bennett summarizes the considerable extent of overlap between these two broad classes of problems, indicating that these are not always separate populations. Any mental health care system is bound to encounter high rates of substance use disorders among its clients. Similarly, anyone who treats substance use disorders ought to be prepared to deal with a full panoply of mental disorders.

In Chapter 10, Nancy Handmaker and Robert Anderson take the next logical step, examining what is known about the treatment of these concomitant problems. They present general ways of proceeding: a parallel approach in which substance use and mental health issues are treated separately by different specialists, and an integrated approach in which the person's various problems are addressed by a single care team. They offer an original and detailed meta-analysis of treatment studies bearing on these two approaches, published here for the first time.

CHAPTER 9

Interrelationship of Substance Abuse and Mental Health Problems

MELANIE E. BENNETT

INTRODUCTION

There is now considerable evidence documenting high rates of substance use disorders and other forms of mental illness around the world. Such research illustrates the enormous toll that both sets of disorders take on individuals and society, and shows how both types of disorders contribute substantially to poor functioning and compromised well-being. We are now starting to understand much about substance use disorders and other forms of mental illness. We have good evidence regarding the nature and course of many types of mental and substance use disorders, and for many we have studied a range of psychosocial and pharmacological treatments with efficacy ranging from promising to clearly beneficial.

Despite these advances, comparatively little attention has been devoted to understanding and treating comorbid mental illness and substance use disorders (Handmaker & Anderson, this volume). While individually these disorders cause a range of problems, when combined they yield an even more negative impact on the lives and functioning of individuals. In the United States, substance abuse and mental illness historically have been viewed as separate and unrelated problems, and the service systems designed to address these disorders developed relatively independently (Grella, 1996; Polcin, 1992; Ridgely, Lambert, Goodman, Chichester, & Ralph, 1998). As a result, approaches to etiology, assessment, treatment, and research differ starkly between the two systems (see Grella, 1996 for a review). The mental health system has traditionally

MELANIE E. BENNETT • Department of Psychiatry, University of Maryland School of Medicine, Baltimore, Maryland 21201

focused on use of psychotropic medications, treatment delivered by medical professionals, and substance abuse not as an illness in its own right but a condition that develops out of attempts to "self-medicate" psychiatric symptomatology (Grella, 1996; Polcin, 1992). This approach has excluded many issues relevant from the substance abuse treatment system perspective, including addressing spiritual factors in treatment, the use of self-help groups in recovery, and medication-free approaches to treatment (Grella, 1996; Polcin, 1992). Such a split in the provision of treatment has yielded poorer provision of services for patients with comorbid disorders in the United States. In some parts of the world, there is a lack of attention to mental and substance use disorders within any health care system or setting. Thus many countries (including the United States) are poorly equipped to deal with the sizeable percentage of patients who are "dual diagnosis"—a term that generally refers to individuals suffering from both mental illness and substance use disorders. The term is somewhat misleading in that many so-called dual diagnosis patients meet diagnostic criteria for more than two disorders (Kessler et al., 1994). Not surprisingly, research from a range of countries shows what clinicians have long known—dual diagnosis has a profound and pervasive impact on the course and severity of both mental illness and substance use disorders.

This chapter reviews rates of dual diagnosis from both the mental illness and the substance abuse perspectives. The first section reviews issues that impact research on prevalence rates of dual diagnosis, followed by an examination of prevalence data for substance use disorders in mental illness, and of mental illness among individuals with substance use disorders. The final section reviews the many ways that dual disorders impacts illness, service utilization, and treatment outcome.

METHODOLOGICAL ISSUES IN DETERMINING PREVALENCE RATES

There are several methodological issues that affect rates of co-occurring mental illness and substance use disorders. To begin with, data on rates of dual diagnosis come from both general population studies and studies of clinical samples. Since the 1980s, several large epidemiological studies have documented the interface of substance abuse and mental illness, providing representative information on rates of dual diagnosis among individuals living in the general population. Due to their large sample sizes and their random sampling of individuals in the community, general population studies are relevant to the population as a whole, and they typically employ structured diagnostic assessments administered by trained interviewers that are highly reliable. Other information comes from studies of clinical samples. Given the constraints on conducting research in treatment settings, clinical studies often utilize less rigorous methods of assessment and less highly trained interviewers. However, such studies are crucial in terms of understanding the full impact of dual disorders on patients and the treatment systems that serve them.

Importantly, general population and clinical samples will provide widely differing estimates of dual diagnosis. Because those with multiple disorders are more likely to seek treatment, prevalence estimates of dual disorders will be higher in clinical samples than in community samples (a condition known as "Berkson's fallacy", Berkson, 1949). Relatedly, the settings from which samples are taken impact prevalence rates of dual diagnosis. Factors such as inpatient or outpatient status and chronicity of illness may affect rates of comorbid substance abuse and mental illness. For example, research on substance abuse in schizophrenia has suggested that more severely impaired inpatients are less likely to have a comorbid substance use disorder than patients who are less ill (Mueser et al., 1990). Another example is findings that different hospital settings cause variations in dual diagnosis rates, with hospital emergency rooms reflecting higher estimates than other settings (Barbee, Clark, Crapanzano, Heintz, & Kehoe, 1989; Galanter, Casteneda, & Ferman, 1988).

Assessment methods can influence rates of dual diagnosis. Structured research interviews are generally accepted as the most reliable method of diagnosis (Mueser, Bellack, & Blanchard, 1992), yet not all studies use such interviews. A related issue concerns the types of substances that are assessed when evaluating dual disorders. Studies typically assess drinking, along with use of a range of illicit drugs including cocaine, heroin, hallucinogens, and stimulants. However, there are other substances that are less frequently considered, either because they are rarely or commonly used in the general population, despite evidence that such substances can have an important relationship to mental health and functioning. For instance, nicotine use is typically not assessed, even though a growing literature suggests that nicotine dependence has links, perhaps biological in nature, to both major depression (Quattrocki, Baird, & Yurgelun-Todd, 2000) and schizophrenia (Ziedonis & George, 1997). In addition, definitions of "dual diagnosis," "comorbidity," and "substance abuse" are far from uniform. Often unstructured assessments of substance use disorders are employed, yielding differing definitions of substance use disorders and making prevalence rates diverse and difficult to compare. For example, studies might assess different substance use patterns, ranging from heavy use to substance abuse to substance dependence, and others do not specify the exact nature of the substance use they are assessing. Among studies that do define the type of substance use problem they are assessing, different diagnostic criteria are often used, making comparison difficult.

Patient demographic variables have been shown to correlate with substance abuse, and differences in patient variables across samples influence prevalence rates. For example, gender and age both correlate with substance abuse: males and those of younger age are more likely to abuse substances. Because studies of comorbidity in schizophrenia often use samples of inpatients who are more likely to be male, the comorbidity rate in schizophrenia may be inflated since males are more likely to have substance use disorders and more likely to be inpatients in psychiatric hospitals. Relatedly, findings cross-nationally with regard to rates of substance use and mental illness are influenced by cultural attitudes and norms regarding substance use, as well as diagnostic conventions and methods of assessments (Gureje, Vazquez-Barquero, & Janca, 1996). Over the last several years, an important trend towards examination of dual diagnosis cross-nationally has taken place, in which many studies utilize similar measures and diagnostic criteria. For example, the development of the Composite International Diagnostic Interview (CIDI) by the World Health Organization (1991) has allowed researchers from around the world to utilize Diagnostic and Statistical Manual of Mental Disorder (APA, 1987) criteria to diagnose a range of Axis I and Axis II disorders in both general and clinical populations. Such research has enabled those studying co-occurring substance use and mental disorders to examine the issue internationally, yielding both a broader perspective on the issue as well as important data concerning how substance use and mental health disorders impact individuals around the world.

PREVALENCE OF SUBSTANCE USE DISORDERS AMONG INDIVIDUALS WITH MENTAL ILLNESS

Epidemiological Studies

The Epidemiologic Catchment Area Study (ECA; Regier et al., 1990) was the first large-scale study of comorbidity in a general population sample. The ECA surveyed more than 20,000 adults in five cities in the United States over four years, and included individuals both in the community and in institutions. Overall, findings showed substantial rates of comorbidity in the general population. Having a psychiatric illness was found to confer more than twice the risk for an alcohol use disorder, with an 11% rate of alcohol use disorder among those in the general population versus a 22.3% rate among those with mental illness. Moreover, those with mental illness had more than four times the risk of meeting criteria for a drug use disorder (a 3.7% rate of drug use disorder in the general population versus a 14.7% among those with mental illness). The ECA study also examined comorbidity of substance use disorders within specific mental disorders. Antisocial personality disorder (ASP) showed the highest comorbidity rate (83.6%), and high rates of comorbidity also were found for bipolar disorder (60.7%), schizophrenia (47%), panic disorder (35.8%), obsessive-compulsive disorder (32.8%), and unipolar depression (27.2%). The ECA results made clear the significant risk faced by individuals with mental disorders for developing substance use disorders.

The National Household Survey (NHS; Kessler et al., 1994) assessed over 8000 non-institutionalized individuals in the United States, ages 15 to 54, across 48 states with the Composite International Diagnostic Interview (CIDI, World Health Organization, 1991). Importantly, the NHS documented even higher rates of substance use disorder among those with mental illness, with greater than 50% of those with mental illness meeting diagnostic criteria for a lifetime substance use disorder. Analyses for individual classes of diagnoses found that many mental disorders conferred at least twice the risk of lifetime alcohol or drug use disorders.

A third large-scale survey, the National Longitudinal Alcohol Epidemiology Study (NLAES; Grant et al., 1994), examined rates of co-occurrence of substance use disorders and affective disorders in a general population sample of over 40,000 adults in the United States. Grant and Hartford (1995) found that those with major depression showed almost three times the rate of alcohol dependence as those without major depression. The associations were even stronger for drug use disorders: individuals with drug dependence were nearly seven times more likely to report lifetime major depression than those without drug dependence (see Bucholz, 1999 for a review).

Results from epidemiological studies in other countries show strikingly similar findings (see Witchen, Perkonigg, & Reed, 1996 for a review). For example, the 7-year Munich Follow-up Study (Wittchen, Essau, von Zerssen, Krieg, & Zaudig, 1992) examined comorbidity of substance use disorders and affective and anxiety disorders in an adult general population sample in West Germany. Overall, 13.5% of the sample met criteria for lifetime dual disorders. Newman and colleagues (1996) conducted a survey of young adults in New Zealand and found substantial rates of comorbid substance use disorders for both anxiety (23.1%) and mood disorders (29.5%). Farrell and colleagues (1998) reported results from the National Psychiatric Morbidity Survey, a British study of comorbidity that surveyed three samples, among them a household sample of over 10,000 people. Substance use was significantly associated with higher rates of psychological morbidity. Such results from epidemiological studies from a range of countries illustrate the frequency with which dual diagnosis affects individuals in the general population.

Clinical Studies

Clinical studies of comorbidity assess either samples of general psychiatric patients or samples of patients with specific psychiatric disorders. Overall, studies of general psychiatric patients in the United States indicate that one-third to three-quarters of general psychiatric patients may meet criteria for comorbid mental and substance use disorders (Ananth et al., 1989; Chen et al., 1992). Mezzich, Ahn, Fabrega, and Pilkonis (1990) conducted a survey of dual substance use and mental disorders in a diverse population of individuals presenting for evaluation and referral to a comprehensive psychiatric hospital over an 18-month period. Results showed substantial rates of dual diagnosis among patients with primary mental health disorders. For example, 33% of patients with major depression were diagnosed with an alcohol use disorder, and 18% were diagnosed with a non-alcohol substance use disorder. Rates were even more striking among patients with severe mental illnesses such as bipolar disorder (45% for alcohol use disorder and 39% for another substance use disorder) and schizophrenia or paranoid disorders (42% and 38% were diagnosed with alcohol and other substance use disorders respectively).

Such trends are also found in other countries. Rabinowitz, Mark, Popper, and Slyuzberg (1996) examined dual diagnosis among discharged psychiatric patients in Israel and found that 13.2% of men and 3.6% of women met criteria for comorbid substance use disorders, with the greatest rate of dual diagnosis found for patients with discharge diagnoses of personality disorder. A study of patients with psychotic disorders in London (Menezes et al., 1996) found a one-year prevalence rate of 36.3% for any substance problem, and 43% of a sample of Taiwanese patients with major depression were found to have a substance use diagnosis (Bai, Lin, Hu, & Yeh, 1998). These and other findings (Kozaric-Kovacic, Folnegovic-Smalc, Folnegovic, & Marusic, 1995) clearly demonstrate the significant rates of dual diagnosis in general clinic samples both in the United States and in other nations.

Other clinical studies have examined samples of patients with specific forms of mental illness. Rates of dual substance use and mental disorder appear to be highest among patients with major mental illnesses including schizophrenia, bipolar disorder, and major depression. Studies have found rates of close to or surpassing 50% in patients with schizophrenia (Dixon, Haas, Weiden, Sweeney, & Frances, 1991; Meuser et al., 1990), and rates among patients with bipolar disorder have been found to range from 18–75% (Goodwin & Jamison, 1990). Lower, but still substantial rates of substance use disorders have been found in samples of patients with major depression (Lewis, Rice, Andreasen, Endicott, & Hartman, 1986; Merikangas, Leckman, Prusoff, Pauls, & Weissman, 1985). In their review of dual anxiety and substance use disorders, Kushner, Sher, and Beitman (1990) found differing rates based on anxiety disorder type. Social phobia had the highest range, followed by agoraphobia and panic disorder. Others have found substantial rates of dual substance use disorders and obsessive-compulsive disorder (Eisen & Rasmussen, 1989) and posttraumatic stress disorder (PTSD; Keane, Gerardi, Lyons, & Wolfe, 1988).

In sum, dual diagnosis occurs with great frequency among those with mental illness. Results from both epidemiological and clinical studies clearly illustrate the fact that dual disorders are a common occurrence in both the general population and among those in mental health treatment. Patients with personality disorders and severe mental illness appear to be at highest risk for comorbid substance use disorders, but those with anxiety and mood disorder often show twice the rate of dual substance use disorders than is found in the general population. As we will see below, this pattern holds for individuals with primary substance use disorders.

PREVALENCE OF MENTAL DISORDERS IN SUBSTANCE ABUSING POPULATIONS

Epidemiological Studies

Mental illness among primary substance abusers has also been examined in many of the large-scale epidemiological studies. Results from the ECA study found that among those with an alcohol disorder, 36.6% had a dual mental disorder, while more than half (53.0%) of those with a drug use disorder were diagnosed with a comorbid mental disorder (Regier et al., 1990). In other words, having an alcohol use disorder puts an individual at an almost three times greater risk of mental illness, while having a drug use disorder confers almost five times the risk of mental illness. Further analyses (Helzer & Pryzbeck, 1988) found that among those with alcohol use disorders, the strongest association was with antisocial personality disorder (odds ratio, OR = 21.0), followed by mania (OR = 6.2) and schizophrenia (OR = 4.0). NCA findings similarly documented high rates of mental illness among those with substance use disorders (Kessler et al., 1997). The majority of participants with an alcohol use disorder had a history of some nonsubstance use psychiatric disorder, and the same held true for those with other drug use disorders (Kessler, 1997; Kessler et al., 1997). Findings from the NLAES (Grant, 1995; Grant & Harford, 1995) highlight the significant association between substance use disorders and major depression. Those with an alcohol use disorder were almost four times more likely to have lifetime major depression than were those without alcohol use disorder. For drug dependence the findings were even more striking: those with drug dependence were almost 7 times more likely to meet a diagnosis of major depression than those without drug dependence. Such findings clearly illustrate that the dual diagnosis issue is significant, whether one looks at it from the mental illness or substance use disorder side of the equation.

Similar findings have been obtained in other countries. Russell, Newman, and Bland (1994) report findings from a large-scale household survey of mental disorders among those with substance abuse or dependence in Edmonton. Over 80% of those with drug abuse or dependence met criteria for some other mental disorder. In their survey of young adults in New Zealand, Newman and colleagues (1996) found that among those with substance use disorders, 45.2% met criteria for either a mood or an anxiety disorder or both. The International Consortium in Psychiatric Epidemiology (ICPE, Merikangas et al., 1998) utilized data from six large-scale epidemiological studies in Europe and North America, all of which used the CIDI to examine rates of mood and anxiety disorders, conduct disorders, and substance use disorders in general population samples. This study had several important findings, chief among them the similarity in rates of dual substance use and mental disorders cross-nationally. Findings from averages across sites showed that 20% of individuals with alcohol problems (similar to DSM-III-R alcohol abuse) and 20% of those with alcohol dependence had a lifetime history of mood disorder. For lifetime prevalence rates of anxiety disorders, the rates were 25% among those with alcohol problems and 32% among those with alcohol dependence. In addition, between 25% and 50% of those with alcohol use disorders also met criteria for either conduct disorder or antisocial personality disorder. Findings with drug use disorders were even more pronounced. Almost 35% of respondents with drug dependence met criteria for a lifetime mood disorder, 45% met criteria for a lifetime anxiety disorder, and 50% met criteria for either conduct or antisocial personality disorder. Importantly, this multi-national study found a relationship between the number of mood/anxiety disorders and the magnitude of comorbidity with substance use disorders. The greater the number of mood/anxiety disorders met, the greater the likelihood that the individuals experienced co-occurring substance abuse or dependence. In addition, findings for drug use disorders showed that degree of comorbidity was related to severity of drug dependence, with those with multiple mood/anxiety disorders showing greater severity of drug dependence.

Clinical Studies

High rates of both Axis I and Axis II disorders have been confirmed in many studies of treatment seeking substance abusers (Herz, Volicer, D'Angelo, & Gadish, 1990; Mirin, Weiss, Griffith, & Michael, 1991; Nace, Davis, & Gaspari, 1991; Penick et al., 1984; Powell, Penick, Othmer, Bingham, & Rice, 1982; Ross, Glaser, & Stiasny, 1988). For example, almost 74% of a sample of cocaine abusers was diagnosed with a lifetime psychiatric disorder (Rounsaville et al., 1991), and 77% of a sample of hospitalized alcoholics was similarly found to have some sort of mental illness (Hesselbrock, Meyer, & Keener, 1985). Ross, Glaser, & Germanson (1988) found that 78% of a sample of patients in an alcohol and drug treatment facility met criteria for some form of mental illness. Rates of current mental disorder in these samples were found to be high as well, ranging from 55.7% in the group of cocaine abusers (Rounsaville et al., 1991) to 65% in the general substance abuse sample (Ross et al., 1988). Milby and colleagues (1996) assessed a sample of patients with opioid dependence on methadone maintenance therapy and found that over half met criteria for at least one anxiety disorder, almost two-thirds met criteria for at least one affective disorder, and over one-third met criteria for both anxiety and affective disorders.

Major depression and personality disorders are particular problems for substance abusers in treatment (Brooner, King, Kidorf, Schmidt, & Bigelow, 1997; Hasin, Grant, & Endicott, 1988; Hesselbrock et al., 1985; Merikangas & Gelrnter, 1990; Rounsaville, Weissman, Wilber, Crits-Christoph, & Kleber, 1982). In their evaluation of over 4000 patients presenting for initial assessment and referral, Mezzich and colleagues (1990) found that almost one-third of those diagnosed with alcohol use disorders met criteria for major depression, as did one-fifth of those with non-alcohol substance use disorders. Moreover, 18% of those with alcohol use disorders and almost 25% of those with substance use disorders met criteria for an Axis II disorder. Morgenstern, Langenbucher, Labouvie, and Miller (1997) assessed prevalence rates of personality disorders in a multisite sample of 366 substance abusers in treatment, and found that over 57% of the sample met criteria for at least one personality disorder. Antisocial personality disorder was the most prevalent, followed by borderline, paranoid, and avoidant personality disorders. Moreover, the presence of a personality disorder doubled the likelihood of meeting criteria for a comorbid Axis I disorder. In addition, high rates of dual anxiety disorders have been found among substance abusers in treatment, including phobias (Bowen, Cipywnyk, D'Arcy, & Keegan, 1984; Hasin et al., 1988; Ross et al., 1988), panic disorder (Hasin et al., 1988; Penick et al., 1984), obsessive-compulsive disorder (Eisen & Rasmussen, 1989), and social phobia (Thomas et al., 1999). Substance abusers also appear to be especially affected by PTSD (Bonin et al., 2000; Davis & Wood, 1999; Triffleman, Marmar, Delucchi, & Ronfeldt, 1995). In an analysis of cocaine-dependent patients in the National Institute on Drug Abuse Collaborative Cocaine Treatment Study, Najavitis and colleagues (1998) found that 30.2% of women and 15.2% of men met DSM-III-R criteria for PTSD.

Such findings have been replicated in other countries. Pozzi and colleagues (1997) studied the prevalence of mental disorders among treatment-seeking individuals with drug use disorders in Italy and found that 32.3% reported lifetime comorbidity. In their survey of 226 individuals with drug dependence in Greece, Kokkevi and colleagues (1998) found a 59.5% prevalence rate of personality disorder, with over 60% of these patients meeting criteria for more than one personality disorder. Moreover, those with personality disorders were at twice the risk for meeting an additional Axis I diagnosis. Tomasson and Vaglum (1995) surveyed a national sample of individuals seeking treatment for substance abuse treatment in Iceland and found that 70% of those with alcohol use disorders and over 90% of those with polysubstance abuse or dependence had co-occurring mental disorders. Moreover, a significant percentage of those with comorbid disorders met criteria for both affective and anxiety disorders, in addition to substance abuse, further illustrating the complex nature of "dual" diagnoses.

In sum, individuals with substance use disorders are at high risk for the co-occurrence of mental disorders. Whether assessed in the general population or while receiving substance abuse treatment, those with primary substance use disorders show high rates of almost all mental disorders, with antisocial personality disorder and major depression being among the most prevalent. From this review it is clear that dual diagnosis is common, both in the general population and among clients in mental health and substance abuse treatment, in countries around the world.

IMPACT OF COMORBIDITY AND IMPLICATIONS FOR CARE

The importance of dual diagnosis lies in its serious and pernicious impact on the course and prognosis of both mental and substance use disorders, as well as the implications dual disorders have for assessment, diagnosis, and treatment outcome. Dual diagnosis has a profound impact on almost every area of patient functioning, clinical care, and research. Research from many countries has shown that patients with dual disorders show more severe symptoms of mental illness (Hays & Aidroos, 1986; Najavitis et al., 1998; Saladin, Brady, Dansky, & Kilpatrick, 1995), more frequent hospitalizations (Carpenter et al., 1985;

Drake & Wallach, 1989, Haywood et al., 1995; Menezes et al., 1996), more frequent relapses (Linzen, Dingemans, & Lenior, 1994; O'Connell, Mayo, Flatow, Cuthbertson, & O'Brien, 1991, Sokolski et al., 1994), and a poorer course of illness (Mueller et al., 1994) than do single diagnosis patients. In addition, these patients show poorer life functioning (Dixon, 1999; Hirschfeld, Hasin, Keller, Endicott, & Wunder, 1990; Newman et al., 1998), higher rates of violence (Fulwiler, Grossman, Forbes, & Ruthazer, 1997; Marzuk, 1996; Soyka, 2000) and suicide (Cohen, Test, & Brown, 1990; Landmark, Cernovsky, & Merskey, 1987; Pages et al., 1997; Potash et al., 2000), increased risk for HIV and AIDS (Carey, Carey, & Kalichman, 1997; Hoff, Beam-Goulet, & Rosenheck, 1997; Thompson et al., 1997), more legal involvement (Clark, Ricketts, & McHugo, 1999), and greater rates of homelessness (Dixon, 1999; Fichter & Quadflief, 1999; Greifenhagen & Fichter, 1997; Koegel, Sullivan, Burman, Morton, & Wenzel, 1999) as compared to those with either mental health or substance use disorders alone.

Dual diagnosis has a significant impact on assessment and diagnosis. For example, substance abuse and withdrawal can resemble mental illness, making it difficult to determine whether psychiatric symptoms are due to a psychopathological process in their own right or represent a substance-induced process (Schuckit, 1983). In addition, dual disorder patients experience an array of impairments, making it difficult to discern which problems are due to which disorders. The overlap of diagnostic criteria between some mental and substance use disorders confounds diagnosis and raises questions as to whether two disorders that co-occur with great frequency truly represent two nosologically separate entities or are better conceptualized as one disorder (Widiger & Shea, 1991). Moreover, symptom overlap may result in failures to diagnose some disorders that are disorders in their own right but are masked by substance abuse (Brady et al., 2000; Brunello et al., 2001; Evans, 2000).

Importantly, treatment is considerably affected by dual diagnosis. Individuals with dual disorders show greater rates of service utilization and cost of health care (Bai, Lin, Hu, & Yeh, 1998; Dickey & Azeni, 1996; Garnick, Hendricks, Comstock, & Horgan, 1997; Merikangas et al., 1996; Ross, Lin, & Cunningham, 1999), and poorer retention in treatment, treatment compliance, and treatment outcome (Lambert, Griffith, & Hendrickse, 1996; Owen et al., 1996; Pages et al., 1998; Tomasson & Vaglum, 1997). Longitudinal studies have shown that symptoms of mental illness are among the best predictors of relapse to substance use following substance abuse treatment (Glenn & Parsons, 1991). That dual disorder patients seek and receive more and higher-cost treatment and yet have worse outcomes has been found across differing health care systems (Ross & Cunningham, 1999). Such findings suggest that individuals with dual disorders access the most expensive treatment options (inpatient hospitalization, visits to emergency rooms) that are short-term in order to manage acute distress, but fail to get the comprehensive and ongoing care that they require. It remains unclear how to address the many and varied problems of individuals with dual disorders, especially in situations in which mental health and substance abuse treatment systems either have failed to coordinate services to deliver the full range of necessary interventions, or are nonexistent within healthcare systems.

CONCLUSION

At present, we know that dual substance use and mental disorders are highly prevalent in countries around the world. We also have a good understanding of the many ways that dual disorders impact illness, functioning, prognosis, and outcome. It is clear that the time has come to broaden the scope of dual diagnosis research. We have relatively little understanding of why substance use and mental disorders co-occur with such frequency, and what are the underlying factors linking these disorders. While a range of theories has been proposed (see Blanchard, 2000 for a review), more specific work is required in order to fully examine the links between mental illness and substance use disorders. Moreover, research examining dual disorders must understand that individuals with dual disorders often have multiple diagnoses, each of which influence functioning and treatment needs. Dual diagnosis is a tremendous clinical and public health problem. Treatment systems must bridge their differences, and develop systems-level strategies for meeting the needs of dual disorder patients.

REFERENCES

American Psychiatric Association. (1987). Diagnostic and Statistical Manual of Mental Disorders (3rd edition, revised). Washington, DC: American Psychiatric Association.

Anath, J., Vandewater, S., Kamal, M., Brodsky, A., Gamal, R., & Miller, M. (1989). Mixed diagnosis of substance abuse in psychiatric patients. Hospital and Community Psychiatry, 40, 297–299.

Bai, Y.M., Lin, C.C., Hu, P.G., & Yeh, H.S. (1998). Risk factors for substance use disorders among inpatients with major affective disorders in Taiwan Chinese. General Hospital Psychiatry, 29(6), 377–380.

Barbee, J.G., Clark, P.D., Crapanzano, M.S., Heintz, G.C., & Kehoe, C.E. (1989). Alcohol and substance abuse among schizophrenic patients presenting to an emergency psychiatric service. Journal of Nervous and Mental Disease, 177, 400–407.

Berkson, J. (1949). Limitations of the application of four-fold tables to hospital data. Biometric Bulletin, 2, 47–53.

Blanchard, J.J. (2000). The co-occurrence of substance use in other mental disorders: Editor's introduction. Clinical Psychology Review, 20(2), 145–148.

Bonin, M.F., Norton, G.R., Asmundson, G.J., Dicurzio, S., & Pidlubney, S. (2000). Drinking away the hurt: The nature and prevalence of PTSD in substance abuse patient attending a community-based treatment program. Journal of Behavior Therapy and Exp Psychiatry, 31(1), 55–66.

Bowen, R.C., Cipywnyk, D., D'Arcy, C., & Keegan, D. (1984). Alcoholism, anxiety disorders, and agoraphobia. Alcoholism Clinical and Experimental Research, 8(1), 48–50.

Brady, K.T., Killeen, T.K., Brewerton, T., & Lucerini, S. (2000). Comorbidity of psychiatric disorders and posttraumatic stress disorder. Journal of Clinical Psychiatry, 61 Suppl 7, 22–32.

Brooner, R.K., King, V.L., Kidorf, M., Schmidt, C.W., & Bigelow, G.E. (1997). Psychiatric and substance use comorbidity among treatment-seeking opioid abusers. Archives of General Psychiatry, 54(1), 71–80.

Brunello, N., Davidson, J.R., Deahl, M., Kessler, R.C., Mendlewicz, J., Racagni, G., Shalev, A.Y., & Zohar, J. (2001). Posttraumatic stress disorder: Diagnosis and epidemiology, comorbidity and social consequences, biology and treatment. Neuropsychobiology, 43(3), 150–162.

Bucholz, K.K. (1999). Nosology and epidemiology of addictive disorders and their comorbidity. Psychiatric Clinics of North America, 22(2), 221–239.

Carey, M.P., Carey, K.B., & Kalichman, S.C. (1997). Risk for human immunodeficiency virus (HIV) infection among persons with severe mental illnesses. Clinical Psychology Review, 17, 271–291.

Carpenter, W.T.J., Heinrichs, D.W., & Alphs, L.D. (1985). Treatment of negative symptoms. Schizophrenia Bulletin, 11, 440–452.

Chen, C., Balogh, R., Bathija, J., Howanitz, E., Plutchik, R., & Conte, H.R. (1992). Substance abuse among psychiatric inpatients. Comprehensive Psychiatry, 33, 60–64.

Clark, R.E., Ricketts, S.K., & McHugo, G.J. (1999). Legal system involvement and costs for persons in treatment for severe mental illness and substance use disorders. Psychiatric Services, 50(5), 641–647.

Cohen, L.J., Test, M.A., & Brown, R.J. (1990). Suicide and schizophrenia: Data from a prospective community treatment study. American Journal of Psychiatry, 147, 602–607.

Davis, T.M., & Wood, P.S. (1999). Substance abuse and sexual trauma in a female veteran population. Journal of Substance Abuse Treatment, 16(2), 123–127.

Dickey, B., & Azeni, H. (1996). Persons with dual diagnoses of substance abuse and major mental illness: Their excess costs of psychiatric care. American Journal of Public Health, 86(7), 973–977.

Dixon, L. (1999). Dual diagnosis of substance abuse in schizophrenia: Prevalence and impact on outcomes. Schizophrenia Research, 35, S93–S100.

Dixon, L., Haas, G., Weiden, P., Sweeney, J., & Frances, A. (1991). Drug abuse in schizophrenic patients: Clinical correlates and reasons for use. American Journal of Psychiatry, 148, 224–230.

Eisen, J.L., & Rasmussen, S.A. (1989). Coexisting obsessive compulsive disorder and alcoholism. Journal of Clinical Psychiatry, 50(3), 96–98.

Evans, D.L. (2000). Bipolar disorder: Diagnostic challenges and treatment consideration. Journal of Clinical Psychiatry, 61 Suppl 13, 26–31.

Farrell, M., Howes, S., Taylor, C., Lewis, G., Jenkins, R., Bebbington, P., Jarvis, M., Brugha, R., Gill, B., & Meltzer, H. (1998). Substance misuse and psychiatric comorbidity: An overview of the OPCS National Psychiatric Morbidity Survey. Addictive Behaviors, 23(6), 909–918.

Fichter, M., & Quadflieg, N. (1999). Alcoholism in homeless men in the mid-nineties: Results from the Bavarian Public Health Study on homelessness. European Archives of Psychiatry and Clinical Neuroscience, 249(1), 34–44.

Fulwiler, C., Grossman, H., Forbes, C., & Ruthazer, R. (1997). Early-onset substance abuse and community violence by outpatient with chronic mental illness. Psychiatric Services, 48(9), 1181–1185.

Galanter, M., Castaneda, R., & Ferman, J. (1988). Substance abuse among general psychiatric patients: Place of presentation, diagnosis, and treatment. American Journal of Drug and Alcohol Abuse, 14(2), 211–235.

Garnick, D.W., Hendricks, A.M., Comstock, C., & Horgan, C. (1997). Do individuals with substance abuse diagnoses incur higher charges than individuals with other chronic conditions? Journal of Substance Abuse Treatment, 14(5), 457–465.

Glenn, S.W., & Parsons, O.A. (1991). Prediction of resumption of drinking in posttreatment alcoholics. International Journal of the Addictions, 26(2), 237–254.

Goodwin, F.K., & Jamison, K.R. (1990). Manic-Depressive Illness. New York: Oxford University Press.

Grant, B.F., & Harford, T.C. (1995). Comorbidity between DSM-IV alcohol use disorders and major depression: Results of a national survey. Drug and Alcohol Dependence, 39, 197–206.

Grant, B.F., Harford, T.C., Dawson, D.A., Chou, P., Dufour, M., & Pickering, R. (1994). Prevalence of DSM-IV alcohol abuse and dependence: United States, 1992. Alcohol Health and Research World, 18(3), 243–248.

Greifenhagen, A., & Fichter, M. (1997). Mental illness in homeless women: An epidemiological study in Munich, Germany. European Archives of Psychiatry and Clinical Neuroscience, 247(3), 162–172.

Grella, C.E. (1996). Background and overview of mental health and substance abuse treatment systems: Meeting the needs of women who are pregnant or parenting. Journal of Psychoactive Drugs, 28(4), 319–343.

Gureje, O., Vazquez-Barquero, J.L., & Janca, A. (1996). Comparisons of alcohol and other drugs: Experience from the WHO collaborative cross-cultural applicability research (CAR) study. Addiction, 91(10), 1529–1538.

Handmaker, N. (). Learning what we knew: Integrated services for "dual diagnosis" patients. In W.R. Miller and C. Weisner (Eds.), Changing Substance Abuse Through Health and Social Systems.

Hassin, D.S., Grant, B.F., & Endicott, J. (1988). Lifetime psychiatric comorbidity in hospitalized alcoholics: Subject and familial correlates. The International Journal of the Addictions, 23(8), 827–850.

Hays, P., & Aidroos, N. (1986). Alcoholism followed by schizophrenia. Acta Psychiatrica Scandinavica, 74(2), 187–189.

Haywood, T.W., Kravitz, H.M., Grossman, L.S., Cavanaugh, J.L. Jr., Davis, J.M., & Lewis, D.A. (1995). Predicting the "revolving door" phenomenon among patients with schizohprenic, schizoaffective, and affective disorders. American Journal of Psychiatry, 152, 856–861.

Helzer, J.E., & Pryzbeck, T.R. (1988). The co-occurrence of alcoholism with other psychiatric disorders in the general population and its impact on treatment. Journal of Studies on Alcohol, 49(3), 219–224.

Herz, L.R., Volicer, L., D'Angelo, N., & Gadish, D. (1990). Additional psychiatric illness by Diagnostic Interview Schedule in male alcoholics. Comprehensive Psychiatry, 30(1), 72–79.

Hesselbrock, M.N., Meyer, R.E., & Keener, J.J. (1985). Psychopathology in hospitalized alcoholics. Archives of General Psychiatry, 42, 1050–1055.

Hirschfeld, R.M.A., Hassin, D., Keller, M.B., Endicott, J., & Wunder, J. (1990). Depression and alcoholism: Comorbidity in a longitudinal study. In J.D. Maser & C.R. Cloninger (Eds.), Comorbidity of mood and anxiety disorders (pp. 293–303). Washington, DC: American Psychiatric Press.

Hoff, R.A., Beam-Goulet, J., & Rosenheck, R.A. (1997). Mental disorder as a risk factor for human immunodeficiency virus infection in a sample of veterans. Journal of Nervous and Mental Disease, 185(9), 556–560.

Keane, T.M., Gerardi, R.J., Lyons, J.A., & Wolfe, J. (1988). The interrelationship of substance abuse and posttraumatic stress disorder: Epidemiological and clinical considerations. In M. Galanter (Ed.), Recent Developments in Alcoholism. New York: Plenum Press.

Kessler, R.C., McGonagle, K.A., Zhao, S., Nelson, C.B., Hughes, M., Eshleman, S., Wittchen, H., & Kendler, K.S. (1994). Lifetime and 12-month prevalence of DSM-III-R psychiatric disorders in the United States. Archives of General Psychiatry, 51, 8–19.

Koegel, P., Sullivan, G., Burman, A., Morton, S.C., & Wenzel, S. (1999). Utilization of mental health and substance abuse services among homeless adults in Los Angeles. Med Care, 37(3), 306–317.

Kokkevi, A., Stephanis, N., Anastasopoulou, E., & Kostogianni, C. (1998). Personality disorders in drug abusers: Prevalence and their association with Axis I disorders as predictors of treatment retention. Addictive Behaviors, 23(6), 841–853.

Kozaric-Kovacic, D., Folnegovic-Smalc, V., Folnegovic, Z., & Marusic, A. (1995). Influence of alcoholism on the prognosis of schizophrenic patients. Journal of Studies on Alcohol, 56, 622–627.

Kushner, M.G., Sher, K.J., & Beitman, B.D. (1990). The relation between alcohol problems and the anxiety disorders. American Journal of Psychiatry, 147(6), 685–695.

Lambert, M.T., Griffith, J.M., & Hendrickse, W. (1996). Characteristics of patients with substance abuse diagnoses on a general psychiatry unit in a VA Medical Center. Psychiatric Services, 47(10), 1104–1107.

Landmark, J., Cernovsky, Z.Z., & Merskey, H. (1987). Correlates of suicide attempts and ideation in schizophrenia. British Journal of Psychiatry, 151, 18–20.

Lewis, C.E., Rice, J., Andreasen, N., Endicott, J., & Hartman, A. (1986). Clinical and family correlates of alcoholism in men with unipolar major depression. Alcoholism: Clinical and Experimental Research, 10(6), 657–662.

Linszen, D.H., Dingemans, P.M., & Lenior, M.E. (1994). Cannabis abuse and the course of recent-onset schizophrenic disorders. Archives of General Psychiatry, 51, 273–279.

Liskow, B., Powell, B.J., Nickel, E.J., & Penick, E. (1991). Antisocial alcoholics: Are there clinically significant diagnostic subtypes? Journal of Studies on Alcohol, 52(1), 62–69.

Marzuk, P.M. (1996). Violence, crime, and mental illness: How strong a link? Archives of General Psychiatry, 53, 481–486.

Menezes, P.R., Johnson, S., Thornicroft, G., Marshall, J., Prosser, D., Bebbington, P., & Kuipers, E. (1996). Drug and alcohol problems among individuals with severe mental illnesses in South London. British Journal of Psychiatry, 168, 612–619.

Merikangas, K.R., Angst, J., Eaton, W., Canino, G., Rubio-Stipec, M., Wacker, H., Wittchen, H.U., Andrade, L., Essau, C., Whitaker, A., Kraemer, H., Robins, L.N., & Kupfer, D.J. (1996). Comorbidity and boundaries of affective disorders with anxiety disorders and substance misuse: Results of an international task force. British Journal of Psychiatry, 168 (suppl. 30), 58–67.

Merikangas, K.R. & Gelernter, C.S. (1990). Comorbidity for alcoholism and depression. Psychiatric Clinics of North America, 13(4), 613–633.

Merikangas, K.R., Leckman, J.F., Prusoff, B.A., Pauls, D.L., & Weissman, M.M. (1985). Familial transmission of depression and alcoholism. Archives of General Psychiatry, 42, 367–372.

Merikangas, K.R., Mehta, R.L., Molnar, B.E., Walters, E.E., Swendsen, J.D., Aguilar-Gaziola, S., Bijl, R., Borges, G., Caraveo-Anduaga, J.J., Dewit, D.J., Kolody, B., Vega, W.A., Wittchen, H., & Kessler, R.C. (1998). Comorbidity of substance use disorders with mood and anxiety disorders: Results of the International Consortium in Psychiatric Epidemiology. Addictive Behaviors, 23(6), 893–907.

Mezzich, J.E., Ahn, C.W., Fabrega, H., & Pilkonis, P. (1990). Patterns of psychiatric comorbidity in a large population presenting for care. In J.D. Maser & C.R. Cloninger (Eds.), Comorbidity of mood and anxiety disorders (pp. 189–204). Washington, DC: American Psychiatric Press.

Milby, J.B., Sims, M.K., Khuder, S., Schumzcher, J.E., Huggins, N., McLellan, A.T., Woody, G., & Haas, N. (1996). Psychiatric comorbidity: Prevalence in methadone maintenance treatment. American Journal of Drug and Alcohol Abuse, 22(1), 95–107.

Mirin, S.M., Weiss, R.D., Griffin, M.L., & Michael, J.L. (1991). Psychopathology in drug abusers and their families. Comprehensive Psychiatry, 32(1), 36–51.

Morgenstern, J., Langenbucher, J., Labouvie, E., & Miller, K.J. (1997). The comorbidity of alcoholism and personality disorders in a clinical population: Prevalence rates and relation to alcohol typology variables. Journal of Abnormal Psychology, 106(1), 74–84.

Mueller, T.I., Lavori, P.W., Keller, M.B., Swartz, A., Warshaw, M., Hasin, D., Coryell, W., Endicott, J., Rice, J., & Akiskal, H. (1994). Prognostic effect of the variable course of alcoholism on the 10-year course of depression. American Journal of Psychiatry, 151(5), 701–706.

Mueser, K.T., Bellack, A.S., & Blanchard, J.J. (1992). Comorbidity of schizophrenia and substance abuse: Implications for treatment. Journal of Consulting and Clinical Psychology, 60(6), 845–856.

Mueser, K.T., Yarnold, P.R., Levinson, D.F., Singh, H., Bellack, A.S., Kee, K., Morrison, R.L., & Yadalam, K.G. (1990). Prevalence of substance abuse in schizophrenia: Demographic and clinical correlates. Schizophrenia Bulletin, 16(1), 31–56.

Nace, E.P., Davis, C.W., & Gaspari, J.P. (1991). Axis II comorbidity in substance abusers. American Journal of Psychiatry, 148(1), 118–120.

Najavitis, L.M., Gastfriend, D.R., Barber, J.P., Reif, S., Muenz, L.R., Blaine, J., Frank, A., Crits-Christoph, P., Thase, M., & Weiss, R.D. (1998). Cocaine dependence with and without PTSD among subjects in the National Institute on Drug Abuse Collaborative Cocaine Treatment Study. American Journal of Psychiatry, 155(2), 214–219.

Newman, D.L., Moffitt, T.E., Caspi, A., Magdol, L., Silva, P.A., & Stanton, W.R. (1996). Psychiatric disorder in a birth cohort of young adults: Prevalence, comorbidity, clinical significance, and new case incidence from ages 11 to 21. Journal of Consulting and Clinical Psychology, 64(3), 552–562.

Newman, D.L., Moffitt, T.E., Caspi, A., & Silva, P. (1998). Comorbid mental disorders: Implications for treatment and sample selection. Journal of Abnormal Psychology, 107(2), 305–311.

O'Connell, R.A., Mayo, J.A., Flatow, L., Cuthbertson, B., & O'Brien, B.E. (1991). Outcome of bipolar disorder on long-term treatment with lithium. British Journal of Psychiatry, 159, 123–129.

Owen, R.R., Fischer, E.P., Booth, B.M., & Cuffel, B.J. (1996). Medication noncompliance and substance abuse among persons with schizophrenia. Psychiatric Services, 47(8), 853–858.

Pages, K.P., Russo, J.E., Roy-Byrne, P.P., Ries, R.K., & Cowley, D.S. (1997). Determinants of suicidal ideation: The role of substance use disorders. Journal of Clinical Psychiatry, 58(11), 510–515.

Pages, K.P., Russo, J.E., Wingerson, D.K., Ries, R.K., Roy-Byrne, P.P., & Cowley, D.S. (1998). Predictors and outcome of discharge against medical advice from the psychiatric units of a general hospital. Psychiatric Services, 49(9), 1187–1192.

Penick, E.C., Powell, B.J., Othmer, E., Binghan, S.F., Rice, A.S., & Liese, B.S. (1984). Subtyping alcoholics by coexisting psychiatric syndromes: Course, family history, outcome. In D.W. Goodwin, K.T. Van Dusen, & S.A. Mednick (Eds.), Longitudinal Research in Alcoholism. Boston: Kluwer-Nijhoff Publishing.

Polcin, D.L. (1992). Issues in the treatment of dual diagnosis clients who have chronic mental illness. Professional Psychology: Research and Practice. 23(1), 30–37.

Potash, J.B., Kane, H.S., Chiu, Y.F., Simpson, S.G., MacKinnon, D.F., McInnis, M.G., McMahon, F.J., & DePaulo. (2000). Attempted suicide and alcoholism in bipolar disorder: Clinical and familial relationships. American Journal of Psychiatry, 157(12), 2048–2050.

Powell, B.J., Penick, E.C., Othmer, E., Bingham, S.F., & Rice, A.S. (1982). Prevalence of additional psychiatric syndromes among male alcoholics. Journal of Clinical Psychiatry, 43(10), 404–407.

Pozzi, G., Bacigalupi, M., & Tempesta, E. (1997). Comorbidity of drug dependence and other mental disorders: A two-phase study of prevalence at outpatient treatment centers in Italy. Drug and Alcohol Dependence, 46(1–2), 69–77.

Quattrocki, E., Baird, A., & Yurgelun-Todd, D. (2000). Biological aspects of the link between smoking and depression. Harvard Review of Psychiatry, 8(3), 99–110.

Rabinowitz, J., Mark, M., Popper, M., & Slyuzberg, M. (1996). Reported comorbidity of mental disorders with substance abuse among psychiatric inpatients in Israel. Journal of Mental Health Administration, 23(4), 471–478.

Regier, D.A., Farmer, M.E., Rae, D.S., Locke, B.Z., Keither, S.J., Judd, L.L., & Goodwin, F.K. (1990). Comorbidity of mental disorders with alcohol and other drug abuse. Journal of the American Medical Association, 264, 2511–2518.

Ridgely, M.S., Lambert, D., Goodman, A., Chichester, C.S., & Ralph, R. (1998). Interagency collaboration in services for people with co-occurring mental illness and substance use disorder. Psychiatric Services, 49, 236–238.

Ross, H.E., & Cunningham, J. (1999). Mental health service use: A comparison of treated and untreated individuals with substance use disorders in Ontario. Canadian Journal of Psychiatry, 44(6), 570–577.

Ross, H.E., Glaser, F.B., & Germanson, T. (1988). The prevalence of psychiatric disorders in patients with alcohol and other drug problems. Archives of General Psychiatry, 45, 1023–1031.

Ross, H.E., Glaser, F.B., & Stiasny, S. (1988). Differences in the prevalence of psychiatric disorders in patients with alcohol and drug problems. British Journal of Addiction, 83, 1179–1192.

Ross, H.E., Lin, E., & Cunningham, J. (1999). Mental health service use: A comparison of treated and untreated individuals with substance use disorders in Ontario. Canadian Journal of Psychiatry, 44, 570–577.

Rounsaville, B.J., Anton, S.F., Carroll, K., Budde, D., Prusoff, & Gawin. (1991). Psychiatric diagnoses of treatment seeking cocaine abusers. Archives of General Psychiatry, 48(1), 43–51.

Rounsaville, B.J., Weissman, M.M., Wilber, C.H., Crits-Christoph, K., & Kleber, H.D. (1982). Diagnosis and symptoms of depression in opiate addicts: Course and relationship to treatment outcome. Archives of General Psychiatry, 39, 151–156.

Russell, J.M., Newman, S.C., & Bland, R.C. (1994). Epidemiology of psychiatric disorders in Edmonton. Drug abuse and dependence. Acta Psychiatrica Scandinavica, 376 Suppl., 54–62.

Saladin, M.E., Brady, K.T., Dansky, B.S., & Kilpatrick, D.G. (1995). Understanding comorbidity between PTSD and substance use disorders: Two preliminary investigations. Addictive Behaviors, 20(5), 643–655.

Schuckit, M.A. (1983). Alcoholism and other psychiatric disorders. Hospital and Community Psychiatry, 34(11), 1022–1027.

Sokolski, K.N., Cummings, J.L., Abrams, B.I., DeMet, E.M., Katz, L.S., & Costa, J.F. (1994). Effects of substance abuse on hallucination rates and treatment responses in chronic psychiatric patients. Journal of Clinical Psychiatry, 55, 380–387.

Soyka, M. (2000). Substance misuse, psychiatric disorder and violent and disturbed behaviour. British Journal of Psychiatry, 176, 345–350.

Thomas, S.E., Thevos, A.K., & Randall, C.L. (1999). Alcoholics with and without social phobia: A comparison of substance use and psychiatric variables. Journal of Studies on Alcohol, 60, 472–479.

Thompson, S.C., Checkley, G.E., Hocking, J.S., Crofts, N., Mijch, A.M., & Judd, F.K. (1997). HIV risk behavior and HIV testing of psychiatric patients in Melbourne. Australia and New Zealand Journal of Psychiatry, 31(4), 566–576.

Tomasson, K., & Vaglum, P. (1995). A nationwide representative sample of treatment-seeking alcoholics: A study of psychiatric comorbidity. Acta Psychiatrica Scandinavica, 92, 378–385.

Tomasson, K., & Vaglum, P. (1997). The 2-year course following detoxification treatment of substance abuse: The possible influence of psychiatric comorbidity. European Archives of Psychiatry and Clinical Neuroscience, 247(6), 320–327.

Triffleman, E.G., Marmar, C.R., Delucchi, K.L., & Ronfeldt, H. (1995). Childhood trauma and posttraumatic stress disorder in substance abuse inpatients. Journal of Nervous and Mental Disease, 183(3), 172–176.

Widiger, T.A., & Shea, T. (1991). Differentiation of Axis I and Axis II disorders. Journal of Abnormal Psychology, 100(3), 399–406.

Wittchen, H., Essau, C.A., von Zerssen, D., Krieg, J., & Zaudig, M. (1992). Lifetime and six-month prevalence of mental disorders in the Munich follow-up study. European Archives of Psychiatry and Clinical Neuroscience, 241, 247–258.

Wittchen, H., Perkonigg, A., & Reed, V. (1996). Comorbidity of mental disorders and substance use disorders. European Addiction Research, 2, 36–47.

World Health Organization. (1991). Composite International Diagnostic Interview (CIDI). Geneva, Switzerland: World Health Organization.

Ziedonis, D.M., & George, T.P. (1997). Schizophrenia and nicotine use: Report of a pilot smoking cessation program and review of neurobiological and clinical issues. Schizophrenia Bulletin, 23, 247–254.

CHAPTER 10

Integrating Substance Abuse and Mental Health Treatment: A Meta-Analytic Review

NANCY S. HANDMAKER AND ROBERT ANDERSON

Co-occurring alcohol and drug use disorders in persons with mental illness are referred to as dual diagnoses or dual disorders. These terms are frequently misnomers, as persons with dual disorders often have three or four diagnoses including serious medical conditions. The prevalence of co-occurring substance use disorders (abuse or dependence) is especially high among persons with severe mental illnesses such as schizophrenia, panic disorder, and affective disorders (Bennett, this volume).

Substance use disorders are associated with a multitude of problems and risks for persons who have severe mental illnesses. Illicit drug use and drinking interact with and exacerbate psychiatric symptoms, causing even small amounts of substances to be disruptive to the psychosocial functioning (e.g., relationships, housing stability) of persons with dual disorders (Drake & Mueser, 2000). Moreover, the use of alcohol and illicit drugs impairs reasoning abilities and judgment. Since most persons with psychiatric disorders already show attendant problems with judgment, attention, and memory, substance use further impairs their already compromised reasoning abilities, diminishing their capacity for independent functioning and decreasing their likelihood of benefiting from treatment (Bellack & DiClemente, 1999). Persons with concomitant mental and substance use disorders (SUDs) experience higher rates of the many adverse consequences that accompany mental illness or SUDs such as homelessness, legal problems, incarceration, poverty, family problems, HIV risk, violence, and suicide (Bennett, this volume).

NANCY S. HANDMAKER AND ROBERT ANDERSON • Department of Psychology, University of New Mexico, Albuquerque, New Mexico 87131

Despite the risks and the serious negative effects, persons with concomitant SUD and mental illnesses are less adherent with treatment than their counterparts who do not use substances. Consequently, they are more likely to experience relapses in both conditions leading to greater utilization of costly, crisis-oriented services in psychiatric hospitals, medical trauma units, and jails. Clinicians struggle with how to increase engagement and retention among this population. Remission in SUDs occur after years of treatment engagement. Researchers and clinicians consistently report that patients with dual disorders require longer periods of treatment engagement than patients who do not have severe mental illnesses in order to achieve stable sobriety (Drake & Mueser, 2000).

Given the high prevalence of SUD in mental illness, the related serious adverse consequences, the social problems and costs for services, this chapter will focus primarily on treatment issues for severely mentally ill populations. We offer a brief summary on the problems encountered by persons with dual disorders when treatment does not address both disorders. Integrated mental health and substance abuse treatment is widely accepted as a model for improving treatment outcomes. However, few studies have compared this approach to others. In this chapter we offer a review of the substance abuse and retention outcomes from studies of integrated substance abuse and mental health treatment.

TRADITIONAL TREATMENT

Historically there has been a lack of coherent treatment programming for persons with dual disorders. For example, in the U.S., substance use disorders and mental illnesses have been treated separately by two different sets of professionals and provider systems. The tendency for substance abuse and mental health treatment to be divided into separate systems is partly rooted in the lack of success of psychoanalytic approaches to effectively treat addictive behaviors. A concept of an addictive personality emerged with the attendant beliefs that alcoholics and addicts had persistent, and pervasive character styles, which led them to be treatment resistant. This assisted the development of self-help groups in the U.S., which provided an alternative view for attaining abstinence. Over time, the mutual-help philosophy became the prevailing basis for treatment within substance abuse treatment systems, and separate educational and professional licensure pathways for alcohol and drug counselors emerged. Other bases for the maintenance of separate treatment systems have been the lack of common administrative structures and separate funding support systems for mental health versus substance abuse (Ridgely et al., 1987).

Within separate systems, persons with co-occurring disorders have enrolled in multiple treatment programs concurrently or sequentially. Two treatment approaches, *parallel* and *sequential*, are associated with separate systems of care, which result from the lack of coordination between mental health and substance abuse providers systems (Rosenthal & Westreich, 1999). In a sequential approach, the clinicians typically hold the belief that one form of treatment must come first. There are instances when pursuing a sequential approach has clinical validity. For example, it is well known that alcohol and illicit drug use cause emotional problems, which remit with prolonged abstinence. Furthermore, evidence suggests that with anxiety disorders (e.g., PTSD) stable sobriety improves outcomes for the concomitant mental condition (Rosenthal & Westreich, 1999). Issues related to treatment sequencing have not yet been adequately addressed. The argument against sequencing is that in actual practice, a sequential approach creates barriers to access and exclusion from treatment (Ridgely et al., 1987). Moreover, where separate systems have co-existed, dually disordered clients have been known to be prematurely terminated from one program due to the complicating effects of a second disorder (e.g., heavy drinking interfering with psychopharmacologic treatment of a depression in a mental health facility) only to be referred back to a provider that previously ejected them for non-compliance (e.g., unwillingness to reduce alcohol consumption in substance abuse treatment agency). In a parallel treatment approach, patients have been directed to engage in separate treatment systems simultaneously. Under these circumstances, the task of integrating treatment into a coherent plan has been placed on the shoulders of the patient, which can be particularly challenging especially when the two systems have maintained different philosophical approaches to care as in the U.S.. Not surprisingly, studies have shown that separate treatment systems have been largely ineffectual in treating dual disorders (Drake et al., 1998; Drake & Mueser, 2000).

A REVIEW OF INTEGRATED TREATMENT APPROACHES

By the end of the 1980s, several investigators (e.g., Ridgely et al., 1987) had reported on the undue problems experienced by persons with dual disorders in accessing care, and on the lack of success among traditional (e.g., parallel and sequential) approaches with this population. The need for a hybrid program which integrated mental health and substance abuse treatment within a unified conceptual and programmatic framework was recognized (Minkoff, 1989). New integrated programs emerged within mental health care service delivery systems with the primary aim of improving the long-term outcomes among persons with dual disorders. Integrated treatment is simply "... a program in which the same clinician (or team of clinicians) provides treatment for both the mental illness and the substance use disorder at the same time" (Mueser et al., 1998, p. 131). Integrated treatment is not a single modality or program of care; rather, the clinician has the responsibility for developing a coherent individualized treatment program that simultaneously addresses "two or more interwoven, chronic disorders" (Drake et al., 1998, p. 590). Individualized patient-specific treatment plans are developed that recognize the interrelatedness of comorbid SUDs and mental illness. Ideally, the clinician (or team) offers the best "fit" of clinical services given the level of functioning and severity of the problems experienced by the patients with the highest degree of integration possible (Rosenthal & Westreich, 1999). Addiction treatment is combined with existing mental health service care into programs that appear "seamless" to dually diagnosed patients.

The earliest approach to integrated treatment simply added substance abuse groups to the usual mental health treatment programs such as medication monitoring, acute care (e.g., crisis services or inpatient hospitalization), and counseling (Kofoed et al., 1986; Hellerstein & Meehan, 1987; Nigam et al., 1992; Hellerstein et al., 1995). The groups emphasized skills for reducing or abstaining from substances and enhancing knowledge while providing peer support. A second early approach was intensive integrated programming that focused on the rapid achievement of stabilization and sobriety through multiple treatment modalities including peer counseling, individual and group counseling, and milieu therapy within inpatient, residential, or day programs.

During the 1990s the Community Support Program (CSP), a demonstration project for young adults with dual disorders (e.g., schizophrenia and mood disorders) led to significant changes in integrated programs (National Institute for Mental Health, 1989). The CSP was initiated to explore the feasibility for combining mental health and substance abuse into integrated programs. Despite the limitations in their research findings, the CSP projects suggested that persons with dual diagnoses are unmotivated to pursue abstinence early in treatment, but long-term, "stage-wise" interventions could engage and retain this seriously at-risk population in treatment. Based on these findings, interventions to engage and retain patients such as assertive community outreach, intensive case management, group and family counseling, within a stage-wise motivational framework have been added to comprehensive integrated treatment. Interventions (i.e., engagement, persuasion, active treatment, and relapse prevention) matched to the patient's stage of recovery, based on Osher and Kofoed's model (1989) are incorporated in most models of integrated treatment.

Since the CSP projects, greater efforts have been made to evaluate the outcomes of integrated treatment programs, but almost 10 years later the question of whether integrated dual-disorders treatment leads to better outcomes than standard mental health treatment remains largely unanswered.

Methodology for the Review

We conducted a quantitative analysis of effect sizes on a subset of the treatment studies recently reported in a comprehensive review by Drake and his colleagues (1998). The general goal of the analysis was to assess the relative efficacy of differing integrated treatment approaches on two outcomes: substance abuse and retention rates for the dually diagnosed. Specifically, we re-analyzed studies contained in Drake and colleagues comprehensive review on dual disorders treatment groups, intensive integrated treatments, and comprehensive integrated treatments. (The CSP demonstration projects were not included in this meta-analysis.) We included studies that contained usable data in at least one of the outcome domains that were of interest to us (i.e., substance abuse outcomes or retention data, either pre-post or between groups).

As long as they reported quantitative data, and adequately applied an integrative treatment, we included the studies regardless of whether they were open clinical trials, quasi-experimental designs, or true experimental designs. We used studies within the selected categories that contained usable data in at least one of the outcome domains that were of interest to us (i.e., substance abuse outcomes or retention data, either pre-post or between groups; see Table 1).

All of the included studies contained dependent variables that were either dichotomous or continuous. However, two studies with dichotomous outcomes that found 'no difference' in substance abuse outcomes did not report specific data. Retention rates were typically reported as either the proportion of treatment-assigned participants who were substantially exposed to treatment, or as the number retained in treatment at various follow-up periods. One

Table 1 Studies considered for the meta-analysis

			Substance Abuse		Treatment Retention	
Study #	Author(s)	Year	Within Group	Between Group	Within Group	Between Group
Dual Disorders Groups						
1	Kofoed et al.	1986	—	—	Yes	—
2	Hellerstein & Meehan	1987	—	—	Yes	—
3	Nigam et al.	1992	Yes	—	Yes	—
4	Hellerstein et al.	1995	Yes	Yes	Yes	Yes
Intensive Integrated Treatment						
5	Ries & Ellingson	1990	Yes	—	—	—
6	Hoffman et al.	1993	Yes	—	—	—
7	Bachman et al.	1997	Yes	—	—	—
8	Mowbray et al.	1995	-	Yes	—	Yes
9	Bartels & Drake	1996	Yes	—	Yes	—
10	Blankertz & Cnaan	1994	Yes	Yes	Yes	Yes
11	Rahav et al.	1995	—	—	Yes	Yes
12	Hanson et al.	1990	Yes	—	Yes	—
13	Burnam et al.	1995	—	Yes	—	—
Comprehensive Integrated Treatment						
14	Detrick & Stiepock	1992	—	—	—	—
15	Durell et al.	1993	Yes	—	—	—
16	Bartels et al.	1995	—	—	—	—
17	Drake et al.	1993	Yes	—	Yes	—
18	Meisler et al.	1997	Yes	—	Yes	—
19	Jerrell & Ridgely	1995	Yes	Yes	—	—
20	Drake et al.	1998	Yes	—	Yes	—
21	Godley et al.	1994	Yes	Yes	—	—
22	Drake et al.	1997	Yes	Yes	Yes	Yes
	Total Studies in Meta-Analyses (k):		15	7	12	5

Note: "Within" comparisons are Pre- versus Post- for integrated treatment; "Between" comparisons are integrated versus non-integrated treatment; "Yes" indicates that suitable data for a given analysis existed.

Table 2 Dependent measures for studies in the substance abuse meta-analysis

Type of Measure	Study Numbers (from Table 1) Within Group	Between Group
Dichotomous:		
"No Improvement/Difference"	7	4
Abstinence	3, 5, 6, 9, 10	10
Abstinence or Mild Use	18	
No Abuse or Dependence	12	
Remission	17	
Decreased Substance Abuse	15	
Continuous:		
ASI Composite Score	4	8
Quantity/Frequency Measures	21	13, 21
C-DISR	19	19
AUS and DUS	20, 22	22

Note: "Within" comparisons are Pre- versus Post- for integrated treatment; "Between" comparisons are integrated versus non-integrated treatment.

Table 3 Dependent measures by treatment setting for studies in the treatment retention meta-analysis

Treatment Setting and Type of Measure	Study Numbers (from Table 1) Within Group	Between Group
Outpatient:		
3 months and 12 months	1	
6 months and 12 months	2	
>6 months	3	
4 months and 8 months	4	4
Day Program:		
6 months and 12 months	12	
Inpatient:		
Days in treatment		8
Residential:		
Completed	9	
>2 months	10	10
In progress or completed	11	11
Community:		
48 months	17	
12 to 48 months	18	
36 months	20	
18 months	22	22

Note: "Within" comparisons are Pre- versus Post- for integrated treatment; "Between" comparisons are integrated versus non-integrated treatment.

study reported days in treatment as the dependent variable. Tables 2 and 3 contain details regarding the variety of dependent measures used.

For all measures in the studies, we used correlations as the effect sizes for the meta-analyses. This is an acceptable method of creating standardized effect size estimates in situations where effect sizes based on experimental data are not available (Hunter, Schmidt & Jackson, 1982; Hedges & Olkin, 1985). When no specific data were reported for substance abuse outcomes, but the author(s) explicitly stated lack of improvement pre-post (i.e., within groups) or no differences between groups, we used a correlation of zero. For pre-post dichotomous variables, it was assumed that the baseline for each variable was that zero percent of the sample had a positive outcome. Continuous variable data were treated according to how they were presented in the original study, with weighted averages being used to calculate correlation coefficients wherever possible.

Using meta-analysis software created by Ralf Schwarzer (Meta-Analysis Programs, Version 5.3), which is available on the internet at http://www.yorku.ca/faculty/academic/schwarze/author.htm), we combined the estimates of correlations and analyzed them in order to estimate (1) the population effect size and (2) the homogeneity of the estimated population effect size. The procedures used are based on Hunter, Schmidt and Jackson (1982) and Hedges and Olkin (1985). Since there is not universal agreement over which estimates of population effect size and level of homogeneity are best, a decision was made to first check for consistency among the various measures. As long as the estimates were reasonably consistent, then we considered the estimates of population effect size (r) and homogeneity (Q statistic) based on Hedges and Olkin's method to be adequate. In addition, we reported the estimated 95% confidence interval for the population and the mean standardized difference score (g statistic) based on Schmidt and Hunter.

Results

Table 4 shows the effect size correlations by study number. Table 5 shows the population effect size estimates, homogeneity (Q-statistics), 95% confidence intervals, and mean standardized difference statistic (g) for all four dependent variables.

For within-group substance abuse outcome, the results indicate a large population effect size overall with significant heterogeneity. This is indicative of the presence of a moderator effect. Hence, even though it appears that there is a large population effect size overall, it is likely that there are sub-populations with markedly different effect sizes that vary due to systematic differences in study characteristics. For substance abuse comparisons between experimental (i.e., integrated treatment) and control (i.e., non-integrated treatment) groups, the results indicate a small population effect size with evidence of marginal heterogeneity.

For the within-group treatment retention analysis, the overall pattern of effect size for pre- to post-treatment retention (i.e., large population effect

Table 4 Estimates of effect sizes R and sample sizes (n) by study number

	Substance Abuse		Treatment Retention	
Study #	Within Group	Between Group	Within Group	Between Group
1			.5427 (32)	
2			.8076 (10)	
3	.8944 (8)		.8944 (8)	
4	.5794 (16)	.0000 (25)	.9121 (16)	.2894 (28)
5	.8551 (17)			
6	.8402 (12)			
7	.0000 (33)			
8		.0000 (391)		.3272 (427)
9	.2842 (39)		.6342 (41)	
10	.6642 (51)	.2853 (88)	.9025 (63)	.2966 (135)
11			.6670 (118)	.1326 (272)
12	.8703 (118)		.5321 (118)	
13		.0000 (192)		
14				
15	.8275 (43)			
16				
17	.7992 (18)		.9999* (18)	
18	.6405 (67)		.9999* (67)	
19	.0973 (132)	.2266 (132)		
20	.2594 (114)		.9238 (203)	
21	.2522 (42)	.0900 (39)		
22	.5612 (74)	.1457 (103)	.9271 (158)	.1153 (217)
	(k = 15)	(k = 7)	(k = 12)	(k = 5)

Note: "Within" comparisons are Pre- versus Post- for integrated treatment; "Between" comparisons are integrated versus non-integrated treatment; *retention rates were 100%.

Table 5 Estimates of population effect sizes (r) and homogeneity

	Substance Abuse		Treatment Retention	
Study #	Within Group	Between Group	Within Group	Between Group
Population Effect Size Estimate (Hedges & Olkin method):	.55	.08	.92	.23
Q-statistic (Hedges & Olkin):	159.79 (p < .0001)	11.07 (p = .0862)	1135.58 (p < .0001)	11.22 (p < .0242)
95% Confidence Interval (Schmidt-Hunter method):	.50 to .60	.01 to .14	.91 to .93	.18 to .29
Mean Standardized Difference (g):	1.60	0.15	2.56	0.49
# of studies (total N)	k = 15 (784)	k = 7 (970)	k = 12 (853)	k = 5 (1079)

Note: "Within" comparisons are Pre- versus Post- for integrated treatment; "Between" comparisons are integrated versus non-integrated treatment.

estimates with substantial heterogeneity) is similar to that of pre-post substance abuse outcomes, but with a higher population effect size estimate. The finding of a higher effect size, of course, is likely due to the way that the effect measures were calculated for within group treatment retention (i.e., any treatment retention above 0% resulted in a positive effect size correlation). For the comparison between experimental and control groups for treatment retention, the results are consistent with a medium population effect size and some variation due to systematic differences in study characteristics.

Discussion and Conclusions

The quantitative review of substance abuse and retention provides almost a historical review of the treatment delivery models for integrated mental health and substance abuse treatment. The earliest studies of the addition of dual-disorders groups had relatively small samples (e.g., range = 8–32), short-term follow-ups, selection bias toward motivated clients, and reliance on self-report, which may have contributed to the rather large pre-post effects of the groups on substance use and retention. Furthermore, the majority of patients dropped out of treatment in one study before the first follow-up. No benefits were observed between the non-integrated and integrated approach on substance use outcomes in the one study that included a comparison group (Hellerstein et al., 1995), but there was better retention in the integrated program at a 4-month follow-up. However, by the 8-month both groups of patients had dropped out of treatment. Nine studies were included in the analyses for the intensive integrated treatment programs. Similar to the dual-disorders findings, small-to-medium effect sizes were observed on retention rates among the integrated programs when there was a comparison group in the study (Mowbray et. al. 1995; Blankertz & Cnaan, 1994; Rahav et al., 1995). Only one study showed an advantage of the integrated program over the non-integrated approach (Blankertz & Cnaan, 1994) on substance abuse outcomes. These studies had large samples, but drop-out rates prior to treatment entry or during treatment were very high. In a large study (Rahav et al., 1995) of residential treatment for people who were homeless or at risk of becoming homeless, only 13% of dually disordered clients remained at follow-up within a therapeutic community (TC) or the community residence (CR). When these data were available and reported, effects on pre-post substance abuse within the intensive treatment programs ranged from moderate to very high. The actual studies suggest that patients improved while in the intensive programs, but attrition and relapse rates were high. Perhaps the patients were unable to tolerate the social and emotional demands of the intensive programs, especially the long-term program in the TC and CR.

The effect sizes for substance abuse suggested that integrated care has only a slight advantage over non-integrated treatment among studies that addressed comprehensive integrated programs. In contrast, retention rates were very good among integrated programs and showed a medium effect compared with non-integrated treatment programs. The programs that included assertive community outreach and case management such as Drake et al. (1997) did well in retaining patients. Presumably these components improve treatment engagement and retention. However, given the heterogeneity of study characteristics and potential moderator effects, research is needed to draw conclusions about the impact of components within an integrated approach.

One possibility for addressing the problems with treatment engagement observed among most of the studies would be to include motivational interviewing (MI) at the beginning of treatment or following discharge from hospitalization. Although the later studies on integrated programs suggested that MI was part of their therapies, no formal interventions were described. When a session of MI or motivational enhancement therapy has been added to treatment, positive results in increasing treatment engagement and adherence with dual disorders have been found. At least four pilot studies have found that MI significantly increased the rates of client engagement with outpatient treatment following discharges from inpatient treatment (Daley & Zuckoff, 1998; Daley, Salloum, Zuckoff, Kirisci, & Thase, 1998; Swanson, Pantalon, & Cohen, 1999; Martino, Caroll, O'Malley, & Rounsaville, 2000). Another study of a small outpatient sample (Graeber, Moyers, Griffith, Guajardo, & Tonigan, 2000) for persons with alcohol use disorders and schizophrenia found that a group that received up to three MI sessions showed a benefit on drinking outcomes (i.e., fewer drinking days) and treatment attendance at a short-term follow-up. Given the consistency in the findings from these pilot studies, further research is warranted to determine the added benefit of MI for the treatment engagement and retention among this population.

Substance abuse treatment approaches that were most frequently included in studies of integrated approaches were education, problem-solving, peer support, case management, and group psychotherapy. With few exceptions (e.g., Jerrel & Ridgely, 1995), empirically-supported approaches such as cognitive and behavioral therapy or 12-step facilitation with specific or manualized therapy protocols were not included as part of the integrated programs. The community reinforcement approach (CRA) is a treatment method that ranks among the highest in treatment efficacy (Miller et al., 1995). CRA is a behavioral intervention derived from behavioral therapies for both severely mentally ill populations (Ayllon & Azrin, 1968) and SUDs (Meyers & Miller, 2001) that employs social, recreational, familial, therapeutic, and vocational contingencies for encouraging or discouraging a behavior (e.g., substance use). Moreover, CRA is consistent with most aspects of an integrated treatment model of community outreach, case management, medication compliance, etc. At least one trial with a severely impaired sample of alcoholic homeless persons, a percentage of whom had comorbid mental illness, suggests that CRA is a promising approach for this population (Smith, Meyers, & Delaney, 1998).

SUMMARY

Dually disordered clients who engage in and remain in treatment over extended periods show significant improvements in substance use problems

(Drake et al., 1998). The studies reviewed suggest that comprehensive integrated treatment models improve retention. Treatment retention appears to be related to the components believed to be important for an integrated model: community outreach, medication management, skills training, and intensive case management tailored for dual disordered clients. Integrated treatment approaches showed only a slight advantage over non-integrated treatment for substance abuse outcomes.

One reason for small differences may be reliance upon treatment methods with relatively weak effects. Empirically-supported treatment methods such as motivational interviewing and the community reinforcement approach show promise for increasing treatment engagement and improving outcomes as part of integrated treatment for people with dual disorders.

REFERENCES

Ayllon, T. & Azrin, N. H. (1968). *The token economy: A motivational system for therapy and rehabilitation*. New York: Appleton-Century-Crofts.

Bartels, S. J. & Drake, R. E. (1995). Long-term course of substance use disorders among patients with severe mental illness. *Psychiatric Services*, 46, 248–251.

Burnam, M. A., Morton, S. C., McGlynn, E. A., Petersen, L. P., Stecher, B. M., Hayes, C., & Vaccaro, J. V. (1995). An experimental evaluation of residential and nonresidential treatment for dually diagnosed homeless adults. *Journal of Addictive Diseases*, 14, 111–134.

Daley, D. C., Salloum, I. M., Zuckoff, A., Kirisci, L., & Thase, M. E. (1998). Increasing treatment adherence among outpatients with depression and cocaine dependence: A pilot study. *American Journal of Psychiatry*, 155, 1611–1613.

Daley, D. C. & Zuckoff, A. (1998). Improving compliance with the initial outpatient session among discharged inpatient dual diagnosis clients. *Social Work*, 43(5), 470–473.

Detrick, A. & Stiepick, V. (1992). Treating persons with mental illness, substance abuse, and legal problems: The Rhode Island Experience. In: Stein, L. I., (ED). *Innovative Community Mental Health Programs*. New Directions for Mental Health Services, No 56. San Francisco: Jossey-Bass, 65–77.

Drake, R. E., Mercer-McFadden, C., Mueser, K., McHugo, G. J., & Bond, G. R. (1998). Review of integrated mental health and substance abuse treatment for patients with severe mental illness: A review of recent research. *Schizophrenia Bulletin*, 24(4), 589–608.

Drake, R. E., & Mueser, K. T. (2000). Psychosocial approaches to dual diagnosis. Schizophrenia Bulletin, 26(1), 105–118.

Godley, S. H., Hoewing-Robertson, R., & Godley, M. D. (1994). *Final MISA Report*. Bloomington, IL: Lighthouse Institute.

Graeber, D. A., Moyers, T. B., Griffith, G., Guajardo, E., & Tonigan, S. (2000, June). *Comparison of motivational interviewing and educational intervention in patients with schizophrenia and alcoholism*. Paper presented at the 2000 Scientific Meeting of the Research Society on Alcoholism, Denver, CO.

Hedges, L. V. & Olkin, I. (1985). *Statistical methods for meta-analysis*. New York: Academic Press.

Hunter, J. E., Schmidt, F. L., & Jackson, G. B. (1982). Meta-analysis. Cumulating research findings across studies. Beverly Hill, CA: Sage.

Jerrell, J. M. & Ridgely, M. S. (1995). Comparative effectiveness of three approaches to serving people with severe mental illness and substance abuse disorders. *Journal of Nervous and Mental Disease*, 183, 566–576.

Kemp, R., Hayward, P., Applewhaite, G., Everitt, B., & David. A. (1996). Compliance therapy in psychotic patients: randomized controlled trial. *British Medical Journal*, 312, 345–349.

Kemp, R., Kirov, G., Everitt, B. et al. (1998). A randomized controlled trial of compliance therapy: 18 month follow-up. *British Journal of Psychiatry*, 172, 413–419.

Martino, S., Carroll, K. M., O'Malley, S. S., & Rounsaville, B. J. (2000). Motivational interviewing with psychiatrically ill substance abusing patients. *The American Journal on Addictions*, 9, 88–91.

McConnaughy, E. A., DiClemente, C. C., Prochaska, J. O., & Velicer, W. F. (1989). Stages of change in psychotherapy: A follow-up report. *Psychotherapy Practice and Research*, 26, 494–503.

Mercer-McFadden, C., Drake, R. E., Brown, N. B., & Fox R. S. (1997). The Community Support Program demonstrations of services for young adults with severe mental illness and substance use disorders. *Psychiatric Rehabilitation Journal*, 20(3), 13–24.

Meyers, R. J., & Miller, W. R. (Eds.) (2001). *A community reinforcement approach to addiction treatment*. Cambridge, UK: Cambridge University Press.

Miller, W. R., Brown, J., Simpson, T., Handmaker, N., Bien, T., Luckie, L., Montgomery, H., Hester, R., & Tonigan, J. (1995). What works? A methodological analysis of the alcohol treatment outcome literature. In R. Hester & W. R. Miller (Eds.), Handbook of alcoholism treatment approaches: Effective alternatives (2nd ed., pp. 12–44). New York: Allyn & Bacon.

Miller, W. R., & Rollnick, S. (1991). *Motivational Interviewing: Preparing People to Change Addictive Behavior*. New York: Guilford Press.

Minkoff, K. (1989). An integrated treatment model for dual diagnosis of psychosis and addiction. *Hospital and Community Psychiatry*, 40, 1031–1036.

Minkoff, K. M., & Drake, R. E., eds. (1991). *Major Mental Illness and Substance Disorder*. New Directions for Mental Health Services, No. 50 San Francisco: Jossey-Bass.

Mowbray, C. T., Solomon, M,, Ribisl, K. M., Ebejer, M. A. Deiz, N., Brown, W., Banla, H., Luke, D. A., Davidson, W. S., & Herman, S. (1995). Treatment for mental illness and substance abuse in a public psychiatric hospital. *Journal of Substance Abuse Treatment*, 12, 129–139.

Mueser, K. T., Bennett, M., & Kushner, M. G. (1995). Epidemiology of substance use disorders among persons with chronic mental illnesses. In A. F. Lehman, & L. Dixon (Eds.) *Double Jeopardy: Chronic Mental Illness and Substance Abuse* (pp. 9–25). New York, NY: Harwood Academic Publishers.

Mueser, K. T., & Noordsy, D. L. (1996). Group treatment for dually diagnosed clients. In R. E. Drake, & K. T. Mueser (Eds.). *Dual Diagnosis of Major Mental Illness and Substance Abuse Disorder: II. Recent Research and Clinical Implications* (pp. 33–51). New Directions for Mental Health Services, No. 70. San Francisco, CA: Jossey-Bass.

Mueser, K. T., Drake, R. E., & Noordsy, D. L. (1998). Integrated mental health and substance abuse treatment for severe psychiatric disorders. *Journal of Practical Psychiatry and Behavioral Health*, 4(3), 129–139.

Mullen, B., & Rosenthal, R. (1985). Basic Meta-analysis: Procedures and Programs. Hillsdale, NJ: Erlbaum.

Osher, F. C., & Kofoed, L. L. (1989). Treatment of patients with psychiatric and psychoactive substance abuse disorders. *Hospital and Community Psychiatry*, 40, 1025–1030.

Owen, R. R., Fischer, E. P., Booth, B. M., & Cuffel, B. J. (1996). Medication noncompliance and substance abuse among patients with schizophrenia. Psychiatric Services, 47(8), 853–858.

Project MATCH Research Group (1997). Matching alcoholism treatments to client heterogeneity: Project MATCH post treatment drinking outcomes. *Journal of Studies on Alcohol*, 58, 7–29.

Regier, D. A., Farmer, M. E., Rae, D. S., Locke, B. Z., Keith, S. J., Judd, L. L., & Goodwin, F. K. (1990). Co morbidity of mental disorders with alcohol and other drug abuse. *Journal of the American Medical Association*, 264, 2511–2518.

Ribisl, K. M., Davidson, W. S., Luke, D. A., Mowbray, C. T., & Herman, S. H. (1996). "The Role of Social Networks and Psychopathology in Predicting Substance Abuse Treatment Outcome in a Dual Diagnosis Sample." Unpublished manuscript.

Ridgely, M. S., Osher, F. C., Goldman, H. H., and Talbott, J. A. (1987). *Executive Summary: Chronic Mentally Ill Young Adults With Substance Abuse Problems: A Review of Research, Treatment, and Training Issues*. Baltimore: Mental Health Services Research Center, University of Maryland School of Medicine.

Rosenthal, R. (1991). Meta-analytic procedures for social research. London: Sage Publications.

Rosenthal, R., & Westreich, L. (1999). Treatment of persons with dual diagnoses of susbtance use disorder and other psychological problems. McCrady, B., & Epstein, E. (Eds.). In *Addictions: A Comprehensive Guidebook* (pp. 439–476). New York: Oxford Press.

Smith, J. E., Meyers, R. J., & Delaney, H. D. (1998). The community reinforcement approach with homeless alcohol-dependent individuals. *Journal of Consulting and Clinical Psychology*, 66(3), 541–548.

Swanson, A. J., Pantalon, M. V., & Cohen, K. R. (1999). Motivational interviewing and treatment adherence among psychiatric and dually-diagnosed patients. *Journal of Nervous and Mental Disease*, 187, 630–636.

PART D

Intervening through Social Systems

Thus far we have explored why it is necessary to move beyond a specialist treatment model (Section A), and have considered ways in which substance abuse can be addressed through health care systems (Section B) and mental health services (Section C). Yet substance abuse is entangled with social problems that extend far beyond health care. It becomes part of a self-perpetuating cycle of unemployment and poverty. Prisons are filled with people whose offenses were committed under the influence of, or were otherwise somehow involved with the use of alcohol and other drugs. Most problem drinkers or drug users directly harm or devastate the lives of at least several others, often their own family members and loved ones. Substance abuse is a principal contributor to domestic violence and to the problems that engage child protective services. School systems struggle with the consequences of substance abuse among students and parents. In the workplace, substance abuse inflicts major problems and costs in the form of impaired productivity, lost work time, errors and accidents, and lost employees.

As a result, most social service systems also serve a clientele among whom substance use disorders are over-represented. It is estimated, for example, that 80% of those imprisoned in the U.S. committed their offenses while intoxicated by alcohol and/or other drugs, or have a diagnosable substance use disorder. These social service systems thus represent important additional opportunities for identifying, addressing, and even preventing substance abuse.

A principal obstacle here, of course, is that many such systems do not regard the addressing of substance abuse to be part of their mission. Resources are already stretched too thin in trying to fulfill the agencies' central mission, and substance abuse seems someone else's concern. Thus, as in health care, social service systems often do little to address the substance use disorders that are so prevalent in the populations they serve. Yet these problems will not go away. Often substance abuse contributed to, exacerbates, and maintains the difficulties that bring people to the attention of social service agencies. A referral for specialist treatment is effective in some cases, but for reasons discussed previously in this book, such referrals are often never completed. Ongoing substance abuse makes the person more difficult to serve, and in turn the unresolved social problems make it less likely that the person will seek, begin, continue with, and succeed in specialist treatment. Thus the cycle continues.

The main themes that run throughout this part are similar to those for Part A and B. There is much that can be done to address substance abuse—often at low cost—within the context of social service agencies. Because people's social problems are intertwined with substance abuse (and other health) problems, it makes sense to integrate services, or at least make them easily accessible through proximity. Often the basic work of a social service system can be applied to address substance abuse. Those who are incarcerated, for example, are already in a "residential program," with a great deal of time on their hands, and little to do that is productive or meaningful. Failing to address substance abuse complicates and compromises the fulfillment of agencies' missions. For all these reasons, it makes sense to address rather than ignore substance abuse within social service systems.

The chapters of this part explore ways in which this can be accomplished. Susan Rose and Allen Zweben (Chapter 11) document the ways in which substance abuse and social problems are inextricably linked. Sonja Frison and Jesse Milby (Chapter 12) discuss how the resources of a social welfare system can be applied contingently to decrease substance abuse. In Chapter 13, Alan Flisher and his colleagues discuss ways of addressing substance abuse within school systems, drawing upon their own South African context for examples. The opportunities for making a difference through correctional systems are the subject of Craig Love's chapter (14). In the U.S., there is a long history of programs for addressing substance abuse among employees, and Paul Roman (Chapter 15) explores opportunities in the rapidly changing landscape of the workplace. Family members affected by a loved one's substance abuse also regularly come into contact with health and social service systems, and represent yet another avenue through which to intervene. Jane Smith and her colleagues (Chapter 16) discuss important recent advances in how to work effectively through family and social support systems, when drinkers or drug users are not themselves motivated for change.

In the final chapter of this part, Mikyta Daugherty and her co-authors examine an enduring global puzzle: Why is it that displaced indigenous peoples of the world so often show substance abuse levels far higher than those of the general population, and why are their patterns of substance use and related problems so similar across vastly different cultures? This chapter particularly reminds us that solutions to substance abuse require thinking in larger social and public health terms, rather than relying upon the treatment of affected people as individual disorders.

CHAPTER 11

Interrelationship of Substance Abuse and Social Problems

SUSAN J. ROSE AND ALLEN ZWEBEN

INTRODUCTION

There is a growing acceptance that substance-related problems are not narrowly confined. That is, problematic alcohol and other drug use, despite level of severity, does not affect just an individual's job performance or personal relationships or health status, but touches many aspects of an individual's life and the lives of those around them. In addition, there is an elevated probability of social problems among those with substance abuse in their everyday experience, including mental health disorders (Kessler et al., 1996; Castanada et al., 1996) homelessness (Fisher & Breakey, 1991), child adjustment and behavior problems (Johnson & Leff, 1999), domestic violence (Greenfield, 1998; Kantor & Asdigian, 1997), child maltreatment (NCASA, 1999), and AIDS (NIAAA, 2000).

A number of trends have contributed to greater numbers of persons with substance abuse problems identified in more diverse settings. These trends include the use of broader definitions of alcohol and drug use problems, the recognition of the multiplicity of social problems experienced by persons abusing substances, and the growing acceptance of alcohol and drug use problems as a public health problem (Rose, Zweben & Stoffel, 1999). Thus individuals with all levels of substance use problems are being identified in child protection programs, voluntary family support agencies, employee assistance programs, health maintenance organizations, inpatient and outpatient psychiatric facilities, health care settings, public financial support programs, schools, faith-based organizations, and vocational rehabilitation settings.

SUSAN J. ROSE AND ALLEN ZWEBEN • Helen Bader School of Social Welfare, University of Wisconsin, Milwaukee, Wisconsin 53201

In addition, recognition of the impact of substance abuse has become more global, with greater acknowledgement of the role of alcohol and drug use in the incidence of mental health disorders and family dysfunction, especially violence and the maltreatment of children, and the spread of disease (AIDS) worldwide. This chapter will focus on social problems experienced by persons with substance use disorders in the areas of interpersonal (family relationships), mental health, and physical (AIDS) functioning, that require more coordinated intervention, discuss the challenges to care related to these complex needs, identify barriers to coordinated care, and suggest system-wide modifications useful in intervention with persons abusing alcohol and other drugs.

FAMILY DYSFUNCTION

The impact of substance abuse on family functioning has been difficult to estimate, and most studies have concentrated on the areas of child maltreatment and domestic violence.

Child Maltreatment

Estimates of the incidence of substance abuse in the 2.9 million annual reports of child maltreatment in the United States have ranged widely from 25 to 90 percent (Tracy, Green, & Bremseth, 1993; Young et al., 1998; NCASA, 1999). In the United Kingdom, where only the most severe incidents of child maltreatment are recorded on the Child Register, approximately 160,000 children are physically and/or sexually abused or severely neglected annually (Department of Health, 1995).

Approximately 10 million children in the US are living in households with an adult substance abuser, and child abuse and neglect are suspected to be more likely in families with a substance abusing parent (Gelles & Cornell, 1990; Murphy et al., 1991), as 675,000 children annually are seriously maltreated by substance-abusing caretakers (Daro & Mitchell, 1994). Through state reporting to the federal Adoption and Foster Care Analysis and Reporting System (AFCARS), it has been suggested that children from families with at least one person with substance use problems come to the attention of child welfare authorities younger than other children, are more likely to be placed in substitute care, to remain in care longer, and to leave care by adoption (Semidei et al., 2001; US Department of Health and Human Services, 1999).

Of recent concern has been the impact of cocaine use among parents of young children. The increase in the use of cocaine among U.S. women of child bearing age in the past ten years, has been associated with an increase in the foster care population nationwide (Barth, 1997). Children born to cocaine addicted mothers entered foster care in greater numbers from 1990 to 1995. Eighty percent of drug-exposed infants entered foster care, and their length of stay in substitute care has been longer that non-drug exposed children (Barth, 1997).

A growing concern has been the use of alcohol and drugs during pregnancy and the subsequent effects on children's development. Because of the lack of common screening methods used by hospitals, the prevalence of infant exposure to alcohol or drugs has been difficult to estimate. One study of 36 urban U.S. hospitals reported that 11 percent of all live births involved *in utero* exposure to illegal drugs (Friere, Griffith & Chasnoff, 1991). A record review of eight hospitals in Philadelphia found that 16.3 percent of women had used cocaine while pregnant (Hurt, 1990). The prevalence of alcohol consumption among pregnant women has increased to 15.3 percent (Ebrahim et al., 1998) after a decline the previous 10 years, and estimates of Fetal Alcohol Syndrome (FAS) vary from 0.5 to 3 per 1000 live births (Stratton et al., 1996). Recent studies in South Africa have reported similar patterns of FAS occurrence and maternal risk as in North American communities, but the prevalence is reportedly higher (May et al., 1999).

Domestic Violence

Recent research suggests that substance use, and alcohol use in particular, is much more likely to be a factor in intimate partner violence than stranger violence (Greenfield, 1998). It has been reported that alcohol was used by 67 percent of persons in a violent encounter with an intimate partner, compared with 31 percent of persons who were violent toward a stranger (Greenfield, 1988). In a recent study, O'Farrell and colleagues reported that addressing both alcohol use and marital problems concurrently reduced the incidence of partner violence in alcohol-complicated marriages (O'Farrell et al., 2001).

It is difficult to determine the prevalence of more generic family problems among persons abusing substances as these individuals more commonly focus on issues which initially bring them to seek help such as marital conflict, domestic violence, and employment problems and they tend not to make a connection between these problems and their substance use (Zweben & Barrett, 1997; Cooney, Zweben & Fleming, 1994). Social workers and other service providers often do not make the connection between stated family problems and substance use because of their lack of knowledge of appropriate screening instruments. In a study of 100 cases from four different agencies, only five cases were initially identified as containing a substance abuse problem; subsequent interviews with these families revealed that 39 of the cases had a substance use disorder (Kagle, 1987).

MENTAL HEALTH DISORDERS

In the general mental health population, it is estimated that nearly 50% of those with severe and persistent mental illness also have a co-occurring substance use disorder (Mueser et al., 1990; Testa et al., 1989). The difficulty of identifying substance use disorders in mental health settings is that patients presenting with symptoms of other Axis I disorders rarely offer information about their alcohol use and are rarely queried about problematic use at intake (Rosenthal & Westreich, 1999). When alcohol screening is conducted in mental health settings, it is primarily through structured history taking and physical examination.

Even moderate amounts of alcohol or drugs can be harmful to people with mental health disorders, mood and anxiety disorders in particular, because psychiatric symptoms may worsen, and individuals can easily experience adverse drug interactions if they are taking medication (Castaneda et al., 1996). In addition substance dependence elevates the risk for all types of affective and anxiety disorders (Kessler et al., 1996). A Canadian study reported that substance users are two to three times more likely than abstainers to have mood disorders and almost twice as likely to have anxiety disorders (Ross et al., 1997).

HIV/AIDS

HIV infection continues to be a world wide epidemic particularly for men and women between the ages of 25–44 (NIAAA, 2001). In the United States it is the fifth leading cause of death of men and women in this age group (SAMHSA, 2000); one million people in the US have been infected, with 450,000 reported deaths from HIV (*New York Times*, July 7, 2001). A higher prevalence rate of HIV has been found in the developing countries; 36 million people (one in five adults) have been infected in Africa and four million in India. Rates of HIV infection nearly doubled last year in Eastern Europe and Russia (*New York Times Magazine*, January 28, 2001). A similar story can be found in Southeast Asia; in Cambodia 3% of the adult population (170,000) have been found to be HIV positive while 800,000 have been infected in Thailand (*New York Times*, July 7, 2001).

Based on studies conducted in the US, substance use disorders (SUD) have been consistently linked with HIV infection. Injection drug users represent the largest HIV-infected substance abusing population in the US with 23% of reported AIDS cases identified as men and women who inject drugs (SAMHSA, 2000). These individuals usually become infected by using contaminated needles. Despite less attention by the popular press, alcohol use has also been closely linked with HIV infection, based on surveys of sexual risk behaviors (Avins et al., 1994). High prevalence rates of HIV infection have been reported among individuals in the 18–29 age group with alcohol use disorders (AUD, i.e. alcohol abuse or dependence) (NIAAA, 2001), with rates of AUD among HIV/AIDS patients between 3 and 12 percent for heterosexuals without serious co-morbid drug use (NIAAA, 2001). Moreover, individuals with AUD are three times more likely to have a sexually transmitted disease (a condition often associated with HIV infection) than those without AUD (SAMHSA, 2000).

HIV infection has been associated with specific lifestyle behaviors of individuals with AUD such as failure to use condoms, frequent or anonymous sex partners, and other factors (e.g., thrill-seeking behavior). Women, for example, are more likely to have sexual relations with less well known or anonymous partners when intoxicated, a behavior closely linked with HIV infection (Testa & Collins, 1997). Among alcohol treatment samples (inpatients and outpatients), approximately 30 percent fail to use condoms as reported in a survey of this population (NIAAA, 2001).

Among persons with serious mental illness (SMI), substance use is closely tied to HIV risk-taking behavior (e.g. frequent sex partners, lack of condom use, etc.). Rates of HIV infection among individuals with SMI such as schizophrenia and major affective disorders range between 4 and 23% (Kalichman et al., 1996). As reported in surveys of persons with SMI, approximately 50 percent currently use alcohol and one-third use other drugs (Kalichman et al., 1996), and more importantly among this population, individuals who drink during sex are least likely to use condoms (Sacks et al., 1994). In short, substance use among the SMI has been found to be the best predictor of unsafe sexual practices accounting for 21% of the variance in one study examining various predictors of HIV risk behaviors in a SMI population (Kalichman et al., 1994).

Among individuals already infected with HIV, continued substance use presents a host of difficulties related to HIV/AIDS. Clinical findings show that increased levels of alcohol consumption further diminish immune functions as evidenced by lower levels of CD4 (white blood cells that are necessary for maintenance of the immune system) cell activity (NIAAA, 2001). HIV kills off these cells, which in turn makes the individual more susceptible to other infections (SAMHSA, 2000). Individuals with AUD also have lower adherence rates on antiretroviral medications; combinations of these medications are necessary to sustain the viability of the immune system (Duran et al., 2001). Finally, alcohol use appears to be a crucial factor in the progression of liver disease among individuals co-infected with HIV and Hepatitis C (NIAAA, 2001).

CHALLENGES TO COORDINATED CARE

Given the multiplicity of needs identified above, coordination of care is critical in any treatment plan for persons with substance abuse problems. While there may be agreement on the need for such coordinated care, the challenges to its implementation are daunting. These challenges include (1) common definitions of the problem that are useable for all providers, (2) development of some common means of screening and assessment, (3) reaching consensus on the goals of care, (4) resolving the use of disparate interventions, and (5) developing relevant interventions, including ways of protecting and sharing clients' confidential information among providers.

Problem Definition

The first obstacle to coordinating care is reaching agreement on the problem and how to define its parameters. US mental health settings rely primarily on the DSM-IV dichotomy of "alcohol abuse" and "alcohol dependence" (APA, 1994), by meeting a set of specific criteria over a period of time, without specific reference to frequency or amount consumed. DSM-IV criteria for other substance abuse utilize the same set of diagnostic indicators for legal and illegal drug use as used for alcohol, with no reference to the reality that one time use of an illegal substance may be problematic to judicial systems without meeting the criteria for either abuse or dependence.

Social service agencies that treat family-based problems, including child maltreatment and domestic violence, may not think in terms of formal diagnosis of substance use disorders. Staff in these agencies may view substance use as indicative of underlying problems, or as simply contributing to the problem for which help is sought (Moncher et al., 1992). Medical staff may view alcohol use problems primarily from a biochemical perspective, as they affect medical care.

The problem in these kinds of disparities becomes magnified from a client's perspective, when many of the "helpers" are not consistent in their definition of the problem. Clients may find it difficult to understand what they should do when only a diagnosis is given, as this has little utility for treatment planning or goal setting. In addition, labeling clients as "alcoholic" or "substance dependent" can cause interactional problems between client and counselor as clients often have difficulty accepting such stigmatizing terms. These clients can be more amenable to discussing an alcohol or a drug problem in terms of how it affects family matters or their medical status, rather than as a "stand alone" issue. For example, in child protection, a parent may be more open to addressing an alcohol or drug problem if it is discussed in terms of how her drug use has impacted her specific parenting skills (e.g., insuring proper supervision, serving meals at similar times each day, etc).

Common Screening and Assessment

Coordination of complex resources for care is also complicated by a lack of common screening methods and assessment methods among various components of the care continuum. Many social service and mental health care systems do not even routinely screen or evaluate for substance use problems, much less agree on how to do so. Googins (1984) reported that only 40 percent of social service agencies included questions about an individual's drinking history (or that of family members) in their intake procedures. Similarly, alcohol use by pregnant women is not routinely identified despite the harm associated with the drinking (Serdula, Williamson, Kendrick, Anda & Byers, 1992). While there are a number of screening instruments available for use in secondary settings, professionals are not always knowledgeable or trained in their use (Van Wormer, 1987).

In a more recent survey conducted in substance abuse treatment settings in New England states of the U.S. (Hall et al., 2000), social workers were reported to have lower skill levels than non social work providers in assessing alcohol and drug problems, but higher levels than nonsocial workers in interpersonal skills, special populations and administration. In particular, knowledge of specific screening tools, as well as familiarity with compliance enhancement techniques (e.g., motivational interviewing) necessary in facilitating successful referral, was sorely lacking (Hall et al., 2000). A clear implication of this study is that issues directly or indirectly related to alcohol and drug abuse such as co-morbid physical (hepatitis, HIV infection, and gastroenteritis) and psychiatric problems could be missed by these social workers. Failure of graduate social work curricula to provide adequate training in substance abuse problems plus the lack of adequate clinical supervision in substance abuse treatment was seen as responsible for these deficiencies (Hall et al., 2000).

Assessment of substance use disorders in mental health has been hampered by confusion around the concept of "dual diagnosis," for which there is no standard definition. As a result, clinical guidelines or methods of determining a dual diagnosis vary widely. For example, in making a "dual diagnosis" some focus on which disorder came first (Evans & Sullivan, 1990) with no further guidelines on how to implement this method. When considering assessment of substance abuse and mental health, social workers have sometimes been directed to compendia of measures that are often not specific to substance abuse (Hilarski & Wodarski, 2001), and commonly used mental health assessment tools contain few questions about substance abuse.

Consensus on Goals

Following from the difficulties in problem definition and common assessment, a significant challenge to coordinating care is the lack of agreement about what the goal of treatment should be for persons in secondary alcohol-specific treatment settings. Conflicting goals among providers act as a substantial barrier.

For example, the overriding goal in child welfare practice is the identification of children at risk of parental maltreatment, and the provision for their safety through a continuum of services from prevention to temporary substitute care, reunification and adoption (Downs, Costin & McFadden, 1996). The identification and treatment of substance use problems is only a facilitative goal in the degree to which such problems interfere with the parents' ability to care for a child. The problems of treating caretakers with substance use disorders while protecting dependent children from harm is problematic for many providers.

This conflict can best be seen by the role of relapse. While relapse is regarded by many professionals as an expectable part of recovery from a substance abuse disorder, it raises significant questions for the care and safety of dependent children when a parent has sole custody of a young child and returns to destructive, dependent substance use for *any* period of time.

In mental health settings, the treatment goals are more often to control the most problematic symptoms of mental disorders, rather than to cure them (Austrian, 2000). The increasing use of medications in treatment of persons with dual diagnosis is an attempt to control symptoms of psychopathology, but if the substance abuse and mental health disorder are not considered together recovery can be compromised.

Disparate Interventions

Related to the definitional discrepancies of alcohol use problems, many organizations use widely differing interventions that reflect widely differing theoretical and cultural orientations to treatment that are not easily blended. In the U.S., some referring agencies mandate abstinence as a condition for treatment participation (e.g., probation and parole agencies) and require regular AA attendance, which may conflict with treatment that promotes client choice and individualized treatment goals, recognizing that AA may not be a good cultural fit. Some social service agencies require the client to stop drinking before family counseling can begin, while others negotiate differences between client and practitioner concerning how problem drinking behaviors will be addressed in the treatment situation. The use of medications in mental health settings may also conflict with a drug-free philosophy of some treatment or recovery. Such conflicting models may dissuade clients from participating in treatment.

In child welfare settings, openness about use and relapse are fraught with difficulty for women who abuse substances. Many women who abuse alcohol or drugs have significant histories of physical and sexual abuse. For example, in a current multi-site substance abuse treatment program women, 65% reported, during their treatment, a lifetime history of physical abuse and 40% reported a lifetime history of sexual abuse (Rose et al., 2001). During the screening phase, however, only 11 percent had reported any abuse. Screening, assessment, or treatment methods that require immediate disclosure of these histories can act as a barrier to care if counselors do not appreciate that women will disclose these issues when they are ready to do so.

Mothers with minor children face particular hazards in seeking and engaging in substance abuse treatment. These women may be acutely aware of the danger in which they have placed themselves and their children in order to use, and are cognizant of the consequences of "telling their story" to mandated reporters of child abuse and neglect (SAMHSA, 1998). The choice may be between obtaining treatment and retaining the custody of their own children. These issues have become more pressing in the U.S. as more states continue to enact "concurrent planning" policies that require workers to pursue termination of parental rights and adoptive placements at the same time in order to dispose of a case within 18 months (Semidei et al., 2001). Only evidence of complete cure (total abstinence) is accepted by some juvenile courts before minor children, especially infants, will be returned to maternal custody. Such policies place an emphasis on the behavior of the mother as opposed to the consequences for the child. If a caretaker can maintain gains in their parenting skills during a "slip" (e.g., provide for supervision of a minor child), attention might be more effectively focused on how a mother cared for her children during the slip, rather than the fact that she resumed drinking.

Social stigma may also deter help-seeking. In Russia, for example, individuals register as "alcoholics" before they can receive treatment. This registry is public record and open to all potential employers (Krupitsky, 2001). Such public exposure, intended to be curative, may actually act as a barrier to obtaining care.

Currently, HIV risk prevention interventions that are offered in primary care and mental health agencies are often not pertinent to the treatment needs of substance users who are high risk for HIV (i.e., use contaminated needles, practice unsafe sex with multiple partners, etc.) despite the fact that a substantial proportion of these individuals are seen in health care settings. What is typically offered in the U.S. for HIV risk prevention is mainly didactic counseling for alcohol and drug use and referral, which in the majority of cases is unsuccessful (SAMHSA, 2000; Kamb et al., 1996). Alternatively, care systems may rely upon treatment methods designed for high-severity cases, which are unsuitable for individuals seeking treatment primarily for health (e.g., sexually transmitted disease) or mental health (psychiatric symptomatology) concerns rather than substance use problems (Drake et al., 1994; Zweben and Barrett, 1997; Kelly, 1997; Kalichman et al., 1996).

At the same time, individuals at risk or already infected with HIV are poorly served by traditional substance abuse treatment programs. Staff often lack knowledge about HIV/AIDS and have negative biases against working with individuals susceptible to HIV infection or those already with HIV (Kelly, 1997). These biases may stem from the stigma associated with HIV or related to religious views of the providers (e.g., substance abuse programs housed in hospitals administered by certain religious groups can be squeamish about addressing condom use). Thus, the potential for conducting opportunistic interventions with individuals at risk for HIV infection is lost in these specialist settings (Kelly, 1997). In addition, substance abuse treatment settings do not have the necessary resources available to address the care needs of those already infected such as employing case managers to assist infected individuals in obtaining medical care and other services related to HIV (SAMHSA, 2000). These clients need early access to medical management with appropriate antiretroviral therapy and medication combinations to prevent a worsening of their conditions (SAMHSA, 2000).

NEW DIRECTIONS IN INTERVENTION

Despite the challenges and barriers, the need for coordinated care to address the complex issues in overlap of substance abuse and social problems is pressing. To bridge the gaps between the ideal and current practice, cross training of service providers, the development of financial incentives for coordination, and increased public support for integration of treatment systems can assist in modification of the current system.

In relation to family and interpersonal arenas, practitioners should receive specific training for helping persons with alcohol and drug use problems with whom they come in contact. Practitioners should learn "state of the art" assessment and intervention methods appropriate for addressing alcohol and drug use problems as part of overall care.

Second, public funding bodies ought to take the lead to provide incentives for coordination of care. Mental health and substance abuse treatment in particular are sometimes funded and administered by separate agencies using different procedures and definitions of appropriate problems to be addressed.

Third, social service professionals and systems should seek to integrate physical as well as mental health care. There is a growing body of outcome literature demonstrating that integrative models addressing substance use in conjunction with HIV risk behaviors can be reasonably employed in mental health and health care settings to prevent and treat HIV infections (Kelly, 1997). This combined model has been employed in various studies conducted in public health settings in the United States, Europe and Australia with individuals vulnerable to HIV (Weinhardt et al., 2000). Recent findings on this integrative model have been encouraging (Weinhardt et al., 2000), and data show that a motivational intervention geared to reducing alcohol or drug use along with HIV-risk reduction skill training can promote positive change.

CONCLUSION

Because substance abuse overlaps with so many other social problems and health/mental health disorders, substantial numbers of individuals with substance use disorder will continue to appear in agencies geared to dealing primarily with medical and social problems such as child abuse, domestic violence, and emergency services. The challenge is to meet these help seekers where they interact with the treatment system and modify the system to more adequately meet their many and complex needs.

REFERENCES

American Psychiatric Association (1994). Diagnostic and Statistical Manual of Mental Disorders.

Avins, W. L., Woods, W. J., Lindan, C. P., Hudes, E. S., Clark, W. & Hulley, S. B. (1994). HIV infection and risk behaviors among heterosexuals in alcohol treatment programs. *Journal of the American Medical Association, 271*, 555–518.

Castaneda, R., Sussman, N., Westreich, L., Levy, R. & O'Malley, M. (1996.). A review of the effects of moderate alcohol intake on the treatment of anxiety and mood disorders. *Journal of Clinical Psychiatry, 57*(50): 207–212.

Daro, D. & McCurdy, K. (1994). *Current Trends in Child Abuse Reporting and Fatalities: NCPCA'S 1993 Annual Fifty State Survey*. Chicago: National Committee for Prevention of Child Abuse.

Dawson, D.A. & Grant, B. F. (1998). Family history of alcoholism and gender: their combined effects on DSM-IV alcohol dependence and major depression. *Journal of Studies in Alcoholism, 59*(1): 97–106.

Dawson, D. A., Grant, B. F., Chou, S. P. & Pickering, R. P. (1995). Subgroup variation in US drinking patterns: Results of the 1992 National Longitudinal Alcohol Epidemiologic Study. *Journal of Substance Abuse, 7*: 331–344.

Department of Health. (1995). *Child Protection: Messages from Research*. London: Her Majesty's Stationery Office (HMSO).

Drake, R. E. & Noordsy, D. L. (1994). Case management for people with co-existing severe mental disorder and substance use disorder. *Psychiatric Annals, 24*: 427–431.

Duran, S. et al. (2001). Self-reported symptoms after initiatio of a protease inhibitor in HIV-infected patients and their impact on adherence to HAART. *HIV Clinical Trials, 2*: 38–45.

Ebrahim, S. H., Luman, E. T., Floyd, R. L. Murphy, C. C., Bennett, E. M. & Boyle, C. A. (1998). Alcohol consumption by pregnant women in the United States during 1988–1995. *Obstetrics & Gynecology, 92*(2): 187–192.

Evans, K. & Sullivan, J. (1990). *Dual Diagnosis*, NY: Guilford.

Fischer, Pamela J. & William Breakey. (1991). "The Epidemiology of Alcohol, Drug, and Mental Disorders Among Homeless Persons." *American Psychologist, 46*: 1115–1128.

Friere, M.C., Griffith, D. R. & Chasnoff, I. J. (1991). In utero drug exposure: Developmental follow-up and maternal-infant interaction. *Seminars in Perinatology, 15*(4): 310–316.

Greenfield, L.A. (1998). *Alcohol and Crime: An Analysis of National Data on the Prevalence of Alcohol Involvement in Crime*. Report prepared for Assistant Attorney General's National Symposium on Alcohol Abuse and Crime. Washington, DC: US Department of Justice.

Hall, M. N., Amodeo, M., Shaffer, H. J. & Vander Bilt, J. (2000). Social workers employed in substance abuse treatment agencies: A training needs assessment. *Social Work, 45*: 141–154.

Hunt, H. (1990). 1000 Babies: Philadelphia 1989 (abstract). *Pediatric Research, 27*: 93.

Johnson, J. L. & Leff, M. (1999). Children of substance abusers: Overview of research findings. *Pediatrics, 103*(5): 1085–1099.

Kalichman, S. C., Kelly, J. A., Johnson, J. R. & Butto, M. (1994). Factors associated with HIV infection among chronic mentally ill adults. *Psychiatric Services, 46*: 275–280.

Kalichman, S. C., Carey, M. P. & Carey, K. B. (1996). Human immunodeficiency virus (HIV) risk among the seriously mentally ill. *Clinical Psychology: Science and Practice, 3*: 130–143.

Kamb, M. L., Dillon, B. A., Fishbein, M. & Willis, K. L. (1996). Quality assurance of HIV prevention counseling in a multi-center randomized controlled trial. *Public Health Reports, 111*: (Supplement 1): 99–108.

Kantor, G. K. & Asdigian, N. When women are under the influence: Does drinking or drug use by women provoke beatings by men? In Galanter, M., ed., *Recent Developments in Alcoholism. Vol. 13. Alcohol and Violence: Epidemiology, Neurobiology, Psychology, and Family Issues* (pp. 315–336). New York: Plenum Press.

Kelly, J. A. (1997). HIV risk reduction interventions for persons with severre mental illness. *Clinical Psychology Review, 17*: 293–309.

Kessler, R.C., Nelson, C. B., McGonagle, K. A., Edlund, M. J., Frank, R. B. & Leaf, P.J. (1996). The epidemiology of co-occurring addictive and mental disorders: Implications for prevention and service utilization. *American Journal of Orthopsychiatry, 66*(1): 17–31.

May, P. A., Viljoen, D., Gossage, J. , Brooke, L. & Croxford, J. An epidemiological analysis of data from children with fetal alcohol syndrome and controls in Wellington, South Africa. *Alcohol Clinical Experimental Research, 23*(5): 111.

Moncher, , M., Schinke, S. & Holden, G. (1992). Tobacco Addiction: Correlates, Prevention and Treatment. In E. Freeman (ed.), *The Addiction Process*. NY: Longman.

Mydans, S. "Fighting AIDS: A new war is killing Cambodians," *New York Times*, July 7, 2001. A 4.

National Center on Addiction and Substance Abuse (NCASA). (1999). *No safe haven: Children of substance-abusing parents*. New York: Author.

National Institute on Alcohol Abuse and Alcoholism (2001). *Alcohol and AIDS: A guide for research issues and opportunities.* National Institutes of Health. US Department of Health and Human Services.

New York Times, July 28, 2001, A4.

New York Times Magazine, July 7, 2001, 26–28.

O'Farrell, T. (2001). "Behavioral couples therapy for alcohol and drug problems: Recent advances" Presented at, 24th Annual Scientific Meeting of The Research Society on Alcoholism, Montreal, Quebec, Canada, June 23, 2001.

Rose, S. J., Zweben, A. & Stoffel, V. (1999). Interfaces between substance abuse treatment and other health and social systems. In B. McCrady & E. Epstein (Eds.) *Addictions: A Comprehensive Guidebook.* New York: Oxford University Press.

Ross, H., Rehm, J. & Walsh, G. (1997). Patterns of alcohol consumption and psychiatric disorder among Ontario adults. *Contemporary Drug Problems, 24*(3): 533–556.

Sacks, M., Dermatis, H., Burton, W., Hull, J. & Perry, S. (1994). Acute psychiatric illness: Effects on HIV risk behavior. *Psychosocial Rehabilitation Journal, 17*: 5–18.

Semidei, J., Radel, L. F. & Nolan, C. (2001). Substance abuse and child welfare: Clear linkages and promising responses. *Child Welfare, 80*(2): 109–128.

Stratton, K., Howe, C. & Battaglia, F. eds. (1996). *Fetal Alcohol Syndrome: Diagnosis, Epidemiology, Prevention, and Treatment.* Washington, DC: National Academy Press.

Substance Abuse and Mental Health Services Administration, Center for Substance Abuse Treatment (2000). *Substance abuse treatment for persons with HIV/AIDS,* Treatment Improvement Protocol (TIP) Series 37, Department of Health and Human Services Adminitration Publication No. 00–3459.

Testa, M. & Collins, R. L. (1997). Alcohol and risky sexual behavior: Event-based analysis among a sample of high-risk women. *Psychology of Addictive Behaviors, 11*: 190–201.

Tracy, E.M., Green, R. K. & Bremseth, M.D. (1993). Meeting the environmental needs of abused and neglected children: Implications from a statewide survey of supportive services. *Social Work Research and Abstracts, 29*(2), 21–26.

US Department of Health and Human Services, Children's Bureau. (1999). *The AFCARS Report, Current Estimates as of January 1999.* Washington, DC: Author.

Young, N. K., Gardner, S. L. & Dennis, K. (1998). *Responding to alcohol and other drug problems in child welfare: Weaving together practice and policy.* Washington, DC: Child Welfare League of America.

Zweben, A. & Barrett, D. (1997). Facilitating compliance in alcoholism treatment. In B. Blackwell (Ed.). *Compliance and the treatment alliance inserious mental illness.* (pp. 277–293). Newark: Gordon & Breach Publishing Group.

CHAPTER 12

Intervening through the Social Welfare System

A Proposed Contingency Management Program with Implications for Workfare Planning

SONJA FRISON AND JESSE B. MILBY

This chapter outlines one area of the U.S. Social Welfare System and discusses the implications of a contingency management program for Welfare to Work (Workfare) participants with substance abuse problems. This type of programming is important for at least two reasons. One, although the prevalence of substance abuse within this system varies, there is a recognition that screening and treatment are often indicated but are not adequately addressed. Also, substance abuse impacts on the individual's ability to obtain and sustain employment, thus creating challenges to the system if the substance abuse is not treated.

To help outline how a substance abuse intervention program may work with the social welfare system, the U.S. social welfare system is discussed as a representation of westernized programming. Second, the need for substance abuse programs for welfare recipients is further outlined, again based on the U.S. system. Third, employment programming is discussed. Fourth, a proposed Workfare program that integrates social service provision and treatment principles is described which could be wholly implemented in an affluent, westernized social welfare system. Lastly, consideration is given to impact of political, cultural, and contextual norms on program implementation in other countries.

SONJA FRISON • Behavioral Medicine Unit/Division of Preventive Medicine, University of Alabama, Birmingham, Alabama 35294

JESSE B MILBY • Department of Psychology, University of Alabama, Birmingham, Alabama 35294

A: THE SOCIAL WELFARE SYSTEM

The social welfare system has been described as "a nation's system of programs, benefits, and services that helps people meet those social, economic, educational, and health needs that are fundamental to the maintenance of society" (Barker, 1995). Social welfare expenditures include cash benefits, services, and administrative costs of public programs for individuals and families. In 1995, approximately, $1,505.1 billion dollars was expended in the U.S. Social welfare system, 21% of the Gross Domestic Product (Bixby, 1999). The largest allocation is in Social Insurance (47%), followed by Education, and then Public Aid. Examples of U.S. social welfare programs include Social Security, Medicare, Unemployment Compensation, Public Housing, and Welfare (TANF). Affluent western countries such as Britain and Canada have similar welfare systems (Shapiro & Young, 1989) which focus on the ability to transition into work and work participation.

Interventions within the social welfare system have often concentrated on individuals receiving either Public Aid, such as TANF (Temporary Assistance for Needy Families) or disability benefits. Welfare in the U.S. has changed significantly due to the Personal Responsibility and Work Opportunity Reconciliation Act of 1996 (PRWORA: P.L. 104–193). This act placed new emphasis on employment within two years of initial receipt of funds while previous programming focused on long-term educational planning (Pavetti & Wemmerus, 1999). The PRWORA requires states to initiate at least 25% of their welfare participants into work from 1997–2001, and at least 50% in 2002, and limits assistance to less than 5 years. Most individuals leave welfare quickly, with almost half off welfare within a year and 90% within 5 years (Pavetti, 1997; Brown, 2001). Recipients typically respond to work initiatives in one of three ways (Pavetti, 1997): (1) those who will find jobs relatively easily; (2) those who find jobs after skill development; and (3) those who have a difficult time finding a job due to issues such as substance abuse, domestic violence, mental health challenges, criminal history, and language barriers (Brown, 2001). Because of the multi-dimensional and inter-related nature of the difficulties, there is little evidence of effective programming (Brown, 2001), particularly for substance abusers.

B: SUBSTANCE ABUSE AND THE WELFARE SYSTEM: TANF AS AN EXAMPLE FOR WORKFARE INTERVENTIONS

Similar issues face substance abusers in other parts of the social welfare system in their transition to work. For example, changes have occurred in the U.S. Social Security system that have impacted recipients of disability income with concomitant substance abuse. In 1997, U.S. Public Law 104–121 removed recipients from Social Security Income and disability programs who had disabilities due exclusively to alcohol and drug addiction. So, why focus on TANF? First, policy changes indicate an increased focus on work participation, which is a point of intervention. Second, there is a clear legislative mandate for states to move recipients off welfare, with incentives for more successful states (Brown, 2001). Lastly, children of parents on TANF may be positively or negatively impacted by the parent's transition, which has been related to the child's outcomes (e.g., Duncan & Brooks-Gunn) and substance abuse prevention for the child.

Studies have found as many as 25% of welfare recipients have drug and alcohol problems that may interfere with or prevent successful employment (Grant & Dawson, 1996; Olsen & Pavetti, 1996; Sisco & Pearson, 1994). The National Household Survey on Drug Abuse found that drug use is 50% more common in welfare recipient households than a comparison group of non-welfare recipients (Delva, Neumark, Furr, & Anthony, 2000). In an agency level study, almost 41% of the participants reported at least one dependence symptom and 4–6% reported experiencing alcohol related social consequences at least once (Weisner & Schmidt, 1993). There is a mixed picture, however, with one large scale study finding similar rates for welfare recipients compared to the general population (Grant & Dawson, 1996). However, the authors concluded that substance abusing recipients need specially designed prevention and treatment services.

Need for Integration

The social welfare system and the treatment system should integrate services to effect change and ensure that these services are necessary and sufficient, which is often not the case (Brown, 2001). For one, Weisner and Schmidt (1995) found that while heavy substance abusers were receiving services throughout the system, only a small number were engaged in treatment. Also, at the local level, there is a trend to make substance abuser's receipt of entitlements contingent on participation in addiction treatment. Additionally, welfare may be the final safety net for substance abusers denied access to other programming based on changes in the federal, state, and local laws. Thus, there is a compelling rationale for more effective partnerships to work with this population.

C: EMPLOYMENT PROGRAMMING AND INTEGRATION

The majority of the U.S. states report to the Welfare Information Network (WIN) that they require assessment of substance abuse and/or participation in treatment for eligibility and/or participation in treatment as a work activity (WIN, 2001). Most draw upon the expertise of vocational rehabilitation specialists, substance abuse treatment programs, and community based organizations to effect change (Brown, 2001). With respect to employment outcomes, one study examined the effects of substance abuse treatment on employment for AFDC (Aid for Dependent Children) participants in Washington state (Wickizer, Campbell, Kruipski, & Stark, 2000). Clients who completed treatment had a 20–90% higher rate (there were several employment outcomes) of being employed than the comparison group. Another study found that women who completed treatment were more likely to be working after discharge than those who failed to complete treatment (Metsch, McCoy, Miller, McAnany, & Pereyra, 1999).

Other attempts at integration include "social purpose business ventures" (Kramer, 2000). These programs focus on developing businesses similar to sheltered workshops where clients with severe physical and/or psychological limitations may work and are completed in collaboration with TANF agencies. Some states have also hired counselors to work onsite in the TANF agencies to readily address substance abuse issues faced by clients (Strawn, 1997).

D: BRIDGING THE GAP: CONTINGENCY MANAGEMENT WITH HOMELESS SUBSTANCE ABUSERS—IMPLICATIONS FOR SOCIAL WELFARE SYSTEM PROGRAMMING

Numerous challenges face participants in the welfare system who are mandated to work. To help illustrate some of the challenges that are faced by substance abusers transitioning out of the welfare system, we will outline work done with homeless cocaine abusers. Homeless and housed poor individuals have some similar characteristics, with homeless individuals faring worse on some outcomes such as mental health diagnoses, substance abuse, and victimization (Toro, Bellavia, Daeschler, & Owens, 1995). Based on this, findings of the Study Series of Homeless cocaine abusers (Milby et al., 1996: 2000) may have implications for further enhancing Workfare programming for harder to employ substance abusers.

The Challenge of Treating Cocaine Dependent, Homeless Persons

Cocaine dependence treatment, like welfare programming for harder to treat clients, has been marked by frustration in finding effective interventions and retention of clients (e.g., Gainey, Wells, Hawkins, & Catalano, 1993). An estimated 1.7 million Americans used cocaine in 1996 (National Institute on Drug Abuse, 1997). Among illicit drug users in the 1996 National Household Survey, 13% reported using cocaine (NIDA, 1997), almost twice the rate for 1990. A body of experimental research reviewed by Higgins (1997) indicated that non-drug reinforcers disrupt acquisition and maintenance of cocaine abuse and had implications for treatment. Higgins and colleagues found robust treatment effects (Higgins, Budney, Bickel, Foerg, Donham, & Badger, 1994) with voucher reinforcement of cocaine abstinence, which was replicated in a cocaine abusing methadone maintenance population (Silverman, Higgins, Brooner, Montoya, Cone, Schuster, & Preston, 1996). All of these effective treatments included urine surveillance, contact daily for several hours or several days per week, and aftercare lasting six months.

Homeless Study Series

In the first randomized, controlled clinical trial (Milby et al., 1996) with dually diagnosed homeless, 176 homeless substance abusers were randomly assigned to usual care vs. behavioral day treatment and assessed by blind interviewers at baseline, 2, 6, 12 mos. for alcohol and drug use, employment, and homelessness. Usual care involved a 12 step oriented, once weekly individual and group therapy and referral to community resources for housing and vocational assistance. Enhanced care provided transportation to and from shelters and lunch, and attendance at a behavioral day treatment for 2 months with abstinence contingent work therapy focusing on refurbishment of housing and abstinence contingent housing for 4 additional months. The Enhanced care group had significantly improved outcomes on 1–2 weekly random toxicologies and all assessments of drug and alcohol use and homelessness. In the second study (Milby et al., 2000), 141 cocaine dependent homeless persons were randomly assigned to enhanced behavioral day treatment from the first trial (DT) or the same day treatment with abstinence contingencies for housing and work (DT+). Abstinence contingent housing was provided free during the first 2 months of day treatment followed by the abstinence contingent work therapy and housing interventions from the first study. Abstinence results for drug use were replicated and showed robust differences favoring DT+ with 72% vs. 34% at 2 months follow up and 49% vs. 17% at 6 months follow up.

Bridging the Gap

Using these previous studies of contingency management programming, a program is outlined to help bridge the gap. For the individual with a substance abuse problem and a longstanding pattern of welfare participation and concomitant poor housing, private sector employment could be a path to recovery and a more stable and satisfying lifestyle. It is possible that successful elements from the two fields of study, social welfare and substance abuse treatment, could be combined to develop innovative, effective interventions to address the issues these clients often face (Olsen & Pavetti, 1997). Schmidt & McCarty (2000) outlined five areas that need to be addressed in service provision for substance abusing, welfare to work recipients: (1) assessment of the need for services; (2) how substance abuse impacts welfare dependency; (3) how welfare programming can be a pathway to treatment; (4) how effective are welfare and treatment integrated programs; and (5) an understanding of system level influences and policy implications. From studies of substance abuse treatment, particularly with cocaine dependent persons, contingency management based approaches, with services to address some of the underlying social issues such as housing, suggest a significant impact on client abstinence rates was possible as well as engagement in treatment and employment (Milby et al., 1996; Milby et al., 2000). To bridge these two approaches, we outline a Workfare program that addresses these areas that could have an impact on assisting dually diagnosed clients transitioning out of the welfare system, clients whose psycho-social situations are often similar to the homeless population.

INTRODUCTION TO THE WORKFARE PROGRAM MODEL

A Workfare substance abuse intervention model like that outlined here could be utilized across numerous sites and includes the integral social welfare system (see Figure 1). After screening, a Phase I motivational intervention and evaluation lasting two months is begun. Phase II is the Intensive Intervention which includes monitoring and assessment of abstinence, abstinence contingent training/work with a stipend, and ultimately graduation if the client maintains abstinence. Phase III is the Assessment Referral, and Recycling Phase which includes urine monitoring and referral back into the abstinence contingent Workfare program, if abstinence is not sustained.

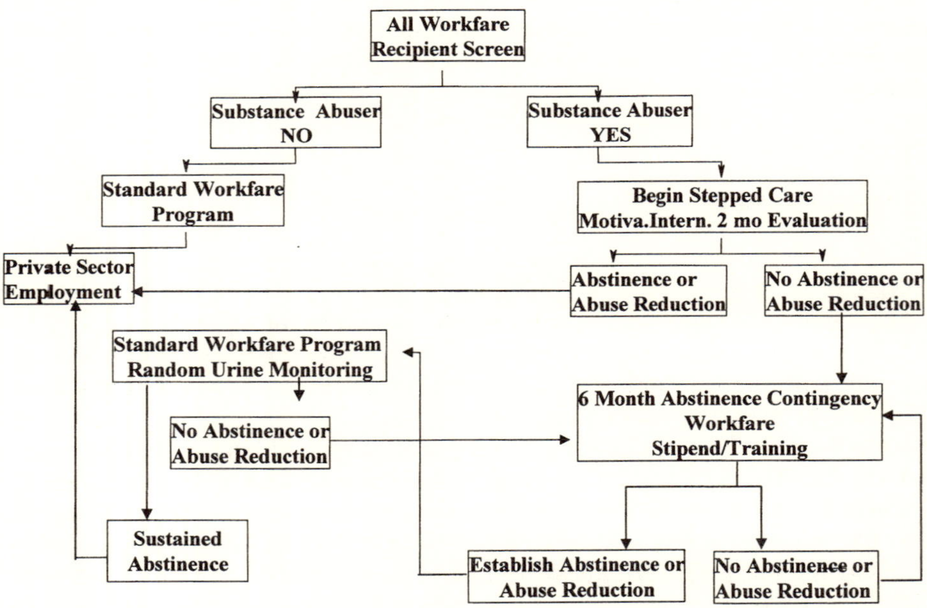

Figure 1 Proposed workfare model to intervene with substance abusing workfare participants.

PHASE I: INITIAL SCREENING AND BRIEF MOTIVATIONAL INTERVENTION

Participants are screened using the Addiction Severity Index (ASI; McLellan, et al., 1991) which can be administered by trained clinicians or non-clinicians in various settings. The drug and alcohol severity indices would be utilized to determine participants' eligibility for the Enhanced Workfare Program. The ASI severity scores range from .0 (indicating no problem) to 1.0 (indicating a severe problem), with .5 indicating eligibility into the Enhanced Workfare Program. Additionally, assessment of employment, legal problems, family/ social, and psychiatric composite scores and severity indices also provide information in those domains of functioning that can both indicate needs for referral to additional services and can monitor client progress during the Workfare program. Based on the ASI, and a random urine screen, Workfare candidates deemed to have a substance abuse problem would be placed into the Stepped Care program.

Brief Motivational Intervention

The motivational intervention utilizes the five principles outlined by Miller and Rollnick (1991): express empathy, develop discrepancy, avoid argumentation, roll with resistance, and support self-efficacy. This type of approach is often used with individuals who may be reluctant to change. Miller and Rollnick state that it can function by "giving a boost" to clients who have determined they want to change but haven't initiated actual change behaviors. The intervention can also create an "openness to change" for clients who are more reluctant. Utilizing principles of motivational interviewing combined with a substance abuse assessment, a brief but effective intervention for problem drinkers has been accomplished in two 1.5 to 2 hour sessions. In the final session, feedback on the client's relative standing in reference to norms for alcohol and drug consumption are presented to the client in a non-confrontive, supportive style. For less motivated clients, the counselor supports efforts to consider or initiate substance use reduction and other life changes which would support abstinence.

Monitoring of Change

Random urine assessment within 2 months following the two session motivational intervention would discover whether sufficient improvement in substance use had occurred to obviate the need for more intensive substance abuse intervention. The assessment would be required and supported by delayed TANF benefits until the assessment was completed. Clients who showed sufficient improvement would be cycled into the general program. Clients who demonstrated insufficient improvement would be transferred to the more intensive abstinence contingent interventions described below.

PHASE II: ABSTINENCE CONTINGENT WORK TRAINING AND WORK ACCESS

Women with Children

Programs providing social welfare system services should include safety nets to address the basic needs of children and the specialized needs of women (Woolis, 1998). For example, substance abusing women are more likely to have been affected by abuse and/or neglect or been victimized in their lifetime (Duncan, Saunders, Kilpatrick, Hanson, & Resnick, 1996; Foa, 1997). This may entail the need for referrals and follow-up to gender sensitive programming in the community. Additionally, child welfare issues also need to be considered in that programs should link, through case management, mothers and children to basic health care for the child, educational opportunities, family oriented housing, and childcare assistance. Therefore, the Phase II intervention has to take into consideration these issues.

The Phase II intervention utilizes regular random urine screens to access the training or work site. Failure to produce a drug-free urine specimen leads to loss of access to the training or work site with consequent loss of financial benefits (excluding wraparound or safety net services for families) until abstinence is shown to be re-established by two consecutive urines free of abused drugs. During the training and work itself, stepped increases in financial incentives are delivered for improved job performance as evidenced by objective indicators of increased job quality, productivity, or both. In addition, incentives are given or removed contingently upon professional demeanor that might include appropriate dress, timely use of breaks, non-confrontation or arguments, etc. with supervisors or fellow workers. Reduction in financial incentives will be provided contingently for the absence of these behaviors during a sustained period.

Overall the system of financial incentives for sustained professional behaviors and those contingent upon production quality, speed and accuracy would be adjusted to financial levels lower than starting salary and wage levels for similar private sector employment. This differential would provide an additional incentive for the Workfare participants to move on to private sector employment where salary and wages would be higher and where there would likely be more freedom from daily supervision and adjusting incentives.

It is anticipated that the nature of supervised Workfare programs would involve work projects for public entities, such as parks, gardens, paths, roads, maintenance of rights-of-ways, maintenance and refurbishing of public buildings, etc. It is likely that such Workfare programs could greatly benefit from the employment of retired experts who could volunteer part-time for nominal pay and health benefits to provide senior expertise and mentorship to complement the full-time staff needed. Such part-time experts could be charged with providing training and small group or one-on-one supervision for Workfare clients learning new skills.

Clients who successfully move through the incentive system to the top of the salary and wage scale could be an excellent source of full time training and supervisory staff for the program. It is anticipated that the useful monitoring of client behaviors and use of performance contingent incentives would require a state-of-the-art computerized data base to track individual client progress and eligibility for incentives. Training in the use and maintenance of the computerized performance-based tracking system could be part of the training provided by the Workfare Program and would better prepare clients for participation in private sector employment where computer data bases are routinely used.

PHASE III: ASSESSMENT, REFERRAL AND RECYCLING

After 3 months, clients who have successfully improved and sustained work performance, while also sustaining abstinence would be transferred back to the usual Workfare program with continued use of random urine testing which would continue for an additional three months or until the participant gained private sector employment. Participants who fail to successfully improve performance and gain maximum financial incentives, or whose continued relapses or failure to sustain required professional behaviors would remain in the intensive program where incentives would continue to provide opportunities to improve skills, productivity, professional demeanor, and sustain abstinence. To obtain financial support, they have to participate and meet minimum requirements to obtain minimum financial aid, which would benefit society and themselves as they would be continuously engaged in useful, self-esteem enhancing work.

WORKFARE MODEL COMPONENTS

There are several underlying factors for the proposed Workfare Program: objective assessment and performance evaluation, contingent incentives, floor level increases, stepped care and stepped performance. These features are all based on the assumption that work is a natural activity that produces increased incentives for increased quality and quantity. The Workfare Model proposed here applies this basic assumption of the reinforcing properties of work in a relatively easily administered, systematic way. The program supports recovery from dysfunction associated with substance abuse and reinforces small steps toward work self-sufficiency.

Objective Performance Assessment and Evaluation

One critical element is the use of objective performance assessment and evaluation. In welfare to work programming, objective follow-up and insuring the client is making the necessary transitions is key to client success. By measuring performance, the program is able to assess the client's functioning throughout and ensure that if there is a worsening in the client's work or work-related behaviors, some level of intervention is initiated, and contingencies and work site performance expectations are adjusted accordingly. The proposed program is structured to utilize objective evaluation of client response to drive changes in the program's structure and response to each individual. For example, objective evaluation of drug use via ASI severity index score and results of urine testing determine whether a welfare client is placed in the first phase of intervention providing motivational assessment feedback to the client followed by three months of monitoring.

Contingent Incentives for Improved Performance

Contingencies are utilized to stimulate reductions in substance abuse and improvements in work and work-related social interaction. For example, clients receive an increase over base level financial support for initiating and sustaining abstinence. Once abstinence is sustained, increased incentives are provided contingent upon pro-social work site behaviors and increased and sustained work quality and quantity.

Incentives Are Built into Floor Level and Increase with Improvement in Functioning

The program provides a floor level of financial support for each client if he/she attends work or training sessions each day, is abstinent and stays on the job. Base level support is reduced for late attendance and leaving the work or training site early without permission. Incremental financial incentives are available contingent upon maintained attendance and initiated and sustained abstinence. For improved work or training performance, further financial incentives are provided. Thus, the system features use of objective measures of performance to provide increasing incentives for each client to improve and function at higher levels.

Stepped Care and Stepped Performance

The proposed program provides three levels of stepped care for substance abusing clients. One is the motivational intervention. If successful, then a lower step involving return to usual Workfare activities but with continuous urine monitoring for several months is utilized. Urine monitoring ceases with indication of sustained abstinence. The final step is the intensive drug treatment program which utilizes abstinence contingencies and client movement to the less intensive step of regular Workfare activities with urine monitoring.

System Provision for Clients who Fail to Obtain Work in the Private Sector

The authors recognize that some portion of the clients may never cycle out of the proposed Workfare Program into private sector employment. The nature of work performed in the Workfare Program is proposed public sector activity such as refurbishing and maintenance of public facilities and therefore Workfare clients who never graduate into private sector employment can still earn a minimum wage or slightly higher by contributing work supporting public facilities. Such productive activities would be required for public benefits and would likely garner increased public respect and recognition for work accomplished and benefit self, family and community.

CONSIDERATION OF THE WORKFARE PROGRAM IN OTHER COUNTRIES

It is noted that the outlined program may readily apply to most U.S. based welfare systems and with some modifications, other affluent westernized Social welfare system. However, one question is how could such a program fit within social welfare system programming in a country with fewer resources and with special populations? Each program within a geographical location will have to consider how to contend with local constraints. Some key elements of the Workfare program to include are: contingencies, floor level increases, and stepped care and stepped performance.

Implementation in Other Countries

Contextual factors such as access, funding, political climate, and cultural factors can impact the implementation of the proposed Workfare program. For example, asylum communities in Australia are greatly impacted by substance abuse, but often don't have access to basic programming (Silove, Steel, McGorry, & Drobry, 1999). Most countries don't have federal programming to deal with substance abuse and it is usually a part of general health programming (WHO, 1999). Also, there are political climate issues such as an example discussed by Weiner (1998) where in the post-socialist era in Eastern Europe, there was a dramatic increase in unemployment as the roles of women changed. Understanding the culture and views on abused substances is important as well. For example in South Africa, the former dop system under apartheid utilized alcohol as wages for work participation. Although this is no longer espoused, there is still some evidence it exists (London, 1999).

An example of a work program that may be modified to address substance abuse dependencies in conjunction with social welfare is one in Botswana and Kenya (Teklu & Asefe, 1999). The authors describe a public works program that entails usage of public work activities to provide employment opportunities. The authors found that this type of work is an acceptable employment strategy for individuals with limited assets, particularly the rural poor, in these countries. However, contextual constraints must be considered. For example, almost 30% of rural Botswanan households produce alcohol for sustenance (Thompson, 1997). Even if this is an overestimate, it reiterates that community norms about alcohol will have to be addressed with key stakeholders and programming developed that is sensitive to the cultural mores of the local system. Also, political norms should be understood. In neighboring South Africa, the social welfare system has undergone dramatic changes to ensure more equal access to social services that in the past have been limited or nonexistent to persons of color (Black Africans) (Letsebe, 1997). These are just examples of how factors need to considered in program implementation in another country.

CONCLUSION

There is a need for interventions to address the multi-faceted challenges of substance abusers within the social welfare system. Although documentation of the prevalence of substance abusers in the social welfare system is variable, there is a recognized need to develop tailored interventions for this highly specialized population. This requires an understanding of the integration of welfare system level demands and effective treatments for harder to employ individuals. Additionally, strategies to employ this program in different settings should be sensitive to cultural and contextual norms. A contingency management approach that has been used successfully with homeless, dually-diagnosed, cocaine-dependent persons is proposed in the context of a Workfare intervention. It is believed that a system that integrates welfare programming requirements with contingency management principles, and is sensitive to local norms, should have an impact on employment, abuse and dependence outcomes for substance abusing Workfare participants.

REFERENCES

Barker, R. L. (1995). Social Welfare. In *The Social Work Dictionary*. Washington, DC: National Association of Social Workers.

Bixby, A. K. (1999). Public Social Welfare Expenditures, Fiscal Year 1995. *Social Security Bulletin, 62*, 86–94.

Brown, A. (2001). *Beyond work first: How to help hard-to employ individuals get jobs and succeed in the workforce.* New York: Manpower Demonstration Research Corporation.

Delva, J., Neumark, Y., Furr, C., and Anthony, C. (2000). Drug use among welfare recipients in the United States. *American Journal of Drug and Alcohol Abuse, 26,* 335–342.

Duncan, G. J., & Brooks-Gunn, J. (2000). Family poverty, welfare reform, and child development. *Child Development, 71,* 188–196.

Duncan, R. D., Saunders, B. E., Kilpatrick, D. G., Hanson, R. F., & Resnick, H. S. (1996). Childhood physical assault as a risk factor for PTSD, depression, and substance abuse: findings from a national survey. *American Journal of Orthopsychiatry, 66,* 437–448.

Foa, E. (1997). Trauma and women: Course, predictors, and treatment. *Journal of Clinical Psychiatry, 58,* 25–28.

Gainey, R. R., Wells, E. A., Hawkins, J. D., & Catalano, R. F. (1993) Predicting treatment retention among cocaine users. *International Journal of Addiction, 28,* 487–505.

Grant, B. F., & Dawson, D. A. (1996). Alcohol and drug use, abuse and dependence among welfare recipients. *American Journal of Public Health, 86,* 1450–1454.

Higgins, S. T. (1997). The influence of alternative reinforcers on cocaine use and abuse: a brief review. *Pharmacology Biochemistry and Behavior, 57,* 419–427.

Higgins, S. T., Budney, A. J., Bickel, W. K., Foerg, F. E,. Donham, R., & Badger, G. J. (1994). Incentives improve outcome in outpatient behavioral treatment of cocaine dependence. *Archives of General Psychiatry, 51,* 568–576.

Kramer, F. (2000). Social purpose businesses: Supported work and training settings for hard-to-place welfare recipients. *Welfare Information Network Design Brief, 1,* 1–18.

Letsbe, M. A. (1997). Social welfare in transition in South Africa: Structures and processes. *International Social Work, 40,* 75–88.

London, L. (1999). The dop system, alcohol abuse, and social capital amongst farm workers in South Africa: A public health challenge. *Social Science and Medicine, 48,* 1407–1414.

Metsch, L. R., McCoy, C. B., Miller, M., McAnany, H., & Pereyra, M. (1999). Moving substance abusing women from welfare to work. *Journal of Public Health Policy, 20,* 36–55.

McLellan, A. T., Kushner, H., Metzger, D., Peters, R., Smith, I., Grissom, G., Pettinati, H., & Argeriou, M. (1992). The fifth edition of the addiction severity index. *Journal of Substance Abuse Treatment, 9,* 199–213.

Milby, J. B., Schumacher, J. E., Raczynski, J. M., Caldwell, E., Engle, M., Michael, M., & Carr, J. (1996). Sufficient conditions for effective treatment of substance abusing homeless. *Drug and Alcohol Dependence, 43,* 39–47.

Milby, J. B., Schumacher, J. E., McNamara, C., Wallace, D., Usdan, S., McGill, T., & Michael, M. (2000). Initiating abstinence in cocaine abusing dually diagnosed homeless persons. *Drug and Alcohol Dependence, 60,* 55–67.

Miller, W. R., & Rollnick, S. (1991). *Motivational Interviewing.* NY: The Guilford Press.

Olson, K., & Pavetti, L. (1997, February). *Personal and family challenges to the successful transition from welfare to work.* Washington, D.C.: The Urban Institute.

Pavetti, L. (1997). New welfare reform: One size fits all? *Forum for Applied Research and Public Policy, 12,* 18–21.

Pavetti, L., & Wemmerus, N. (1999). From a welfare check to a paycheck: Creating a new social contract. *Journal of Labor Research, 20,* 517–537.

Schmidt, L. A., & McCarty, D. (2000). Welfare reform and the changing landscape of substance abuse set-vices for low income women. *Alcoholism-Clinical and Experimental Research, 24,* 1298–1311.

Shapiro, R. Y., & Young, J. T. (1989). Public opinion and the welfare state: The United States in comparative perspective. *Political Science Quarterly, 104,* 59–89.

Sisco, C. B., & Pearson, C. L. (1994). Prevalence of alcoholism and drug abuse among female AFDC recipients. *Health and Social Work, 19,* 75–77.

Silove, D., Steel, Z., McGorry, P., and Drobry, J. (1999). Problems Tamil asylum seekers encounter in accessing health and welfare services in Australia. *Social Science and Medicine, 49,* 951–956.

Silverman, K., Higgins, S. T., Brooner, R. K., Montoya, I. D., Cone, E. J., Schuster, C. R., & Preston, K. L. (1996). Sustained cocaine abstinence in methadone maintenance patients through voucher-based reinforcement therapy. *Archives of General Psychiatry, 53*, 409–415.

Strawn, J. (1997). Substance abuse and welfare reform policy. *Welfare Information Network Issue Notes, 1*, 1–6.

Substance Abuse and Mental Health Services Administration. (2001). *Summary of findings from the 2000 National Household Survey on Drug Abuse* (DHHS Publication No. (SMA) 01-3549). Rockville, MD: SAMHSA.

Teklu, T., & Asefe, S. (1999). Who participates in the labor intensive public works in Sub-Saharan Africa? Evidence from rural Botswana and Kenya. *World Development, 27*, 431–438.

Thompson, B. (1996, December). Global binge: A report on alcohol abuse worldwide. *World Vision's Today*. Retrieved from http://worldvision.org.

Toro, P., Bellavia, C., Daeschler, C., & Owens, B. (1995). Distinguishing homelessness from poverty: A comparative study. *Journal of Consulting and Clinical Psychology, 63*, 280–289.

Weiner, E. (1998). Assessing the political and economic reform of the post-socialist era: The case of Czech and Slovack women. *East European Quarterly, 31*, 473–502.

Weisner, C., & Schmidt, L. (1993). Alcohol and drug problems among diverse health and social service populations. *American Journal of Public Health, 83*, 824–829.

Weisner, C., & Schmidt, L. (1995). Expanding the frame of health services research in the drug abuse field. *Health Services Research, 30*, 707–726.

Welfare Information Network. (2001). *State plan information report: Hard to serve provisions.* Retrieved from http://www.welfareinfo.org.

Wickizer, T. M., Campbell, K., Krupski, A., & Stark, K. (2000). Employment outcomes among AFDC recipients treated for substance abuse in Washington State. *Milbank Quarterly, 78*, 585–608.

Woolis, D. D. (1998). Family works: Substance abuse treatment and welfare reform. *Public Welfare, 56*, 24–31.

World Health Organization. (1999). Global status report on alcohol. Geneva: World Health Organization.

CHAPTER 13

Intervening through the School System

ALAN J. FLISHER, ANDRAÉ BROWN, AND WANJIRŨ MUKOMA

WHY INTERVENE THROUGH THE SCHOOL SYSTEM?

The 1993 World Bank Development Report identified school-based interventions as one of the most cost-effective approaches to health and development (World Bank, 1993). Several arguments support this conclusion.

Many countries have high enrollment rates for both male and female adolescents. This population is relatively accessible for intervention programs. This stands in contrast to the relative inaccessibility of health services in many parts of the world. In South Africa, for example, several provinces have less than one psychiatrist per million population (Flisher, Riccitelli, Jhetam, & Robertson, 1997). However, 97% of children aged 10–14 years attend school (National Institute for Economic Policy, 1996). Thus, intervening through the school system can reduce inequalities in access to health services.

The accessibility of the adolescent population also has the advantage of economic efficiency. Additional economic benefits also accrue from the fact that program developers can use existing infrastructure and involve educators (who are already in place) in the delivery of the program. Also, evaluation studies (including those that collect data at several time points) can be conducted relatively cheaply since there are minimal barriers to locating study participants.

There are additional arguments that are specifically relevant for substance abuse. Globally, school students have been found to have high rates of substance use. The Health Behaviour in School-Aged Children (HBSC) Study recently

---

ALAN J. FLISHER AND WANJIRŨ MUKOMA • Department of Psychiatry and Mental Health, University of Cape Town, Cape Town, Republic of South Africa ANDRAÉ BROWN • Department of Professional Psychology and Family Therapy, Seton Hall University, South Orange, New Jersey 07079

published data from 27 European countries and the USA and Canada (Gabhainn & François, 2000). Among their findings were that most counties report daily smoking rates of under 10% at age 13 years and under 30% at age 15 years. However, large increases are noted in every country between 13 and 15. In both Northern Ireland and Wales, for example, rates are 1% at age 11, 9% at age 13 and 20% at age 15). The rates of reported drunkenness on two or more occasions also increased sharply across age groups, from up to 12% of 11-year-olds, to 37% of 13-year-olds, and 67% of 15-year-olds. Cannabis was not included in this study. However, the National Youth Risk Behavior Survey in the USA found that 26% of high school students had used cannabis in the previous 30 days (Centers for Disease Control and Prevention, 1997). In the developing world, the World Health Organisation has reported an increase in the use of tobacco, alcohol and other drugs (World Health Organisation, 1997). In a study of substance use by students aged 13–14 years in Cape Town (South Africa), Dar es Salaam (Tanzania) and Harare (Zimbabwe), it was found that for males in the previous year, 23.5% in Cape Town had smoked cigarettes, 17.1% in Dar es Salaam had used solvents and 14.7% in Harare had used alcohol (Flisher, Butau, Mbwambo et al., in press). A marked increase in lifetime prevalence rates from Grades 8 to 11 has been observed for male school students in Cape Town (Flisher, Parry, Evans, Muller, & Lombard, in press). For example, among black males the lifetime prevalence rates increased from 21.9% to 50.7% for tobacco, from 34.7% to 55.4% for alcohol and from 10.5% to 23.0% for cannabis.

These high rates provide sufficient rationale for interventions in the school system. Such interventions are especially necessary as adolescence is a critical period for the acquisition of health risk behavior such as substance abuse. If substance abuse is avoided in adolescence, it is very unlikely that it will commence at a later stage. There is evidence from international studies, for example, that almost all adults who smoke cigarettes commenced doing so in adolescence (World Health Organisation, 1997). Interventions offered to young people can thus yield amplified benefits since their effects may be manifest throughout the life span.

Finally, the school is an important agent for child and adolescent socialization and development. Specifically, the school environment shapes relationships, cognitive skills and behavior. Schools can thus provide the necessary context for important issues such as addictive behavior to be raised and processed in a manner that remains informative, respectful, contemporary, and supported by both peers and responsible adults. In other words, the social ecology of the school can be exploited in the interests of addressing addictive behaviors.

DISCRETE PROGRAMS

Discrete programs refer to interventions that: (a) focus on one or more specific addictive behaviors; and (b) exist independently of and isolated from other programs and activities in the school. The early programs that were offered until the mid 1980's focused on providing information and on social and personal development in the domains of stress management, decision making and values clarification (Gilvarry, 2000). More recently, social influence approaches have dominated, which usually involve social and communication skills, problem solving and social resistance training (Gilvarry, 2000). Many such programs also aim to promote norms negative to substance use by strategies such as depicting drug use as socially unacceptable, identifying short-term negative consequences of substance use, providing evidence that substance use is not as widespread among peers as children may think, encouraging children to make public commitments to remain drug free, and using peer leaders to teach the curriculum (Botvin, 1986; Klepp, Halper, & Perry, 1986; Hawkins, Kosterman, Marguin, Catalano, & Arthur, 2000).

Evidence for the effectiveness of discrete programs has been disappointing (Tobler, Lessard, Marshall, Ochshorn, & Roona, 1999). Even the most widely used prevention program in the US, DARE (Drug Abuse Resistance Education), has been shown to have no or almost no impact on addictive behavior (Clayton, Cattarello & Johnstone, 1996; Ennett, Tobler, Ringwalt, & Flewelling, 1994; Harmon, 1993). Botvin, Baker, Dusenbury, Botvin, and Diaz (1995) suggest that a failure to detect beneficial effects may be related to brevity of initial interventions, inadequate booster sessions, faulty program intervention models and insufficient implementation. Also, many evaluations have had methodological shortcomings such as lack of randomization, short follow-up periods and poor fidelity in program delivery (White & Pitts, 1998). Such shortcomings can result in a failure to detect positive program effects.

In recent years, several reports have appeared that present methodologically sophisticated evaluations of sound programs that demonstrate positive outcomes. Three examples are presented below.

- Botvin and his colleagues (Botvin et al., 1995) developed and evaluated their Life Skills program, which embeds social influence resistance training in the broader context of social competence. The intervention consisted of 15 classes in 7th grade with boosters in 8th and 9th grades. Their study involved 3,597 predominately white 12th graders at 56 schools who were randomly allocated to receive the program with annual provider training workshops and ongoing consultation, the prevention program with videotaped training and no consultation, or "treatment as usual". Follow-up data were collected six years after baseline using school, telephone, and mail surveys. Results indicated that adolescents in the two intervention groups had significant reductions in both drug and polydrug usage. There were up to 44% fewer drug users and 66% fewer polydrug users for both groups receiving interventions compared to the "treatment as usual" group.
- The Midwestern Prevention Project (Pentz, Dwyer, MacKinnon et al., 1989) differed from Botvin et al's (1995) Life Skills program in that it aimed to address multiple social environments affecting adolescents. Community components of the intervention included mass media

programming, health policy and community organization. The school component consisted of 10 classroom sessions and 10 homework assignments which focused on social influence resistance training, a normative change curriculum, and parent education and organization. The program was introduced into 42 schools in the Kansas City metropolitan area. Students in the 6th and 7th grades (N = 5,065) received either the full intervention or a delayed intervention (mass media intervention only). One year after the program, the net increase in the prevalence rates for tobacco, alcohol and cannabis use was half that of the delayed intervention schools (Pentz et al., 1989). Even though this program was broader in scope than the Life Skills training of Botvin et al. (1995) in that it included a substantial community component, the design of the study precluded any conclusions about whether any specific component was efficacious or contributed to the positive outcome in the intervention group.

- The Class of 1989 Study (Perry, 1999; Perry, Kelder, Murray, & Klepp, 1992; Perry et al., 1993) was designed as a substudy of the Minnesota Heart Health Program (MHHP), to test the efficacy of the Minnesota Smoking Prevention Program. All 6th graders enrolled in public schools were invited to participate in a baseline survey in 1983 and that grade was surveyed annually until their graduation in 1989. Two parallel communities were identified, one of which served as the intervention community and the other as control. The school-based intervention utilized trained peer leaders to facilitate and prevent tobacco use by influencing the social and psychological factors that encourage the onset of smoking. Students in the program received educational components of the consequences of smoking, identified the consequences and reasons for smoking, learned of normative behaviours for adolescents, the role of peer and societal influences, and resistance skills training. The intervention community also participated in the MHHP populationwide intervention which focused on the restructuring of the adult social and physical environment with regard to heart-healthy behaviors and values through cardiovascular screenings, food labelling education, adult and community risk education and organization, continuing education for health professionals, and mass media education. There were no significant differences at baseline in the cohort sample. However, there were significant differences for smoking prevalence and intensity between communities for this sample at all of the follow up years. At graduation 14.6% of the intervention community were smoking as compared to 24.1% from the reference community (Perry et al., 1992). In this study, the community component was included as an aspect of the intervention that was shown to be efficacious. However, again there are no data that cast light on what aspects of the intervention package were instrumental in reducing cigarette smoking.

Key results of these studies are consistent with the conclusions of recent reviews (Gilvarry, 2000; Hawkins et al., 2000; Tobler et al., 1999; White & Pitts,

1998). Specifically, despite the dissapointing results of earlier efforts, there are grounds to believe that discrete school-based programs can be effective in reducing student substance use. However, they are more likely to be effective when they foster the development of social competencies in an interactive manner; include both specific resistance skills and general life skills; include booster sessions in subsequent years; and include broader community-based components such as parent education, community organization and support, and health policy. However, despite the body of knowledge that has developed in the past few years, several important challenges remain.

First, there needs to be a more precise definition of what components of discrete programs account for positive outcomes. In both the Midwestern Prevention Project (Pentz et al., 1989) and the Class of 89 Study (Perry et al., 1992), for example, it was not possible to determine the extent to which the community components contributed to the positive outcomes. Would the same outcomes have been achieved if the focus has been confined to classroom-based interventions? This is a key issue that needs to be resolved before such program can be rolled out on a massive scale. If it is the case that the community aspects contributed little to the outcome, it would not make sense to continue with this approach. Of course, similar arguments apply to the classroom-based components of the program.

Second, many of the discrete programs have been offered to predominately white, middle class students in the United States. These results may not be generalizable to other populations, which may include students of lower socioeconomic status and other ethnic, cultural and national backgrounds. This is important, as the reasons for substance use may be population-specific. It is possible that in poorer communities, for example, lack of educational opportunities and jobs and the resultant poor connection to educational institutions are more pertinent in the etiology of substance use than (say) peer pressure. If the etiology is different, the most effective interventions may also be different.

Third, many of the evaluations of discrete programs that have been evaluated have been developed and implemented by researchers from universities or research institutions that have access to large amounts of funding. The evaluations can be considered as "efficacy" evaluations as opposed to "effectiveness" evaluations. The former focuses on the measurable effects of a specific intervention. The latter refers to whether interventions are feasible and have measurable beneficial effects across broad populations and in real-world settings. Thus, effectiveness evaluations go beyond an examination of outcome in demonstration projects such as the three that were highlighted above. They examine the outcome of such projects when implemented on a wide scale. This is a key issue for discrete programs. In the case of school-based interventions targetting cigarette smoking, for example, mimimum guidelines for school-based smoking prevention programs have been proposed (Glynn, 1989). These guidelines specify the amount of time that should be set aside over several years and the classroom methods that should be employed. In addition, they urge parental and community involvement. In practice, many schools even in well resourced countries like the United States will not be willing or able to devote the time and resources that are necessary to comply with these minimal guidelines (Nutbeam, 1997). In schools that prioritize health promotion, the focus may fall on other issues such as alcohol use or unsafe sexual behavior. In schools in poor countries, where tobacco companies have recognised that there are large untapped markets, the likelihood of schools implementing the kind of program that will influence youngsters to refrain from smoking is negligible.

HEALTH PROMOTING SCHOOLS

If there are grounds to believe that discrete school-based intervention program can be effective in reducing substance use among school students, why is it necessary to consider alternative approaches, such as health promoting schools?

First, since the publication of the work of Jessor and Jessor (1977), increasing evidence for the covariation between substance use and other risk behaviours has accumulated. Students who engage in substance use are more likely to engage in other risk behaviors such as risky sexual behavior, interpersonal violence and suicidality. This has been documented in several countries, using a spectrum of analytic strategies, and with diverse community- and school-based samples (Wallace, Flisher, & Fullilove, 1997). A number of explanations have been advanced for the covariation. They may share common aetiologies; represent interchangeable ways of achieving the same goals; be related through intervening variables; and occur simultaneously in the social ecology of adolescence (in that the behaviors may be learned and performed together) (Flisher, Ziervogel, Chalton, Leger, & Robertson, 1996). In addition, risk behavior (including substance use) is associated with psychopathology (Deykin, Levy, & Wells, 1987; Flisher, Kramer, Hoven et al., 2000; Kandel & Davies, 1982).

Whatever the reasons for these associations, they imply that intervention programs should be *comprehensive* and not just focus on specific risk behaviors such as use of a particular substance or even substance use in general. The comprehensiveness applies not just to a focus on diverse outcomes but also to the risk factors for such adverse outcomes. If, for example, a youngster uses cigarettes to boost self-esteem, and through an intervention program develops strategies to reduce tobacco consumption, she may then seek other ways of boosting self-esteem. Similarly, both alcohol use and sexual promiscuity may be manifestations of depression. If a student's alcohol intake is reduced following a program that focuses on this issue, he could still be left grappling with both his unsafe sexual behavior and depression.

A second reason that it is necessary to consider other approaches to school-based intervention besides discreet programs is that risk and protective factors for substance use (and other adverse outcomes) are located in the school context. Substance use is associated with poor school performance (Flisher et al., in press b; Hawkins et al., 2000), intention to drop out of school (Nutbeam,

Smith, Moore, & Bauman, 1993), absenteeism (Flisher et al., in press b), a lack of connectedness to school (Resnick, Harris & Blum, 1993), and poor school climate (Ahmed, 1999). These findings suggest that efforts to reduce substance use will be maximally effective if the school environment is addressed.

These considerations were partly instrumental in the development of health promoting schools as an approach to address substance use and other aspects of the health of school-going children and adolescents. Legitimised by the Ottawa Charter (World Health Organisation, 1986), health promotion is today widely accepted as a philosophy and strategy for improving the health of populations around the world. A health promoting school is defined as:

> A place where all members of the school community work together to provide students with integrated and positive experiences and structures which promote and protect their health. This includes both the formal and informal curricula in health, the creation of a safe and healthy school environment, the provision of appropriate health services and the involvement of the family and wider community in efforts to promote health.
>
> (World Health Organisation, 1996, p. 2)

The curriculum is thus one of the experiences and structures that promote and protect health (World Health Organisation, United Nations Educational, Scientific and Cultural Organisation, & United Nations Children's Fund, 1992). In particular, it should:

- view health holistically, "addressing the interrelatedness of health problems and the factors that influence health, within the context of the human and material environment and other conditions of life" (World Health Organisation et al., 1992, p. 4);
- utilise all opportunities for health, which includes drawing on services outside the school;
- serve to harmonise the health messages from the various sources that influence students, which include the media, the health system, family, peers and the school; and
- empower children and youth "to act for healthy living and to promote conditions supportive for health" (World Health Organisation et al., 1992, p. 4).

Practice is generally guided by the principles of the Ottawa Charter of Health Promotion (World Health Organisation, 1986). A health promoting school seeks to provide its students with the optimal educational and health outcomes through the school curriculum, school ethos, policies and involvement of the wider community. The health promoting school embraces a comprehensive approach to improving child and adolescent health by including a broad spectrum of activities within the school and broader community. It endeavours to promote health and well being as well as to protect children and adolescents from vulnerabilities that may put this at risk, such as substance use. The strategy is enshrined within the socio-ecological model of health.

In a recent review of health of evaluations of health promoting schools (Mukoma & Flisher, 2000), we were able to locate only two studies in which substance use was addressed as part of the evaluation of a health promoting school (Jamison, Ashby, Hamilton et al., 1998; Moon, Mullee, Rogers et al., 1999). These programs addressed substance use and a broad range of other behavior by creating vibrant participatory health promoting school physical and social environments within and outside the classroom, and collaborating with other schools and local communities. The strategies employed included: changing teaching approaches; devising policy for substance use; keeping parents and the community better informed about activities in the school; holding health days or health weeks; developing a life skills program; and providing an award to motivate schools to become health promoting (Jamison et al., 1998; Moon et al., 1999).

Whether the health promoting school approach is effective in preventing the development of or a reduction in substance is a moot issue. Concerns have been raised over the absence of convincing evaluations as to the efficacy of this strategy. Indeed, evaluations of health promoting schools by Jamison et al. (1998) and Moon et al. (1999) report at the most only minimal favorable changes in smoking behavior and attitudes. In a summary of the intervention reported by Jamison et al. (1998), Hamilton (1997, pp. 9, 10) reports that there

> ... was no single unambiguous pattern of difference between the pilot and reference schools at the aggregate level. In particular, there was little evidence of measurable positive change over time in learning gains among pilot schools as distinct from those in reference ... schools. The exceptions were, first, in the realm of self-esteem, where overall, pilot schools tended to have slightly higher self-esteem. Secondly, in the primary phase, pupils in the pilot schools were increasingly less likely to be bullied than those in the reference schools.

Students at the intervention school were less likely to smoke or drink alcohol than those at the reference schools. However, the authors state that these could largely be explained by demographic differences between the schools (Jamison et al., 1998).

Moon et al. (1999) included a range of outcome measures. They found for current smoking behavior, the use of low risk drugs and the attitude "using drugs is exciting", the intervention schools generally performed better than the controls for males and females in grades 8 and 11. However, the only statistically significant difference was for grade 8 males for smoking uptake, which was lower in intervention schools compared to those in control schools. There were no differences between the schools for drinking alcohol or intention to smoke at the age of 20 years.

These dissapointing results should be regarded in the light of their methodological shortcomings. Even though both studies employed a quasi-experimental research design with comparison schools, the statistical treatment of the data was superficial and unsophisticated. In addition, data for each student were not linked—rather, aggregate scores at the time points were compared. Finally, the duration of the intervention was limited, and it is possible that for comprehensive programs such as health promoting schools a longer duration is required before a positive impact on health-related behavior can be detected. These problems reflect the immaturity of the field of evaluations of health promoting schools. Indeed, our review was able to unearth only eight interventions involving health promoting schools that had been evaluated, including the two (Jamison et al., 1998; Moon et al., 1999) that included substance use as outcome measures. Although none of the eight interventions were in the developing world, the feasibility of the HPS approach in this context has been demonstrated (Flisher, Cloete, Johnson et al., 2000).

It is clearly an ethical and scientific priority to conduct evaluations of the health promoting schools that exist in many parts of the world. Such evaluations should be of high methodological quality. For example, they should randomly assign schools or communities to the intervention or delayed intervention (control) groups; take measurements before and after the intervention; and measure impact as the changes in outcome indicators for the intervention and control groups. In addition, the evaluations should address all aspects of evaluation: inputs (which refer to what resources are dedicated to the program); process (what services the program actually delivered); outputs (which are about the delivery and implementation of activities); and outcome (whether the program produced the intended benefits). Finally, health promoting school targets change at the individual, school, family and community levels. However, our review (Mukoma & Flisher, 2000) identified a tendency to focus more on individual level outcomes such as knowledge, attitudes and behavior. Clearly, the field of evaluation research is more mature when it comes to assessing these individual-level indicators as compared to school- and community-level indicators. However, individual-level outcomes do not do justice to the more systemic changes that are associated with health promoting schools.

CONCLUSION

This chapter describes the two basic approaches to school interventions, discrete programs and health promoting schools, and discusses their relevance for addressing substance abuse problems in youth. Despite the paucity of data supporting their effectiveness, health promoting schools have been established in many countries in both the developed and developing world and several regional networks have been established. It has been endorsed and supported by the World Health Organisation. However, it has not taken root in the United States. Indeed, Nader (2000) comments that school health efforts in the United States, which are characterised by specified components targeting specific health targets, are ripe for being dismissed, devalued and compartmentalised.

Even though health promoting schools have not taken root in the United States, there is a tendency for the discrete programs in that country and elsewhere to expand their scope to include aspects that may be associated with health promoting schools in Europe and elsewhere. The Midwestern Prevention

Project (Pentz et al., 1989) and the Class of 89 Study (Perry et al., 1992), for example, both had community components that extended beyond a narrow focus on a school-based behavioral intervention. In addition, the Class of 89 Study (Perry et al., 1992) included outcomes other than substance use such as physical activity and food choices (Perry, 1999). Thus, the clear distinction between discrete programs and health promoting schools may become increasingly artificial.

It is probable that discrete programs that address the proximal determinants of a specific behavior (such as cigarette smoking) are more likely to demonstrate positive outcomes on that particular behavior. In contrast, health promoting schools, which do not focus on specific behaviors to the same extent but rather address broader aspects of the school community, are less likely to demonstrate positive outcomes when it comes to specific behaviors. Rather, one might expect that positive impacts are observed for a range of outcomes at the individual, family, school, and community levels. However, these positive impacts may have a smaller effect size, to the extent that they fail to achieve statistical significance. This leads to the *prevention paradox* (Rose, 1981), which states that a prevention measure that brings much benefit to the population offers little to each participating individual. The population benefit derives from the fact that the small changes in each individual have a multiplicative effect when distributed over a large population. It has been estimated, for example, that a 10 mm of mercury lowering of the blood pressure distribution as a whole corresponds to a 30% reduction of the total mortality attributable to hypertension (Rose, 1985).

In this context, a major challenge for those developing school-based programs addressing substance is abuse to adopt the advantages of the discrete programs approach with those of the health promoting schools approach. Thus, ways need to be found to embed discrete programs in the framework of health promoting schools. In other words, the two approaches should be regarded as complementary. While discrete programs can zero in more intensively on the use of selected substances, other activities within the health promoting school can provide infrastructural support through the creation of healthy school and community environments and healthy policies.

REFERENCES

Ahmed, N. (1999). School climate and substance use. M.Phil. (Public Health) dissertation, University of the Western Cape, 1999.

Botvin, G. J. (1986). Substance abuse prevention research: Recent developments and future directions. *Journal of School Health, 56*, 369–374.

Botvin, G. J., Baker, E., Dusenbury, L., Botvin, E. M., & Diaz, T. (1995). Long-term follow-up results of a randomised drug abuse prevention trial in a white middle-class population. *Journal of the American Medical Association, 273*, 1106–1112.

Centers for Disease Control and Prevention (1997). Youth risk behavior survey 97. Atlanta, GA: Centers for Disease Control and Prevention (Compact disc).

Clayton, R. R., Cattarello, A. M., & Johnstone, B. M. (1996). The effectiveness of drug abuse resistance education (Project DARE): 5-year follow-up results. *Preventive Medicine, 25*, 307–318.

Deykin, E. Y., Levy, J. C., & Wells, V. (1987). Adolescent depression, alcohol, and drug abuse. *American Journal of Public Health, 77*, 178–180.

Ennett, S. T., Tobler, N. S., Ringwalt, C. L., & Flewelling, R. L. (1994). How effective is drug abuse resistance education? A meta-analysis of project DARE outcome evaluations. *American Journal of Public Health, 84*, 1394–1401.

Flisher, A. J., Butau, T., Mbwambo, J., Kaaya, S. F., Kilonzo, G. P., Aarø., L. E., Eide, A., Lombard, C., Muller, M., Parry, C. D. H., & Klepp, K-I. (in press a). Substance use by students aged 13–14 years in South Africa, Tanzania and Zimbabwe. *African Journal of Drug and Alcohol Studies.*

Flisher, A. J., Cloete, K., Johnson, B., Wigton, A., Adams, R., & Joshua P. (2000). Health promoting schools: lessons from Avondale Primary School. In: D. Donald, A. Dawes & J. Louw (Eds.) Addressing childhood adversity: Psychosocial interventions in South Africa (pp. 113–130). Cape Town: David Phillip.

Flisher, A. J., Kramer, R. A., Hoven, C. W., King, R. A., Bird, H. R., Davies, M., Gould, M. S., Greenwald, S., Lahey, B. B., Regier, D. A., Schwab-Stone, M., & Shaffer, D. (2000). Risk behavior in a community sample of children and adolescents. *Journal of the American Academy of Child and Adolescent Psychiatry, 39*, 881–887.

Flisher, A. J., Parry, C. D. H., Evans, J., Muller, M., & Lombard, C. (in press b). Substance use in Cape Town, South Africa: prevalence rates and correlates. *Journal of Adolescent Health.*

Flisher, A.J., Riccitelli, G., Jhetam, N., & Robertson, B.A. (1997). A survey of professional activities of psychiatrists in South Africa. *Psychiatric Services, 48*, 707–709.

Flisher, A. J., Ziervogel, C. F., Chalton, D. O., Leger, P. H., & Robertson, B. A. (1996). Risk-taking behaviour of Cape Peninsula high-school students: Part IX. Evidence for a syndrome of adolescent risk behaviour. *South African Medical Journal, 86*, 1090–1093.

Gabhainn, S. N., & François, Y. (2000). Substance use. In C. Currie, K. Hurrelmann, W. Settertobulte, R. Smith & J. Todd (Eds.). Health and health behaviour among young people (pp. 97–114). Geneva: World Health Organisation (Health Policy for Children and Adolescents (HEPCA) Series No. 1).

Gilvarry, E. (2000). Substance abuse in young people. *Journal of Child Psychology and Psychiatry, 41*, 55–80.

Glynn, T. J. (1989). Essential elements of school-based smoking prevention programs. *Journal of School Health, 59*, 181–188.

Hamilton, K. (1997). Evaluation of the European Network of Health Promoting Schools (ENHPS). Paper presented at the British educational Research Association Annual Conference, Sept. 11–14, University of York.

Harmon, M. (1993). Reducing the risk of drug involvement among early adolescents: An evaluation of drug abuse resistance education (DARE). *Evaluation Review, 17*, 221–239.

Hawkins, J. D., Kosterman, R., Maguin, E., Catalano, R. F., & Arthur, M. W. (2000). In R. T. Ammerman & M. Hersen (Eds.). Handbook of prevention and treatment with children and adolescents. Intervention in the real world context (pp. 203–237). New York: John Wiley & Sons, Inc.

Jamison, J., Ashby, P., Hamilton, K., Lewis, G., MacDonald, A., & Saunders, L. (1998). The health promoting school: Final report of the ENHPS Evaluation Project in England. London: Health Education Authority.

Jessor, R., & Jessor, S. L. (1977). *Problem behavior and psychosocial development: A longitudinal study of youth.* New York: Academic Press.

Kandel, D., & Davies, M. (1982). Epidemiology of depressive mood in adolescents. *Archives of General Psychiatry, 39*, 1205–1212

Klepp, K-I., Halper, A., & Perry, C. L. (1986). The efficacy of peer leaders in drug abuse prevention. *Journal of School Health, 56*, 407–411.

Moon, A. M., Mullee, M. A., Rogers, L., Thompson, R. L., Speller, V., & Roderick, P. (1999) Helping schools to become health-promoting environments—an evaluation of the Wessex Healthy Schools Award. *Health Promotion International, 14*, 111–121.

Mukoma, W., & Flisher, A. J. (2000). A review of evaluations of health promoting schools. In: K-I. Klepp (Ed.), The Adolescent Reproductive Health Network (ARHNe). Health System and Health Promotion Research in Eastern and Southern Africa. Report of the fourth ARHNe workshop, Nairobi, Kenya, October 1–6, 2000 (pp. 55–60). Oslo: Institute for Nutrition Research, University of Oslo.

Nader, P. R. (2000). Health promoting schools: Why not in the United States? *Journal of School Health, 70*, 247.

National Institute of Economic Policy (1996). *Children, poverty and disparity reduction: Towards fulfilling the rights of South Africa's children.* Pretoria: Reconstruction and Development Program, Office of the Deputy President.

Nutbeam, D. (1997). Promoting health and preventing disease: An international perspective on youth health promotion. *Journal of Adolescent Health, 20*, 396–402.

Nutbeam, D., Smith, C., Moore, L., & Bauman, A. (1993). Warning! Schools can damage your health: Alienation from school and its impact on health and well-being. *Journal of Paediatrics and Child Health, 29*, 25–30.

Pentz, M. A., Dwyer, J. H., MacKinnon, D. P., Flay, B. R., Hansen, W. B., Wang, E. Y. I., & Johnson, C. A. (1989). A multi-community trial for primary prevention of adolescent drug abuse: Effects on drug use prevalence. *Journal of the American Medical Association, 261*, 3259–3266.

Perry, C. L. (1999). Creating health behavior change. How to develop community-wide programs for youth. Thousand Oaks, CA: SAGE Publications, Inc.

Perry, C. L., Kelder, S. H., Murray, D. M., & Klepp, K-I. (1992). Community-wide smoking prevention: Long-term outcomes of the Minnesota Heart Health Program and Class of 1989 study. *American Journal of Public Health, 82*, 1210–1216.

Perry, C. L., Williams, C. L., Forster, J. L., Wolfson, M., Wagenaar, A. C., Finnegan, J. R., McGovern, P. G., Veblen-Mortenson, S., Komro, K. A., & Anstine, P. S. (1993). Background, conceptualisation and design of a community-wide research program on adolescent alcohol use: Project Northland. *Health Education Research, 8*, 125–136.

Resnick, M. D., Harris, M. J., & Blum, R. W. (1993). The impact of caring and connectedness on adolescent health and well-being. *Journal of Paediatrics and Child Health, 29*, 3–9.

Rose, G. (1985). Sick individuals and sick populations. *International Journal of Epidemiology, 14*, 32–38.

Rose, G. (1981). Strategy of prevention: lessons from cardiovascular disease. *British Medical Journal, 282*, 1847–1851.

Tobler, N. S., Lessard, T., Marshall, D., Ochshorn, P., & Roona, M. (1999). Effectiveness of school-based drug prevention programs for marijuana use. *School Psychology International, 20*, 105–137.

Wallace, R., Flisher, A. J., & Fullilove, R. (1997). Marginalization, information and infection: The correlation of ghetto risk behaviors and the spread of disease to majority populations. *Environment and Planning A, 29*, 1629–1645.

White, D., & Pitts, M. (1998). Educating young people about drugs: A systematic review. *Addiction, 93*, 1475–1487.

World Bank (1993). *Investing in health. World development report.* Oxford: Oxford University Press.

World Health Organisation (1997). *Action for adolescent health: Towards a common agenda. Recommendations of a joint study group.* Geneva: World Health Organisation.

World Health Organisation (1986). *The Ottawa charter for health promotion.* Geneva: World Health Organisation.

World Health Organisation (1996). *Regional guidelines: development of health-promoting schools. A framework for action.* Geneva: World Health Organisation.

World Health Organisation, United Nations Educational, Scientific and Cultural Organisation, & United Nations Children's Fund (1992). *Comprehensive school health education. Suggested guidelines for action.* Geneva: World Health Organisation.

CHAPTER 14

Substance Abuse Treatment and Corrections

CRAIG T. LOVE

SUBSTANCE ABUSE AND CORRECTIONS

Prevalence of Substance Use Disorders among Offenders

It would be difficult to find a subpopulation with higher rates of substance use disorders than offenders. In the United States in1999, there were a total of 43.8 million contacts between police and U.S. citizens in their jurisdiction including traffic stops and other matters (Bureau of Justice Statistics, 2001) resulting in about 15 million arrests (Bureau of Justice Statistics, 2000a). In cities participating in an Arrestee Drug Abuse Monitoring (ADAM) program (Bureau of Justice Statistics, 2000b), an average of 65.8% of male arrestees and 64.2% of female arrestees tested positive for an illicit drug at arrest. Still more offenders are problematically involved with drugs and alcohol but do not test positive at the time of arrest (Bureau of Justice Statistics, 2000a). In sum, the vast majority of those incarcerated, at least in the United States, show a diagnosable substance use disorder.

In the U.S., this is quite a few people. By midyear 2000, there were 1,931,859 people in U.S. prisons and jails (Beck and Karberg, 2001). That represents an incarceration rate of 702 people per 100,000 population behind bars, one of the highest rates in the world. The population of incarcerated Americans has increased by an average of 5.6% per year in each of the past 10 years.

CRAIG T. LOVE • Center for Alcohol and Addiction Studies, Brown University, Providence, Rhode Island 02912

Defining Terms

Systems for dealing with criminal offenders vary widely across nations. In this chapter, the term *criminal justice system* is used to refer collectively to the law enforcement and judicial systems that detect, apprehend, and sentence offenders. While being processed through the criminal justice system, offenders may be detained in holding facilities, which in the U.S. are termed *jails* and in the U.K. *remand prisons*. Once adjudicated, offenders are typically referred into the society's *correctional* system designed variously to punish, deter, and prevent recidivism to crime. Correctional systems usually include *probation* (in-community monitoring in lieu of incarceration), *incarceration* in prison, and *parole* (in-community monitoring after completion of part or all of a sentence of incarceration.

Sentencing Policy

A common response to the influx of drugs into a society is an attempt to regulate that activity through rigorous enforcement of laws created to restrict the use of substances declared illegal (Tullis, 1995). A prominent example, the U.S. "war on drugs", yielded an increase in police and military action against importation as well as possession, distribution and use of identified illicit substances. Like other societies, the U.S. government has taken a two-pronged approach to the growing drug problem—reducing demand and eliminating supply. The vast majority of U.S. resources, however, have been directed toward the supply side of the problem.

By making the possession and sale of drugs illegal, primary responsibility for reducing drug use is placed upon the criminal justice system. A major side effect of this strategy is that various components of the criminal justice and correctional systems become collection points for individuals who use and are dependent on illicit drugs. The use of alcohol and other drugs further contributes to the likelihood of committing other criminal offenses, compounding the problem.

When there is a large accumulation of offenders with substance use disorders, the correctional system affords major opportunities for treating these problems and preventing their recurrence. This usually represents a major shift in the role of corrections that affects nearly all components of the system. Sentencing policy affects the extent to which such treatment occurs in the community (through diversion programs, probation, and parole) or in prisons.

SUBSTANCE ABUSE TREATMENT IN CORRECTIONAL SETTINGS

Does It Work? The Effectiveness of Substance Abuse Treatment

One key issue is the extent to which substance use disorders can be treated effectively in correctional settings, or in general. The latter issue is easier to address, given the large outcome literature that has clearly established the efficacy of a range of options for the treatment of alcohol (Hester & Miller, in press) and other drug use disorders (Carroll, 1998). Recent studies continue to provide evidence that substance abuse treatment within correctional settings can and does work (Lipton, 1998; Martin et al., 1999; Griffith et al., 1999; Knight et al., 1999; Pearson and Lipton, 1999; Wexler et al., 1999). Research methods in such studies have been greatly improved over the past 20 years. There is no empirical reason to believe that offenders, as a group, should be less responsive to evidence-based treatment methods. There is a broad consensus that punishment and incarceration alone have no beneficial effect on an offender's substance use disorder. Given the very high rates of such disorders among offenders, and their close linkage with future offenses, there would seem to be a responsibility (to society, as well as to the offender) to provide effective treatment.

Lipton (1998) presents a reasonable argument for including substance abuse treatment in prisons. A large number of individuals who are imprisoned are also substance abusers who have often had little help with their addictions. According to Lipton, providing substance abuse treatment in prison "provides a propitious opportunity for treatment. It is propitious because these persons would be unlikely to seek treatment on their own, without treatment they are extremely likely to continue their drug use and criminality after release, and there are now cost-effective technologies to effectively treat them" (p. 39). Lipton and all other studies identified here conclude that the residential in-prison treatment programs result in reduced re-arrest rates and drug use in comparison to inmates who do not receive such a program. Their follow-up time periods span a reasonable (3-year) window of observation. For example, 43% of the participants in the "Key Crest" residential therapeutic community program remained arrest free for 3 years but only 30% of the comparison group did so (Martin et al., 1999). It is important to note that inmates who participated in both in-prison treatment and aftercare were most likely to be successful in avoiding criminal justice involvement as well as substance use (Wexler et al., 1999). The combination of substance abuse treatment and aftercare is also cost effective (Griffith et al., 1999).

The Pendulum of Opinion

Unfortunately, the pendulum of public and correctional opinion can swing widely with regard to the merits of treating (rather than simply punishing) offenders, independently from the scientific evidence. In the United States and other nations there have been waves of unwarranted "nothing works" belief, fueled in part by a few influential literature reviews. When I first entered the system in 1974, the U.S. state and federal prison systems were in the throes of a major investment in treatment. That changed as the economy waned, and conservative political policies prevailed, justified in part by citation of a review that had reached negative conclusions (Lipton, Martinson, and Wilkes, 1975).

Even then, there were many studies describing various levels of success in prison-based treatment programs. Martinson et al. (1974) offered a detailed critical analysis, pointing out that very few of the studies were methodologically adequate to provide any meaningful evaluation of the programs. Their scathing criticism of the level and quality of research in corrections-based treatment were warranted, but unfortunately their review further dampened the enthusiasm of prison officials for providing treatment. Their review was interpreted (incorrectly) as a statement that nothing works, a view that was perpetuated in part by preliminary release of their data (Martinson, 1974). At the same time, the political winds in several nations shifted toward a "war on crime" to ensure that offenders were punished. In the 1980s state and federal legislatures in the U.S. passed tough new sentencing laws that established mandatory minimum terms to be served for various offenses. For example, any offense committed with a gun automatically added at least 5 years to a federal sentence, and more years if it was a repeated offense. "Good time" (a reduction in sentence because of good behavior and/or program involvement) was markedly reduced.

Another significant influence was the publication by Norval Morris (1974) of *The Future of Imprisonment*, a little book that had a great impact on correctional administrators' perspectives about indeterminate sentencing. At the time Professor Morris' book was published, many prison inmates were serving indeterminate sentences in which they were released at the discretion of the parole and/or prison system on the basis of their progress in treatment programs. If inmates did well in the program and good reports were sent by the treatment provider, offenders were considered rehabilitated and were released from prison to parole. Professor Morris objected to this practice on moral grounds. He suggested that it was unethical to coerce someone into treatment with the enticement of earlier release. Instead, Morris advocated "humane incarceration."

Now coming full circle in the 21st century, correction systems are showing renewed interest in treatment. There is clear recognition of the high percentage of offenses that involve alcohol and illicit drugs. This movement is supported, if not driven by, the growing evidence that substance abuse treatment can prevent future recidivism. Since the early 1990's substance abuse treatment in prison systems has increased, but has not yet provided an adequate number of treatment slots to meet the needs of inmates. In a recent review of this issue, Mumola (1999) reported that only 15% of prison inmates with a demonstrable need for treatment are receiving it. In the United Kingdom, the Home Office that coordinates both prisons and probation has launched an aggressive and well-funded program called "What Works," to implement evidence-based treatment methods throughout the British correctional system.

Treatment during Incarceration

Prison based treatment programs in general offer some advantages not seen in the community. For example, it is more possible to offer longer term programs (6 months to 1 year) than are available in the free community where funding sources limit treatment terms to a few days of outpatient treatment or a few months of residential treatment. The prison inmates are in the institution and require minimal additional costs (Love et al., 2000). In fact, reviews of the treatment literature suggest that there is an optimal correctional residential program length of 1 year (Wexler and Love, 1995).

Most in prison treatment services are offered in one of the following formats:

> "**residential**"—all inmates housed in a unit are in the program, program events held in the dorm and the daily routine emulates a therapeutic community (Wexler et al., 1999; Wexler and Love, 1995). This is the most intensive program.
> "**day treatment**"—inmates are engaged in the program for a substantial portion of the day at a program location such as the education department but the inmate participants live in a dorm in a different building.
> "**outpatient**"—a few sessions per week offered to inmates in the prison program area outside the inmate's dorm. This is the least intensive program.

While this evidence suggests that future investment of funds for treatment in prisons is warranted, the active ingredients in treatment that make these programs work are not yet clear. Type and format of treatment have not been systematically compared within a corrections population. In two ongoing studies of in-prison substance abuse treatment efficacy, we conducted focus groups with inmates who completed a residential cognitive behavioral treatment, dropped out, or completed and returned. Those who completed the program identified a particular topic or, more often, a particular staff member with whom they could relate. That individual or topic, they said, stimulated them to move toward recovery. It remains to be clarified which aspects of corrections-based treatment favor retention and favorable outcomes.

TREATMENT OUTSIDE OF INSTITUTIONS

Given the large proportion of offenders with alcohol and other drug problems, it does make sense to provide treatment during incarceration. After all, prisons are one place where a large number of drug and alcohol abusers are located. Since many of the offenders commit crimes under the influence of drugs and alcohol or to support their purchase, a reduction in the demand for drugs would reduce the level of crime and create a more positive life for the offender. Further, incarcerated offenders are relatively idle and available for a variety of treatment regimes. In fact, it is possible to offer some of the most intensive treatments available, including therapeutic communities for as long as 12 months or more (Wexler et al., 1999).

However, prison is an unreal environment in which the offender is pressed to adapt and survive by particular means. It is also a tense environment in which many aspects of the quality of life are out of the offender's control. Further, the prison offers a far greater structure (daily schedule, rules for daily living) than is normally part of the offender's experience outside of the prison environment. Ultimately the offender must learn new skills and cope with emotional and other problems in the natural community environment. When released, he or she needs to readjust to freedom (loss of structure), establish social and economic supports, and apply social and refusal skills in entirely different social environments. Given the complexity and intensity of the adjustment required of an individual who has already evidenced many failures in adjustment, it seems unlikely that a treatment effect achieved during incarceration will automatically carry over to the community.

There is already evidence that in-prison treatment is far more successful in reducing return to prison when an aftercare component is added (Martin et al., 1999; Wexler et al., 1999). Programs that include transition to the community, job training, job placement, housing assistance, and reintegration into the family are more likely to result in a positive outcome because they provide the offender support in facing the most challenging aspects of his/her return to the community (Alemagno, 2001). Further, inmates participating in focus groups in our current study have suggested that ex-offenders be assisted in practicing their new skills and knowledge through booster sessions after they have returned to the community. According to our focus groups of returnees and successful releases, in-prison treatment participants believe that the treatment helped them, but they need assistance in making a successful transition from prison to the community.

As we noted above, a segmented corrections system like that found in the U.S. is often poorly suited for this type of transition. For reasons of operational convenience, jails and prisons often process releases after the busy daytime hours, putting the offender back on the street in the middle of the night. It then falls to a separate system to provide in-community support. A meaningful continuity of care in the criminal justice system requires a high level of coordination among the various parts of the system. This is severely hampered when police, jails, prisons, courts, and probation all respond to different jurisdictions with conflicting goals.

Probation is a logical criminal justice component to conduct case management and monitoring of offenders in substance abuse treatment and associated services. A significant obstacle, however, can be the often overwhelmingly large caseload of a probation officer (sometimes 200–300 cases in U.S. systems).

Parole, like probation, is another logical place in the criminal justice system for administering case management and other support services for substance abusing offenders. Parole encompasses the particularly vulnerable period of transition from prison to the community, a high-risk time for recurrence of substance use and problems. The transition from incarceration to parole is a logical time for offering treatment and other forms of support.

SOME ISSUES AND OBSTACLES TO TREATMENT IN CORRECTIONAL SYSTEMS

Blurring of Roles

Substance abuse treatment of offenders is not without its practical problems, of course. As with criminal justice more generally, correctional systems and those who work in them have a responsibility to society. Those who provide treatment and case management are likely to have other roles as well. Sometimes treatment is offered by the same staff who are charged with custodial functions for inmates. A counselor who provides treatment may also be called upon to be armed and subdue attempted escapees, or to participate in gang control activities that require aggressive acts against inmates. Probation officers are interested in their supervisee's welfare, but also have a responsibility to enforce limits and the orders of the courts. This complex blurring of roles can be confusing for both staff and offenders.

The Milieu of Prisons

Prisons by design provide very little privacy and confidentiality. Most treatment programs in prisons are offered in a group setting. This is done in part to accommodate, with limited resources, more of the large group of offenders in need of treatment. Very little in-prison substance abuse treatment is offered as individual counseling. In many prisons, it is extremely difficult to meet privately with an individual inmate. Meetings may take place in a corner of a noisy common room, under conditions not conducive to treatment. Availability is constrained by schedules, guard coverage, lock downs, and the particular circumstances of each offender, leading to at best irregular treatment or case management.

Security considerations also affect how treatment is delivered. For example, a high security prison unit may require that inmate movement be minimized. As a result, the treatment program is offered in the inmate's living unit where inmate interaction is limited, and the program is highly supervised by correctional officers (limiting the openness of discussions), or in some cases inmates remain in their cells during treatment. When counts are held, or there is a security risk at the institution, treatment is suspended until the issue is settled or the count completed.

The Complexity of Correctional Systems

The administrative organization and coordination (or lack thereof) of a nation's correctional and criminal justice system(s) greatly affect the ability to address substance use problems effectively. The U.S. system provides a daunting example of obstacles that can be posed by structural issues. Perhaps no criminal justice system is more complex than this array of quasi-independent subsystems within jurisdictions and specialized enforcement entities (Bureau of Justice Statistics, 2000a,b; Tonry, 1999). In fact, to call it a system is something of a misnomer, in that "system" suggests implies feedback loops whereby each part supports the others, a condition sadly lacking in the U.S. criminal justice structure. Most offenders are passed from one component to another, usually in a single direction (e.g., police to prosecutor to courts to prison to parole) with little communication or coordination. This is because there are several levels of government, each with their own responsibilities and jurisdictions. Most US governmental entities include an executive, judicial, and legislative branch. The latter branch creates the laws that are enforced and interpreted by the executive and judicial branches, respectively, and the U.S. constitution requires the independent operation of each branch. Each governmental entity in turn has a multitude of independent agencies whose jurisdiction is defined by geography or function (e.g., city police, county sheriff, state police, railroad police, Federal Bureau of Investigation, border patrol) and each is administered separately, with policies and procedures rarely coordinated with other agencies. A crowded prison and jammed court docket may have little to no influence on the policies and procedures of local or state police who may decide to escalate enforcement of a particular law, creating more arrests and more cases for courts and prisons. The federal government, states, counties, cities, and towns each have separate courts, jails, and law enforcement personnel. Rarely are there combined facilities or programs. Law enforcement officials or courts have no authority to enforce laws outside of their jurisdiction, which itself may be defined by geography or function. Probation is usually administered by the various courts, separate from the corrections system overseeing jails and prisons.

Planning and Programming without Data

Another common problem is that decisions about programming are made without the benefit of, and sometimes in clear contradiction of scientific evidence of effectiveness. Prevention and treatment programs may be implemented without, or at least long before the availability of evaluation data. When this happens, offenders are widely exposed to interventions of unknown efficacy, which raises serious ethical issues. As discussed earlier, if the authority of society's correctional systems is used to coerce offenders to receive treatment, there should be clear and persuasive evidence of likely benefit. Yet there are numerous and recent examples of offenders coerced into interventions that, when outcomes were properly evaluated, proved to be ineffective or even harmful.

Instead, programs and systems may be implemented on a faddish basis. For example, there are currently over 400 drug courts in operation in the U.S. (Belenko, 1998) that are providing a different approach to the criminal justice system and law enforcement. While there is some encouraging evidence that drug courts can be effective (Belenko, 1998), the overall impact is still far from clear, and the implications of drug courts on the court system and jurisprudence in general have not been clearly addressed (Hoffman, 2000). Most evaluations of drug courts (like those for therapeutic communities) compare participants who complete the program with those who drop out. This clearly biases outcomes, in that non-completers may drop out of the drug court because they are not ready to go into recovery and are not serious about changing their lives. Comparing these self-selected drop-outs with those who complete the program stacks the deck in favor of the treatment group looking much better.

The Content of Treatment

In designing treatment programs for correctional settings, it makes sense to use what works—treatment methods that have a strong track record of efficacy. There is no particular reason to expect that offenders will respond differently than others to treatment approaches. The common finding that mandated and voluntary clients respond similarly to treatment suggests that offenders' outcomes are similar to those of non-offenders in treatment. While there have been reports of differential treatment response based on sociopathy (e.g., Kadden, Cooney, Getter & Litt, 1989), larger studies have not replicated even this finding (Project MATCH Research Group, 1997).

There are also ethical reasons why only evidence-based methods should be used in treating offenders. If the force of law and the courts is used to coerce offenders into treatment, then there should, at very least, be persuasive evidence that the treatment is unlikely to do harm to the person or to society. When coercion is involved, there is a higher responsibility to provide treatment that is likely to be beneficial to the offender, to society, or both.

Substance abuse treatment in correctional settings increasingly includes cognitive-behavioral methods, emphasizing skills for resistance, coping, and prosocial functions. One cognitive behavioral model emphasizing coping skills was developed by Monti, Kadden and their colleagues (Kadden et al., 1992; Monti, Abrams, Kadden & Cooney, 1989), and a more corrections-tailored model was developed in the Canadian prison system (Gendreau, 1996; Gendreau, Coggin & Paparozzi, 1996; Gendreau, Little & Coggin, 1996).

The Role of Coercion in Corrections-Based Treatment

For some time it has been found that compulsory drug treatment, particularly when connected to the criminal justice system in the form of legal coercion, can be very efficacious (Lukefield and Tims, 1988). Anglin (1988) found that legally or otherwise coerced treatment was just as effective as voluntary treatment. Individuals who are mandated to treatment may be more likely to adhere to and complete it. However, drop-outs in corrections-based programs still occur, ranging from 20–25% (Hiller, 1999; Wexler et al., 1999) to 50% or more (Martin et al., 1999). It is unclear, then, that even inmates feel coerced to complete treatment. They may enter treatment with the hope of making a good impression, but continuation appears to be a function of other influences. In one ongoing study, we asked the warden of the institution how inmates were coerced into the program. He indicated that those inmates who did not participate in programs were assigned to live in the less than desirable unit (dorm). We then asked the inmates the same question in focus groups, and were told that all dorms in the institution are less than desirable. They reported entering the program to impress the parole board, to kill time, or to try to improve their chances of release. Regardless of program format or type, most inmates who continued and completed treatment indicated that they did so because someone or something in the program got their attention. It may be the case that while coercion influences initial contact with treatment, continuation and completion are more a function of choice influenced by other circumstances.

Internal or External Providers?

Should treatment be provided by employees of the correctional system or by outside agencies? Some systems contract with public or private agencies in the community to provide services to inmates. Others use in-house staff to provide these services.

There are advantages to both approaches. The use of outside contractors is attractive to the inmates because they have "outsiders" with whom they can interact. Further, the staff are less likely to have their positions as treatment providers compromised by having to provide other staff functions for the institution. Another advantage of using outsourced treatment providers is that local community based agencies are usually more able than prison systems to attract staff who are knowledgeable about and well qualified to treat substance use disorders.

There are also disadvantages in outsourcing. The treatment providing staff may not understand the nuances of security maintenance, and may have difficulties sustaining appropriate boundaries for staff-inmate relationships. The use of outside contractors can exacerbate the common conflict between treatment and security personnel in the institution. Prison staff may dismiss treatment providers as outsiders who don't understand prisons and do not appreciate the custodial aspects of prisons. In this situation, prison staff can significantly undermine and sabotage treatment provision. In a for-profit health care market like the U.S., there can be unique disadvantages of hiring outside contractors. A contract tends to go to the lowest bidder, encouraging the provider to economize by thin staffing, and by hiring low-cost staff who are less experienced and temporary until a better paying job can be found.

An advantage of using in-house staff rests on their knowledge of the correctional environment and their ability to work with the prison bureaucracy to obtain resources. In addition, prison staff may have a better understanding of the dynamics of the prison population. They are less likely to be manipulated and disrupted by inmates and understand the avenues of remedy when an inmate acts out or attempts to manipulate them.

The use of prison staff to serve as treatment providers does not necessarily reduce the differences between security and treatment philosophies in place in the prison. The differences may be reduced if some individuals are promoted from correctional officer to counselor positions, but this also can have its disadvantages in that qualifications for the two positions are usually quite different. Resentments can be exacerbated if individuals are hired directly from the outside into higher-paying counselor positions.

As noted earlier, in-house treatment providers are subject to being called out of their duties for other prison functions. Also, it may be more difficult for in-prison treatment staff to facilitate the transition from prison to community that seems to be most effective (Martin et al., 1999; Wexler et al., 1999).

SUMMARY

There is strong evidence that substance abuse treatment in prisons can be effective in reducing the likelihood that an offender who is drug involved returns to prison. This is particularly true when the intervention includes a community based aftercare component. To some extent, the programs can also reduce the likelihood of the offender's return to substance abuse. One cost effectiveness study (Griffith et al., 1999) demonstrated that substance abuse treatment with aftercare is cost effective, particularly for the most serious offenders. It is thus an excellent idea to provide treatment to drug and alcohol abusing offenders who are incarcerated, as well as to those who are not.

That is not to say that prison and correctional aftercare are the ideal places in which to provide substance abuse treatment. The added costs of incarceration totaled over $24 billion in state and federal correctional spending in 1995 (Bureau of Justice Statistics, 2000a) for an average cost of $18,000 to incarcerate each inmate per year, rendering the prison treatment venue far more expensive than community based treatment. Further, there is evidence that the experience of incarceration has social costs that make prisons an even less desirable location for treatment. Once individuals have the experience of a friend or loved one going to prison, the social control impact of incarceration is reduced with those remaining behind (Clear and Rose, 1999).

Clearly prisons should not be the first choice venue for substance abuse treatment. There are substantial administrative and jurisdictional complications, and prisons are is not well suited to provide the continuity of care that has proven to be most effective. It is unlikely that any nation's prisons are ideally suited for substance abuse treatment. A truly continuous treatment program will require extensive planning efforts including the development of cooperative systems of care and information exchange among agencies. In any event, to intervene in prison is to intervene very late. Far preferable are prevention and treatment in the community. Indeed, prison is the treatment venue of last resort.

REFERENCES

Alcoholics Anonymous (1952). *Twelve Steps and Twelve Traditions.* New York: Alcoholics Anonymous World Services.

Alcoholics Anonymous (1976). *Alcoholics Anonymous (3rd ed.).* New York: Alcoholics Anonymous World Services.

Alemagno, S.A. (2001). Women in jail: Is substance abuse treatment enough? *American Journal of Public Health, 91,* 798–800.

Anglin, M.D. (1988). The efficacy of civil commitment in treating narcotic addiction. In C. Lukefeld and F. Tims (Eds.) *Compulsory Treatment of Drug Abuse: Research and Clinical Practice. NIDA Research Monograph 86.* Washington, D.C.: US Department of health and Human Services.

Beck, A.J., and Karberg, J.C. (2001). Prison and jail inmates at midyear 2000. *Bureau of Justice Statistics Bulletin.* Washington, D.C.: US Department of Justice.

Belenko, S. (1998). Research on drug courts: A critical review. *National Drug Court Institute Review, 1,* 1–42.

Bureau of Justice Statistics (2000a). *Sourcebook of Criminal Justice Statistics 1999.* Washington, D.C.: US Department of Justice.

Bureau of Justice Statistics (2000b). *1999 Annual Report on Drug Use Among Adult and Juvenile Arrestees.* Washington, D.C.: US Department of Justice.

Bureau of Justice Statistics (2001). *Contacts between Police and the Public: Findings from the 1999 National Survey.* Washington D.C.: US Department of Justice.

Carroll, K.M. (1998). Treating drug dependence: Recent advances and old truths. In W.R. Miller & N. Heather (Eds.). *Treating addictive behaviors* (2nd ed.). New York: Plenum Press.

Clear, T.R., and Rose, D.R. (1999) When neighbors go to jail: Impact on attitudes about formal and informal social control. *National Institute of Justice Research Preview.* Washington, D.C.: US Department of Justice.

Gendreau, P. (1996). Offender rehabilitation: What we know and what needs to be done. *Criminal Justice and Behavior, 24,* 144–161.

Gendreau, P., Goggin, C., and Law, M.A. (1996). Principles of effective assessment for community corrections. *Federal Probation, 60,* 64–70.

Gendreau, P., Little, T., and Goggin, C. (1996). A meta-analysis of the predictors of adult offender recidivism: What works! *Criminology, 34,* 575–607.

Glasser, W. (1976). *Positive Addictions.* New York: Harper and Row.

Griffith, J.D., Hiller, M.L., Knight, K., and Simpson, D.D. (1999). A cost-efectiveness analysis of in-prison therapeutic community treatment and risk classification. *The Prison Journal: An International Forum on Incarceration and Alternative Sanctions, 79,* 352–368.

Hester, R.K., and Miller, W.R. (in press). *Handbook of alcoholism treatment approaches: Effective alternatives* (3rd ed.). Boston: Allyn & Bacon.

Hiller, M.L., Knight, K., and Simpson, D.D. (1999). Risk factors that predict dropout from corrections-based treatment for drug abuse. *The Prison Journal: An International Forum on Incarceration and Alternative Sanctions, 79,* 411–430.

Hoffman, M.B. (2000). The drug court scandal. *North Carolina Law Review.* 78N.C.L. Rev. 1437.

Kadden, R., Carroll, K., Donovan, D., Cooney, N., Monti, P., Abrams, D., Litt, M., and Hester, R. (1992). *Cognitive-Behavioral Coping Skills Therapy Manual: A Clinical Research Guide for Therapists Treating Individuals With Alcohol Abuse and Dependence.* National Institute on Alcohol Abuse and Alcoholism, Project MATCH Monograph Series, Vol. 1. Washington, D.C.: US Department of Health and Human Services.

Kadden, R.M., Cooney, N.L., Getter, H., and Litt, M.D. (1989). Matching alcoholics to coping skills or interactional therapies: Posttreatment results. *Journal of Consulting and Clinical Psychology, 57,* 698–704.

Knight, K., Simpson, D.D., and Hiller, M.L. (1999). Three-year reincarceration outcomes for in-prison therapeutic community treatment in Texas. *The Prison Journal: An International Forum on Incarceration and Alternative Sanctions, 79*, 337–351.

Laundergan, J.C. (1982). *Easy Does It: Alcoholism Treatment Outcomes, Hazelden and The Minnesota Model.* Center City, MN: Hazelden.

Lipton, D.S. (1998). Treatment for drug abusing offenders during correctional supervision: A nationwide overview. *Journal of Offender Rehabilitation, 26*, 1–45.

Lipton, D.S., Martinson, R., and Wilks, J. (1975). *The Effectiveness of Correctional Treatment: A Survey of Treatment Evaluation Studies.* New York: Praeger.

Love, C., Shepard, D.S., Daley, M., White, K., and Petersen, C. (2000, November). *The cost-effectiveness of substance abuse treatment for inmates in Connecticut prisons.* Paper presented at the American Public Health Association meeting, Boston, MA.

Lukefeld, C.G., and Tims, F.M. (1988). Compulsory Treatment: A review of findings. In C. Lukefeld and F. Tims (eds.). *Compulsory Treatment of Drug Abuse: Research and Clinical Practice. NIDA Research Monograph 86.* Washington, D.C.: US Department of Health and Human Services.

Marlatt, G.A., and Gordon, J.R. (1985). Relapse prevention. In G.A. Marlatt and J.R. Gordon (eds.). *Relapse Prevention.* New York: Guilford.

Martin, S.S., Butzin, C.A., Saum, C.A., and Inciardi, J.A. (1999). Three-year outcomes of therapeutic community treatment for drug-involved offenders in Deleware. *The Prison Journal: An International Forum on Incarceration and Alternative Sanctions, 79*, 294–320.

Monti, P.M., Abrams, D.B., Kadden, R.M., and Cooney, N.L. (1989). *Treating alcohol dependence.* New York: Guilford Press.

Nowinski, J., Baker, S., and Carroll, K. (1992). *Twelve Step Facilitation Therapy Manual: A Clinical Research Guide for Therapists Treating Individuals With Alcohol Abuse and Dependence. National Institute on Alcohol Abuse and Alcoholism, Project MATCH Monograph Series, Vol. 1.* Washington, D.C.: US Department of Health and Human Services.

Martin, S.S., Clifford, B.A., Saum, C.A., and Inciardi, J.A. (1999). Three-year outcomes of therapeutic community treatment for drug-involved offenders in Delaware: From prison to work release to aftercare. *The Prison Journal: An International Forum on Incarceration and Alternative Sanctions, 79*, 294–320.

Pearson, F.S., and Lipton, D.S. (1999). A meta-analytic review of the effectiveness of corrections-based treatments for drug abuse. *The Prison Journal: An International Forum on Incarceration and Alternative Sanctions, 79*, 384–410.

Tonry, M. (1999, September). Reconsidering indeterminate and structured sentencing. *Sentencing & Corrections: Issues for the 21st Century.* Papers from the executive sessions on sentencing and corrections No.2. Washington, D.C.: US Department of Justice.

Tullis, L. (1995). *Unintended Consequences: Illegal Drugs & Drug Policies in Nine Countries.* London: Lynne Reinner Publishers.

Wexler, H.K., and Love, C.T. (1995). Therapeutic communities in prisons. In F. Tims, G. DeLeon, and N. Janechill (eds.). *The Therapeutic Community as a Treatment.* National Institute of Drug Abuse Research Monographs, 144. Washington, D.C. Supt. of Documents: US Government Printing Office.

Wexler, H.K., Melnick, G., Lowe, L., and Peters, J. (1999). Three-year reincarceration outcomes for Amity in-prison therapeutic community and aftercare in California. *The Prison Journal: An International Forum on Incarceration and Alternative Sanctions, 79*, 321–336.

CHAPTER 15

Missing Work

The Decline in Infrastructure and Support for Workplace Alcohol Intervention in the United States, with Implications for Developments in Other Nations

PAUL M. ROMAN

INTRODUCTION: LESSONS TO BE LEARNED

There is a worldwide search for settings in which to intervene with alcohol and drug problems before there has been substantial damage to individuals or their surrounding social and physical environments. The pioneering movement in the United States to utilize the workplace as a setting for alcohol problem intervention of this genre showed great promise in the 1970s and 1980s. Despite these powerful beginnings, the impact of workplace interventions on alcohol and drug abuse and attention to them by policy makers and scientists have declined markedly in recent years in the US. What has happened? Why has this happened? What can be learned from it?

It is not unusual to document the failure of attempted substance abuse interventions (Ennett et al., 1994; Mauss, 1991; Mauss et al., 1988). The history of substance abuse interventions is marked by repeated efforts to penetrate and harness the energies of major social institutions, such as the educational system, the family, leisure and recreation, and health care. Such institutional penetration and harnessing is distinct from "add-on" programming where external agencies supply staff and resources to augment what is already underway in an institutional setting. Usually efforts to integrate alcohol problem intervention

PAUL M. ROMAN • Center for Research on Behavioral Health and Human Services Delivery, University of Georgia, Athens, GA 30602

into the ordinary flow of activity fail. It is commonly concluded that if the intervention is going to succeed, augmented resources supported by external agencies must be added. Explanations for these shortfalls frequently center on the inadequacy of resources rather than institutional resistances.

The subject of this chapter is an instance where there was initial success in integrating an alcohol problem intervention through harnessing existing institutional energies, but then momentum slowed and faltered. The goal of this chapter is to describe and explain these developments, suggesting lessons to those outside the USA whose focus is upon the identification of alcohol problems and constructing interventions to ameliorate them in either the workplace or in other arenas.

While the decline of workplace utilization for employee alcohol problems has received almost no attention from the alcohol interventionist community, the importance of employed people as a target population can hardly be overstated. From an epidemiological perspective, it is clear that members of the workforce and their dependents easily comprise the largest segment of the population affected directly and indirectly by alcohol abuse. This generalization has worldwide application. Further, there can be no doubt that industrialization and the conduct of work within organizational and bureaucratic boundaries is quickly becoming the norm in many if not most of the world's nation-states. This underlines the diffusion and growth of the human resource management systems that were the foundation for the originally successful workplace intervention effort in the US.

Beyond some potential lessons from US experience for those championing other organizational bases for intervention and the importance of the workplace, this issue is embedded in an irony. This irony in turn may offer a further lesson. The evidence of workplace neglect of employee alcohol problems has emerged while the original vehicle for implementing such interventions has flourished. Over the past two decades workplace-based employee assistance programs (EAPs) have vastly grown in number in the USA, to the point that they can easily be called institutionalized practices (Blum et al., 1992; Hartwell et al., 1996). Further, EAPs are diffusing throughout much of the world with few apparent barriers, with particular growth in the United Kingdom and in nations with a British colonial heritage, including Ireland, Canada, Australia, and New Zealand. There are well developed descriptive materials on EAPs in South Africa (Maiden, 1999; Harper, 2000). Evidence of EAPs or structures very similar to them can also be found in Japan, Korea, Hong Kong, Taiwan, Thailand, Poland, Czech Republic and throughout South America, Scandinavia, and Western Europe (Masi, 2000; Heck, 1999; Klingemann et al., 1992). Unfortunately, a research-based literature centered on programs outside US boundaries does not yet exist, and much of the US database is moving toward obsolescence.

Drawing on these observations and several other bodies of evidence, this analysis asserts that the potential for workplace referrals of substance abusing employees remains, but the infrastructure for such use is being seriously neglected by policy makers, researchers and alcohol problem interventionists. The core of the chapter attempts to explain the observed developments by suggesting that constructive attention to alcohol and other substance abuse problems may be eclipsed when there are opportunities to use these resources for dealing with other, less stigmatized problems as well as problems that are less difficult to treat.

Contrary to other program themes common among substance abuse interventionists around the world, this analysis suggests caution about the concept of "mainstreaming." Specifically, it is argued that when the treatment of alcohol and drug problems is combined and intermingled with the treatment of other human difficulties, there is no assurance that ample attention to substance abuse issues will be sustained. Approaches that mainstream substance abuse treatment into broader interventions have many advantages over specialized programming, especially in terms of efficient service delivery as well as opportunities for comprehensive case management. It is also believed that mainstreaming will reduce stigma and integrate the treatment of alcohol and drug dependencies as "diseases like any other," the historic battle-cry of the constituencies fighting for this recognition. From the experience documented here however, it can be argued that mainstreaming can highlight the varying stigmas associated with different behavioral problems. The empirical indicators of this are the reluctances of the public, referral agents and treatment specialists to approach the stigmatized problems when they have options to direct their energies elsewhere. Thus it is further clear that close attention must be paid to including structures of advocacy and support within mainstreaming efforts in order to maintain a level of focus on alcohol and drug issues that reflects the prevalence of these problems within the target population.

FOCUSING AT THE ORGANIZATIONAL AND INSTITUTIONAL LEVEL

It is not unusual for substance abuse researchers to lament about inadequacies in the diffusion of interventions (Lamb et al., 1998). Once inadequate diffusion is identified, subsequent studies usually follow one of several traditional directions.

First is the effort to define those treatments that are the most "effective," with an assumption either stated or assumed that clients will be attracted to treatments that "work." Second is the study of what "motivates" clients to seek treatments, i.e. the factors which not only bring them to treatment but which generate a "readiness" to accept the direction that treatment has to offer. A third and related arena of study is treatment access, or bringing the opportunities for treatment into close proximity for those that need care. This bundle of issues not only includes questions about adequate levels of service, but also appropriate geographic distribution of treatment opportunities (Institute of Medicine, 1990).

More recently concern has begun to be centered on the issues of "moving from research to practice" (Lamb et al., 1998). Here the issues move away from the treatments and clients and begin to focus upon practitioners and the institutional settings where they work. The concern in this chapter about workplace programming is at this level, focusing on questions of the rise and fall of support for such programming at the managerial, organizational and institutional level. Such a focus defines the difference between the relatively new field of health services research and the more traditional foci of treatment research.

An underlying assertion, albeit unpopular for its pessimistic tone, is that the identification and treatment of alcohol and drug problems are a long way from being institutionalized within the basic structure of culture and values in the US. By definition, this limits the extent to which treatment of these problems can be realistically mainstreamed into both broader systems of service delivery.

Because the constructive management of substance abuse problems was so recently non-existent and/or embedded in systems of punishment and isolation, any indicator of progress can be interpreted as a "great leap forward." Because of this frame of reference, substance abuse specialists throughout the world seem overly optimistic about the amount of change that has occurred and the permanence of the perceived change. This optimism must be tempered by strong evidence of pervasive stigma throughout the service delivery system as well as in the broader culture.

Carefully collected national data in the US demonstrate that there is higher social acceptance of schizophrenics and seriously depressed persons than alcohol dependent persons (Martin et al., 2000). Fifty-six percent of a national sample of adult respondents reported that they were "definitely or probably" unwilling to interact with a person who was described in a hypothetical vignette as alcohol dependent, as compared to 48% unwilling to interact with a person described as schizophrenic and 37% unwilling to interact with a person described with the symptoms of major depression. These data clearly infer the kinds of behavior to be expected when opportunities arise for referral to treatment or post-treatment re-integration of an alcohol dependent individual.

Thus the lessons from the US for other nations is this: Until there is a level playing field with other human problems and disorders, it is essential that supportive infrastructure be developed and maintained to assure continuing attention to alcohol and drug problems in those settings where the opportunities to do so are present. The effective design of these infrastructures and strategies for their maintenance are key questions for health services research, but the experience with workplace programming in the US that is documented below clearly indicates that these infrastructures are essential.

It is suggested that these experiences generalize beyond the workplace, because there are a number of critical settings where mainstreaming is a structural fact rather than an intended consequence, and the social reactions and referral behaviors taken toward persons with alcohol and drug problems may have crucial implications.

Workplace approaches parallel efforts to enhance similar activity in four other settings that also embed "intimate impersonal contacts" with those potentially in need of changing their drinking behavior. This ingredient has been found to be critical in workplace intervention success (Trice & Beyer, 1984; Blum & Roman, 1995). Parallel settings embedding such contacts include primary medical care, welfare services, school systems and the criminal justice system. These institutional settings have in common the opportunity for others to obtain personal information and observe behavior in relatively intimate settings, but without creating the "sticky strings" of intimate personal relationships. People who enter these settings either voluntarily or involuntarily are expected to share a good deal of "private" information in order to fulfil their needs for services, and/or they come to share such information as they spend lengthy periods of time receiving care, being educated, working or passing time.

While the contacts involve sharing of much private information, they are also impersonal in terms of established boundaries of roles and identities. Norms and rules are clear about inappropriate degrees of intimacy and diffuse relationships between supervisors and subordinates, doctors and patients, social workers and clients, teachers and students, and criminal justice employees and their charges. These impersonal features of intimate relationships in institutional settings offer a sharp distinction with family and friendship relationships wherein privacy is also surrendered. This distinction describes why family members and friends are so notoriously inept as agents in the alcohol or drug problem referral process, with a major crisis usually required to provide the impetus to "do something." By contrast, the bounded relationships within the institutional settings can be much more effective at setting the stage for the beginnings of intervention.

Here is where we approach the key issues. Given the intervention potential within these intimate impersonal relationships, why do each of these five settings fall far short of this potential? To elucidate the arguments that have already been set forth, we turn to the story of EAPs in the US and some research evidence about their attention to alcohol problems.

THE BACKGROUND

In the early 1970s, a rapidly growing community of newly federally funded alcohol problem interventionists were hailing the workplace as the new frontier for making huge advances in solving America's alcohol problems (Roman, 1975). From an interventionist's perspective, the logic of this strategy is compelling: the workplace embeds not only a distinctive job-performance based definition for identifying alcohol problems but also the opportunity to retain control over the client through treatment and aftercare.

To address its initial charter as well as create a distinctive identity after it was founded in 1970, the leadership of the new National Institute on Alcohol Abuse and Alcoholism (NIAAA) saw promise in industrial alcoholism programs which been around in small numbers since the early 1940s. There was great excitement that a workplace focus could transform alcoholism programming from the limits of its prior identity and generate new and powerful constituency support. "Project 95" as it was dubbed by NIAAA, was oriented toward the 95 percent of American alcoholics who are in positions of employment and respectability, contrasted with the disaffiliated 5% on Skid Row that were believed to be the core of the alcoholism movement's cultural identity.

The EAP was more or less invented as NIAAA's version of the industrial alcoholism program, but with a critical change in design that has had dramatic implications over time. This change was that EAPs were designed to stretch beyond alcohol problem referrals in two distinctive ways: First, EAPs would receive **any** referral of an employee whose supervisor believed that she had a performance problem that was linked to a personal problem, or **any** self-referral of an employee who perceived that he had a problem that would benefit from EAP assistance. By casting this large net, the EAP was seen to generate alcohol problem referrals without stigmatizing the program and without requiring that supervisors select out particular types of employees for referral. Supervisors could "do their jobs" and just look for performance problems, not attempt to diagnose illness.

Key to making this program design effective in identifying substance abusers was the presence of a program coordinator who was specifically trained in substance abuse intervention and who could subtly enhance substance abuse referrals through supervisory training and publicity without detracting from the broad emphasis of the EAP. Thus, this program design was seen as having an ideal match with the ongoing process of supervisory management and job performance monitoring. As shall be seen however, the program design did not assure that an emphasis on substance abuse would be sustained.

As NIAAA promoted the diffusion of EAPs, it did not emphasize their mainstreaming design, but instead focused on their efficacy in identifying alcohol problems through the utilization of routine supervision and job performance evaluation practices. In service of "Project 95", EAPs were oriented to alcohol problems that were not dealt with properly or in adequate numbers in the past, namely the great numbers of "hidden alcoholics" in the American workplace. Through establishing identification and referral services in the workplace, opportunities for assistance were brought "close" to employed people. Greater utilization on the part of employed people with insurance coverage was expected on the basis of this proximity. This would in turn lead to a greater demand for privately-based treatment for alcohol problems, which was seen as upgrading the quality and quantity of alcohol treatment services by harnessing the entrepreneurial spirit of the private for-profit sector.

Through the 1970s, the NIAAA provided a substantial amount of support for demonstration projects wherein different models of EAP-type service delivery were developed. Through this project support, considerable funding was directed to the National Council on Alcoholism (NCA) which harnessed the interest and influence of many recovering alcoholics in executive and managerial positions in the workplace. Thus through both direct and indirect federal funding, EAP development which included a strong alcohol intervention emphasis proceeded with considerable energy.

Since such projects required a governmental base, NIAAA (and, somewhat later, NIDA) specifically devoted personnel and resources to workplace issues. Through these offices, encouragement for research as well as demonstration projects flowed, and the two types of funding were often combined. Academics were also given many opportunities for involvement in consultation and training as the government encouraged the continuing development of the workplace as a significant base for substance abuse referrals.

At the beginning of the 1980s, funding for demonstration efforts came to a close, and the newly-elected conservative administration essentially withdrew all federal support for behavioral health service delivery as well as strongly discouraging social research. Since much of the federal support had helped sustain a substance abuse focus within EAPs, these changes clearly had an impact on the focus of EAPs. No longer was there the possibility of grant support for service delivery, subsidized attendance of EAP staff at NIAAA conferences and workshops, or indirect federal support for a national EAP association.

The withdrawal of these incentives coincided with the rise of public and workplace interest in work-family conflict issues and the promotion of these dimensions of EAPs' service delivery potential began to be emphasized. Programs moved much more toward a model of receiving self-referrals and toward providing companies with responses to emergent issues such as employees infected with HIV virus or, in more recent years, downsizing and workplace violence.

What has happened to the level of interest within the funding agencies? The removal of support for demonstration projects had an overall impact on both NIAAA and NIDA in terms of transforming them into research institutes. This identity was underlined by their absorption into the National Institutes of Health in 1990. This did not produce the outcome that some had expected, namely a disappearance of behavioral science research or of research oriented toward issues of treatment and prevention. But over time the emphasis on workplace research has gradually deteriorated to the point that research about EAPs as a mechanism for substance abuse intervention has practically disappeared.

EVIDENCE OF DECLINE OF EAP UTILIZATION FOR ALCOHOL PROBLEMS

Because there is practically no research currently underway that focuses upon workplace interventions for alcohol problems, evidence about declining use is largely inferential. Using two data sources that are described in greater detail below, we have found that when examining a national sample of persons who have used EAP services in their workplaces in 1993 and in 1997, there is a significant decline in the reported abstinence from alcohol within the overall user population. This inference is distal, but it is contrary to secular trends in alcohol use and thus may be a sound indicator of a significant drop in EAP utilization for alcohol problems.

Second, within the panels in our national data set, we note a decline over time in supervisory satisfaction with the outcome associated with EAP referrals that they have made of subordinates. Alcohol and drug problem referrals tend to be significantly more likely the result of supervisory action rather than self-referral, and thus this points inferentially toward a drop in what might be both the quality and quantity of EAP services for substance abusing employees.

Third, at the University of Georgia and Georgia Institute of Technology we have been conducting a longitudinal study of a carefully drawn national sample of 400 private substance abuse treatment centers. In 1995 the administrators of these centers were asked in personal interviews about the number of EAPs with which they have referral relationships, revealing an average across the entire treatment center sample of 7.05 EAPs. This question was repeated in 1998, showing a dramatic drop to an average of 2.53 EAPs. Equally dramatic are data indicating the mean proportion of referrals from workplace sources. In early 1996, this proportion was 21.1%, but by 1998 it had dropped to 8.75%.

Fourth, an examination of the publications and conferences directed toward EAP workers indicate little if any emphasis on substance abuse issues other than information or instruction about conformity to federal regulations regarding the testing of certain categories of employees for alcohol and drugs.

Fifth, informal interviews with EAP workers indicate that nearly all have moved to a model emphasizing short-term counseling rather than referral into the community. In these interviews it is reported that few employees with alcohol or drug problems are now referred to the EAP. These short-term counseling efforts are alleged by some to serve as means for reducing use of community treatment resources and thus reducing overall health care costs. Such efforts may be effective (Bien, Miller, & Tonigan, 1993), but they have not been subject to empirical study in EAP settings.

THE DISAPPEARING AND LOST INFRASTRUCTURE

As mentioned, the research activity associated with workplace interventions has largely disappeared, with the exception of a small set of studies funded by the Center for Substance Abuse Prevention that are currently being phased out. It is reasonable to assume that there is a significant relationship between the amount of research conducted on workplaces as referral sources for substance abuse treatment and the vitality of that area of activity. There is clear evidence that a moderately active research network existed over the past two decades, but has now practically ceased to exist.

A review of the CRISP database that includes research grants previously funded by the National Institutes of Health (NIH) indicates 25 major studies concerned with EAPs that were funded between 1972 and 1999. All of these studies were funded by either the NIAAA or NIDA. Nearly all of the principal investigators are deceased or have left active research careers.

This level of activity has dropped dramatically. Despite what appears to be an obvious relevance for alcohol, drug abuse, and mental health concerns, a search of the NIH's inventory of currently funded research studies (including only those classified as "R01" grants) reveals only a single research project which includes mention of employee assistance or EAP in its abstract. In this instance, the study is not directly concerned with substance abuse, but with the extent to which the presence of EAPs reduces workplace injuries (PI, Dr. Ted Miller, Pacific Institute of Research and Evaluation, Bethesda, MD).

The literature about EAPs is not growing, either in relation to substance use or utilization for other personal problems. A review of current social science and management databases indicates very few publications since 1998 topically identified as focused upon "employee assistance" or EAPs. Among the few that are found, sound empirical data are typically absent, with most studies involving a single organizational case or samples of questionable generalizability. In 1999 an impressive-looking volume entitled *The Employee Assistance Handbook* appeared (Oher, 1999). While there is some mention of research techniques that might be utilized to evaluate EAPs, this large volume is otherwise devoid of reviews of research findings or the evaluation of evidence about various EAP practices. Perhaps needless to say, the near-absence of funded research offers a ready explanation for the lack of growth in research literature about EAPs.

THE REMAINING INFRASTRUCTURE AND POTENTIAL PAYOFFS

A substantial infrastructure to support EAP services for substance abusers is still in place. We draw upon two data sets to demonstrate this potential. The first is a series of national sample surveys of employed persons conducted by the University of Georgia and Georgia Institute of Technology in 1993 and 1997, with a new survey currently in the field in 2001. These data demonstrate the accessibility of EAPs to the workforce, the extent of employee utilization of them, and satisfaction with such use.

The 1993 data indicate that 47.4% of respondents reported that their organization provided an EAP, a figure that increased significantly to 57.8% in 1997. When asked in 1993 if respondents would seek help for themselves or a family member from the EAP if they had a problem of the type dealt with by an EAP, 48.5% reported that this was "very likely," and 10.2% indicated that such utilization was "very unlikely." Comparable figures of 45.3% and 12.6% were found for these two response categories when the same question was asked in 1997.

A more specific question centered on whether respondents would use their EAP if they or a member of their family developed a problem with drugs. In 1993, 40.8% reported they would be "very likely" to use EAP services under these circumstances, while 15.1% indicated they would be "very unlikely" to do so. The 1997 data were nearly identical, with 41.1% reporting utilization of the EAP to be "very likely" and 17.3% indicating it would be "very unlikely"

The 1993 data indicated that 12.8% of the respondents had used the EAP for assistance for a problem of their own. Of these, 52.4% reported that the EAP services were "very helpful" and 9.7% reported that they were "not helpful at all." The level of individual use was essentially unchanged at 12.7% in 1997, with a nearly identical 52.8% reporting that EAP services were very helpful and 5% indicating that they were not helpful at all.

In 1993, 8.6% of the respondents reported that they had used EAP services for assistance with a problem affecting a family member. Of these, 44.7% reported that the EAP services were "very helpful" while 10.6% indicated that they were "not helpful at all." In the 1997 survey, this usage changed little, with 7.8% reporting utilization for a family member, 50% reporting the services to be "very helpful" and 6.1% indicating that they were not helpful at all.

The 1993 survey indicated that 19.7% of the respondents with supervisory responsibilities had utilized EAP services for a problem affecting a subordinate. Of these respondents, 41.8% reported that the EAP services were "very helpful" and 6.6% indicated that they were "not helpful at all." In the 1997 survey, this figure had dropped slightly, with 15.7% of the supervisors reporting that they had used the EAP to deal with a subordinate's problem. Those reporting that the services were "very helpful" also dropped to 35% while only 3.8% indicated that the services provided "were not helpful at all."

It is possible to calculate overall utilization rates from the above data. Cross-tabulating these respondents to eliminate multiple users, the data indicate that 21.8% of the 1993 sample had used the EAP either for themselves, a family member, or for a subordinate among those who were supervisors. A similar figure of 20.8% is found in the parallel analysis for 1997.

These data are impressive to the extent that they demonstrate extensive access to EAPs across American workplaces. The data indicate that nearly half of the respondents express a readiness to use the EAP if needed, and about 40 percent would specifically use the EAP for assistance with a drug problem. Further, these national data indicate that EAPs are apparently quite accessible, and are used for personal problems, problems among family members, and problems with workplace subordinates. While an interpretation should be cautious, these data indicate that satisfaction with services is least when supervisors refer subordinates to EAPs. Further, there is a modest trend in the direction of declining satisfaction with these services.

These employee surveys do not provide information on the types of problems dealt with through the EAP, and we can consider their relevance to employee substance abuse only inferentially. However, the potential of EAPs in dealing with employee substance abuse is documented in a second data set which is based upon 6,400 first-time referrals to a sample of 84 EAPs from whom data were collected in 1990–1992. These data are used to describe characteristics of the caseload of employed substance abusers that were referred to workplace EAPs.

Of the 6,400 EAP referrals, a total of 1,185 or 18.5% were found to score 2 or more on the CAGE index, generally accepted as a measure of alcohol problems. Of these, 45.1% scored 2, 33.4% scored 3 and 21.4% scored 4. The latter group, comprising 254 cases or 4% of the total EAP caseload, would be regarded as severely alcohol dependent.

Of this total group, 73.9% were white, 20.1% were African-American and 6% were in other ethnic categories. Of this group, 47.6% were married, 21.2% had never married, and 29.3% were separated or divorced. Modal income was $31,000 per year, with 14.2% over $50,000 and 7.1% under $15,000. Modal education level was high school graduate, with 5.4% having a master's or doctorate, and 4.3% less than high school.

The most common route of referral of these individuals to the EAP was a self-referral, reported by 40.8%. Another 28.6% entered the EAP via a formal or informal supervisory referral, 11.4% came by peer referral and 7.4% by family referral.

Following the initial evaluation, the EAP coordinator provided a prognosis for the individual's recovery. For this group, 17.3% were given an "excellent prognosis," 50.1% were assigned "good," 26.5% "fair" and 6.1% "poor." Of greater workplace relevance, the EAP coordinator also gave a prognosis for the individual's resumption of adequate job performance. Here 29.9% were rated "excellent," 45.6% were rated "good," 19.4% were rated "fair" and 5% were rated "poor."

Perhaps of the greatest interest, and demonstrating EAP efficacy, is follow-up data indicating that 75.8% of those in this group were still employed at a one-year follow-up, indicating a reasonable pattern of rehabilitation. For those working, 26% indicated that they had an "excellent" pattern of job performance, with 51.1% saying their performance was above average, 20.5% indicating an average performance, and 2.5% below average.

WHAT NEEDS TO BE DONE

The infrastructure surrounding workplace intervention is partially in place but partially needs to be reconstructed. Of equal importance is training EAP operatives in the basics of substance abuse intervention. From the perspective of the substance abuse treatment system, the problematic issues include:

1. Educating the key personnel in these referral sources to identify the signs and symptoms of alcohol and drug dependency.
2. Educating these personnel in the steps that can be taken to refer these individuals to substance abuse treatment.
3. Motivating these personnel to actually take these referral steps, i.e., creating an orientation that substance abuse treatment has legitimacy, i.e., that it is congruent with their own professional commitments to the outcomes that are sought for the client.

While not applying to all of these referral sources, a fourth issue is to motivate the agents in these settings to minimize their own efforts to engage in behavior change with these substance abusing clients, and to appropriately refer them to experts. The brief interventions currently being used by EAP specialists have not been researched and are not understood. They may have greater efficacy than would be expected, but it is unlikely that they would work well if the specialists are not receiving any form of substance abuse-specific training.

Finally, it is critical for the leaders in substance abuse intervention to re-open the dialogue that they once had with key leaders in business and industry. These channels have been closed for decades, perhaps on the assumption that stigma had disappeared and that EAPs could be counted upon to take care of themselves. More evidence is needed to confirm the strengths and weaknesses of the current infrastructures, but it is clear that other nations can learn much from what happens when governmental support for substance abuse intervention is withdrawn.

This description and data presentation may be seen as a "case study" from which those in other nations can learn. There is inferential and anecdotal information that many of the same trends seen in the US are evident in other nations, namely that EAPs have emerged with an initial focus on alcohol and drug abuse, but have been quickly drawn to other concerns. Given the extent to which the patterns of work organization and systems of human resource management in newer and newly emerging economies take on features of Western capitalism, there is every reason to expect that a similar pattern of trends away from a substance abuse emphasis will occur.

Earlier in this chapter it was suggested that an emphasis on substance abuse within work-based problem intervention programs cannot be sustained without an infrastructure that emphasizes the importance and value of dealing with substance abuse through these mechanisms. A parallel argument applies to any other effort which taps into educational, religious, criminal justice, welfare or health care systems where there is an effort to couple an emphasis on substance abuse with the kinds of people-processing activities that have already been institutionalized. It is exciting to see data which indicates that professionals and service providers in these systems will attend to substance abuse issues when they are given special training or support to do so, but it is risky and probably fallacious to assume that the interest and activity toward substance abuse will continue after these supports are reduced or removed.

The case presented here offers some tentative prescriptions for how attention to workplace substance abuse might be rejuvenated in the US. There is no suggestion that these same suggestions would work in another culture or nation, but at the same time there is optimism that the overall strategy has merit. Research and international consultation can serve to produce blueprints for how these systems might be adapted in a particular culture and nation. The critical point is that in the US and around the world, we are far from the day when substance abuse interventions "can take care of themselves" within our existing institutions.

REFERENCES

Bien, T. H., Miller, W. R. & Tonigan, J. S. (1993). Brief interventions for alcohol problems: A review. *Addiction* 88: 315–336.

Blum, T. C. & Roman, P. M. (1989). Employee assistance programming and human resources management. In K. Rowland & G. Ferris, eds. *Research in Personnel and Human Resources Management*, Vol. 7, Greenwich, CT: JAI Press.

Blum, T. C. & Roman, P. M. (1995). *The cost effectiveness and preventive implications of employee assistance programs.* Washington, DC: Monograph No. 5 of the Center on Substance Abuse Prevention, US Department of Health and Human Services.

Blum, T. C., Martin, J. K. & Roman, P. M. (1992). A research note on EAP prevalence, components and utilization. *Journal of Employee Assistance Research* 1: 201–229.

Ennett, S., Tobler, N., Ringwalt, C. & Flewelling, R. (1994). How effective is drug abuse resistance education? A meta-analysis of project DARE outcome evaluations. *American Journal of Public Health* 84: 1394–1401.

Evans, B. L. & Trice, H. M. (1995). Acceptance and implementation of EAP core and non-core tasks. *Journal of Drug Issues* 25: 379–385.

Goffman, E. (1963). *Asylums.* New York: Doubleday.

Hartwell, T., Steele, P., French, M. T., Potter, F. J., Rodman, N. F. & Zarkin, G. A. (1996). Aiding troubled employees: the prevalence, cost and characteristics of employee assistance programs in the United States. *American Journal of Public Health* 86: 804–808.

Harper, Tracy. (2000). South Africa, pp. 313–325 in D. Masi (ed.) *International Employee Assistance Anthology*, 2nd edition. Washington, D.C.: Dallen, Inc.

Heck, P. (1999). The evolving role of EAPs in managed behavioral health care: a case study of DuPont. pp. 291–304 in J. Oher (ed.). *The employee assistance handbook.* New York: John Wiley and Sons.

Institute of Medicine. (1990). *Broadening the base for treatment of alcohol problems.* Washington: National Academy Press.

Klingemann, H., Takala, J. & Hunt, G. (eds.). (1992). *Cure, care or control: alcoholism treatment in sixteen countries.* Albany: State University of New York Press.

Lamb, S., Greenlick, M. & McCarty, D. (1998). *Bridging the gap between practice and research: forging partnerships with community based drug and alcohol treatment.* Washington, D.C.: National Academy Press.

Martin, J., Pescosolido, B. & Tuch, S. (2000). Of fear and loathing: the role of "disturbing behavior" labels and causal attriutions in shaping public attitudes toward persons with mental illness. *Journal of Health and Social Behavior* 41: 208–233.

Masi, D. (ed.) (2000). *International employee assistance anthology*, 2nd edition. Washington, D.C.: Dallen, Inc.

Mauss, A. (1991). Science, social movements and cynicism: appreciating the political context of sociological research in alcohol studies. pp. 187–204 in P. Roman (ed.). *Alcohol: the development of sociological perspectives on use and abuse.* New Brunswick, NJ: Publications Division of the Center on Alcohol Studies, Rutgers University.

Mauss, A., Hopkins, R., Weisheit, R. & Kearney, K. (1988). The problematic prospects for prevention in the classroom: should alcohol education programs be expected to reduce drinking by youth? *Journal of Studies on Alcohol* 49: 51–61.

McClellan, K. (1989). Counseling as part of an EAP. *Employee Assistance Quarterly* 4: 67–70.

Roman, P. M. (1975). Secondary prevention of alcoholism: the potential of occupational programs. *Journal of Drug Issues* 8: 345–365.

Roman, P. M. (1981). From employee alcoholism to employee assistance: an analysis of the deemphasis on prevention and on alcoholism problems in work-based programs. *Journal of Studies on Alcohol* 42: 244–272.

Roman, P. M. & Blum, T. C. (1985). The core technology of employee assistance programs. *The ALMACAN* 8: 11–18.

Roman, P. M. & Blum, T. C. (1995). Contrasts and complements between employee assistance and health promotion programs in the workplace, in D. DeJoy & M. Wilson (eds.). *Critical issues in worksite health promotion*. Boston: Allyn-Bacon.

Scott, W. R. (1998). *Institutions and organizations*. Beverly Hills, CA: Sage Publishers.

Trice, H. & Beyer, J. (1984). Work-related outcomes of constructive confrontation strategies in a job-based alcoholism program. *Journal of Studies on Alcohol* 45: 393–404.

CHAPTER 16

Intervening through Social Support Networks

JANE ELLEN SMITH, DENISE LAFRAMBOISE, AND JOYCE BITTINGER

THE NEED TO WORK THROUGH CONCERNED SIGNIFICANT OTHERS

Individuals with alcohol and drug disorders are notorious for being unmotivated as far as addressing their substance abuse problems (Institute of Medicine, 1990). Researchers estimate that more than 80% of people with addictions are not ready to take preliminary steps to change (Snow, Prochaska, & Rossi, 1992). Fortunately there are now specific interventions that can successfully work with people's ambivalent feelings about modifying their addictive behavior, such as motivational interviewing (Miller & Rollnick, 1991). Once these individuals are willing to question their problem behaviors, a host of empirically-backed treatments are available; *none* of which can be utilized though if the substance-abusing individual never presents for treatment.

Interestingly, people who abuse alcohol or drugs often report that the decision to finally pursue treatment was prompted either by the direct influence of concerned significant others (CSOs), or by CSOs acting in concert with courts, employee assistance programs, or informal social networks (Cunningham, Sobell, Sobell, & Kapur, 1995). These CSOs' persuasive efforts are motivated, in part, by the desire to help a loved one. Additionally, CSOs hope to get relief from some of their many alcohol- or drug-related stressors, such as domestic violence, sexual problems, social embarrassment, financial or legal difficulties, and disrupted relationships with the children (Jacob, Krahn, & Leonard, 1991; Paolino & McCrady, 1977; Romijn, Platt, Schippers, & Schaap, 1992; Velleman et al., 1993). Chronic exposure to these stressors results in symptoms of depression, anxiety, somatic complaints, and anger for the CSOs themselves (Brown,

JANE ELLEN SMITH, DENISE LAFRAMBOISE, AND JOYCE BITTINGER • Department of Psychology, University of New Mexico, Albuquerque, New Mexico 87131

Kokin, Seraganian, & Shields, 1995; Collins, Leonard, & Searles, 1990; Spear & Mason, 1991).

LOCATING CSOs OF SUBSTANCE ABUSING INDIVIDUALS

It is estimated that for every individual with an alcohol problem, there are five others who suffer directly (Paolino & McCrady, 1977). And given that 60–80% of illicit drug users either live with their parents or engage in daily contact with them (Stanton, 1982), one could surmise that the "suffering" applies to these families as well. At first glance this may seem disheartening. But one must consider that empirical evidence (presented below) supports the fact that many CSOs can be trained to influence the drinker or drug user to enter treatment. So the positive "spin" is that there is no shortage of potential CSOs with whom to work as an indirect method for reaching the substance abusing individual; the "identified patient" (IP).

Although a number of the CSO interventions to be reviewed typically have been delivered in the context of addiction or mental health facilities, there is no reason why this practice cannot be modified to suit the needs of particular communities. However, operating outside of these specialty centers does present at least one obstacle: where and how to locate potential CSOs. As a starting point, one should recall that CSOs often experience a host of psychological and physical symptoms as a result of the stressors in their lives. In reality, many individuals are regularly being seen within a variety of public agencies for problems that could largely be the result of having a loved one at home who is abusing substances. Examples of possible locales for identifying these CSOs follow.

Religious Settings

A large 20-year survey reported that 40% of Americans had sought a clergy member for assistance with personal problems (Veroff, Kulks, & Douvan, 1981). Is it conceivable that a significant number of these individuals were the CSOs of people with addiction problems? The evidence suggests it is, since the clergy often counsel people with the types of emotional problems experienced by distraught CSOs (e.g., depression, anxiety, marital conflict; Larson et al., 1988). So it is safe to assume that the clergy are having contact with at least some of these CSOs, and could be instrumental in working with them to get resistant substance abusers into treatment.

Domestic Violence Shelters and Emergency Departments

Substance abuse and domestic violence go hand-in-hand. For violent crimes in which the offender was a current or former intimate partner of the victim, two-thirds of the offenders were under the influence of alcohol during the attack (Greenfeld, 1998). When female cases in an emergency department were divided into those who were intentionally injured by a male partner and those who were not, the male perpetrators were four times as likely to have used illicit drugs (Kyriacou et al., 1999). Unfortunately, inquiries about the violence (let alone the associated substance abuse) are rarely made by health care practitioners, and the victims do not routinely volunteer this information (B. Miller, Wilsnack, & Cunradi, 2000). So an opportunity is being missed in emergency departments and domestic violence shelters to begin working with the readily accessible CSOs (of substance abusers in the majority of cases) in an effort to influence their IPs to enter treatment. Perhaps emergency department staff could begin administering a screening protocol that has been developed for health care practitioners to assess physical abuse (Council on Scientific Affairs, 1992; also see chapter by Schermer in this volume). Victims of violence in either setting could then be given brief alcohol and drug screening instruments to complete for the perpetrators (see next section).

Health Care Facilities

Not only do the CSOs of drinkers or drug users often find themselves in emergency rooms, but so do the individuals with the substance abuse problems themselves. A survey in England showed that increased alcohol consumption was associated with increased emergency health care (Cryer, Jenkins, Cook, & Ditchburn, 1999). Given that one would expect a sizeable number of CSOs to accompany their IPs to the emergency room, it might be reasonable to have the medical staff probe CSOs about the potential role of substance abuse if the IP him- or herself was uncooperative. A variety of screening instruments are available (see Babor & Higgins-Biddle, 2000) which could easily be modified so that CSOs could describe their IPs' use. Intervention options could then be offered to CSOs if indicated.

Interestingly, elevated usage of non-emergency medical resources is found for families in which there is a substance abusing individual when compared to families in which there is not, and this difference remains when the alcohol treatment costs are excluded (Holder & Blose, 1986). The implication is that family members are seeking medical care for conditions related to the IP's use. This provides further support for the suggestion that health care practitioners should screen CSOs for family addiction problems, and intervene accordingly.

The Workplace

Employee Assistance Programs have been recognized as a resource for employees with addiction problems for some time now, but they are actually a viable mechanism for identifying the CSOs of substance abusing individuals as well (see chapter by Roman in this volume). The same may be said for the new Employee Wellness Programs (EWPs), which provide health risk appraisals upon reviewing an individual's lifestyle (Cook, Back, & Trudeau, 1996). It would be easy to add pertinent questions to these appraisals about family lifestyle concerns as well, and in that manner eventually gain access to IPs through the CSOs. One innovative EWP program is also offering substance abuse awareness classes to supervisors and workers (Lapham, Chang, & Gregory, 2000). These would be ideal opportunities to describe programs for CSOs with the objective of IP engagement.

Education Systems

CSOs can be reached through educational systems in several ways. Periodically teachers observe cognitive, social, and emotional behavior patterns that are suggestive of a drug-abusing home environment (Greenberg, 1999/2000). In the course of investigating the situation, the teacher ideally would locate a non-using family member or guardian to serve as a CSO. It may also be possible to reach the CSOs of substance-abusing individuals through special classes offered to the community. For example, alcohol and drug issues relevant to CSOs could be covered in courses more broadly entitled "parenting" or "violence/trauma" classes (Ananth, 1999). And since most colleges now have programs devoted to substance abuse issues on campus (Wechsler, Kelley, Weitzman, San Giovanni, & Seibring, 2000), these could be enhanced to meet the needs of CSOs as well. For instance, freshmen orientation could contain basic information regarding how the CSOs of peers with substance abuse problems should respond.

The Legal System

It is important to note that CSOs do not necessarily have to be family members or friends of the individual with the substance abuse problem, albeit they typically are. With this said, one might look to the legal system to identify non-traditional CSOs. Importantly, such CSOs would have to be willing to try to influence a substance-abusing individual to seek treatment or reduce use without resorting to punitive means. Child welfare workers might be good candidates, as they often are involved in family cases in which parental substance use has resulted in children being removed from the home (Hohman & Butt, 2001). Of course, the feasibility of such a plan would depend on the quality of the relationship between the child welfare worker and the parents. Family advocates are possible candidates, since in their role as coordinators of family services within the community and the court, they have the potential to develop healthy relationships with families involved in legal difficulties (Tiktin & Mazorol, 1999). Lastly, given the extremely high rate of drug abuse among juvenile arrestees, there is a need for novel intervention models (Terry, VanderWaal, McBride, & Van Buren, 2000). Perhaps one option would be to train "recovered" and "rehabilitated" juveniles to be CSOs for their peers.

PROGRAM OPTIONS FOR CSOs

Overview

Historically there have been limited options for CSOs who want to impact their loved one's addiction problem. The traditional programs will be reviewed first, followed by the more recently developed ones. They are clustered according to their basic belief about the CSO's role:

1. Lovingly Detach from the Substance Abusing Individual and Take Care of Yourself

(a) Al-Anon/Nar-Anon

Description. Since the 1950s, innumerable CSOs have turned to Al-Anon or Nar-Anon (Al-Anon Family Groups, 1984) when seeking outside assistance for their distress over a substance abusing loved one. In fact, Al-Anon is considered to be the largest program in the world for the family members of heavy drinkers (Whitfield, 1984). Al-Anon and Nar-Anon are programs for CSOs that are modeled after A.A. (Alcoholics Anonymous) and N.A. (Narcotics Anonymous). They are rooted in a disease model of alcoholism and addiction. Al-Anon members are encouraged to accept several principles: (1) family members must practice "loving detachment," which entails not trying to change the behavior of the substance abuser, (2) CSOs must work on their own independence and self-esteem, and (3) CSOs must accept the fact that they need the spiritual strength of a higher power (Al-Anon Family Groups, 1984).

Al-Anon meetings appear similar in format throughout the world. A partner's version of the A.A. Serenity Prayer opens the meeting, which is followed by the chair reading an adapted version of the 12 steps. The chair reminds members that the substance abuser is *not* the subject of the meeting's discussion. An invited speaker may present a short talk. There is open discussion of personal experiences and coping strategies (Barber & Gilbertson, 1997).

Empirical Support. As explained in subsequent sections, involvement of CSOs in Al-Anon has not routinely resulted in the entry of drinkers into treatment, particularly when contrasted with other procedures' success rates (Barber & Gilbertson, 1996; Miller, Meyers, & Tonigan, 1999; Sisson & Azrin, 1986). One study randomly assigned 23 wives of drinkers to either 8 weeks of Al-Anon or to a delayed treatment. A total of 48% of the drinkers had begun treatment by the 1-year follow-up, but since the control condition had also been treated by then, it was impossible to determine if differences were due to Al-Anon (Dittrich & Trapold, 1984). Some have argued that the overall lack of treatment engagement for Al-Anon is not surprising, since 12-step programs do not typically advocate engagement efforts. Still, when Al-Anon was specifically modified to add this objective, it was not successful at accomplishing it (Meyers, Miller, Smith, & Tonigan, 2001; Miller et al., 1999). Participation in Al-Anon *does* often result in improved psychosocial functioning for CSOs (Barber & Gilbertson, 1996; Dittrich & Trapold, 1984; Meyers et al., 2001; Miller et al., 1999).

In summary, although there is some empirical evidence of Al-Anon's ability to improve the psychosocial functioning of CSOs, it does not appear to be instrumental in decreasing the substance use of IPs or in getting them to enter treatment. Also, it does not appear to be a viable treatment choice for CSOs who are unwilling to emotionally detach from their IPs.

2. Prepare for a Single, Dramatic Confrontation in an Effort to Get the Substance Abusing Individual into Treatment

(a) Johnson Institute Intervention

Description. The Johnson Institute intervention involves orchestrating a confrontational "surprise party" with members of the substance abusing individual's social network (Johnson, 1986). A therapist oversees the planning stages for this meeting, including the writing of testimonials. These letters contain a profession of love for the IP, a statement about the stress caused by the substance use, and either a request or a mandate for the IP to get help. Oftentimes CSOs are encouraged to commit to strong consequences (e.g., divorce, employment termination) should the IP choose not to enter treatment. The CSOs then practice the presentation of the testimonials, and in theory follow through with the group confrontation.

Empirical Support. Studies of the Johnson Institute intervention have demonstrated that for families who actually confronted the drinker, the rate of treatment engagement was high (Liepman, Nirenberg, & Begin, 1989; Logan, 1983; Loneck, Garrett, & Banks, 1996a; Miller et al., 1999). Unfortunately, the percentage of families who followed through with the planned confrontation typically was low. Specifically, when Liepman and colleagues (1989) trained 24 "social networks" of drinkers in the intervention, only 29% of them carried out the confrontation. So although there was an 86% engagement rate for the seven families who completed the intervention, the overall success rate was only 24%. A more recent study found a similarly low engagement rate (30%) using the Johnson intervention (Miller et al., 1999).

In summary, the Johnson Institute intervention may not be suited for many families or friends, simply because the method is objectionable to them due to its perceived aversiveness (Barber & Gilbertson, 1997). Furthermore, there is some evidence that relapse is more likely for individuals who receive more confrontational approaches (Loneck, Garrett, & Banks, 1996b).

3. Learn Skills and Strategies to Influence the Substance Abusing Individual's Drinking/Drug Use, to Get that Person into Treatment, and to Take Care of Yourself

(a) Thomas's unilateral family therapy

Description. A more recent approach for responding to CSOs of problem drinkers, unilateral family therapy (UFT), focuses not only on getting IPs into treatment and decreasing their drinking, but also on providing CSO support. It involves teaching CSOs skills to improve their coping and to facilitate sobriety for the substance user. UFT begins with an assessment of the IP's drinking habits and the CSO's reaction. "Role induction" modules are used to explore better ways to respond to the drinking. UFT incorporates either a programmed confrontation, reminiscent of the Johnson intervention, or a timed "programmed request" to encourage the IP to enter treatment. As far as the CSO's own well-being, time is devoted to discussing emotional problems and the need for some independence from the IP (Thomas & Ager, 1993).

Empirical Support. In the first of two studies to examine UFT, 62% of drinkers whose CSOs were in the UFT condition either entered treatment or reduced their drinking by a minimum of 53% (Thomas, Santa, Bronson, & Oyserman, 1987). The no-treatment controls showed neither of these improvements. In the second study, Thomas and Ager (1993) demonstrated significantly higher rates of treatment engagement for IPs if their CSOs received UFT. This was reduced to a trend at 18 months. With regard to other measures of success, drinkers with CSOs in the UFT group decreased their alcohol use across follow-ups by 68%, as compared to only 20% for controls. CSOs also experienced some improvements in psychological functioning, but it was unclear whether these findings were statistically significant.

Thomas's UFT findings should be interpreted cautiously due to nonrandom group assignment. Also, outcome strength was not always clear, since the percent of treatment-engaged individuals was often combined with the percent who had reduced their drinking. Generalizability issues must be raised as well, since this form of UFT has routinely been done only with spouses as CSOs, and with drinkers (as opposed to illicit drug users) as the IPs.

(b) Pressures to change

Description. The Australian "pressures to change" (PTC) program is a somewhat similar UFT approach that utilizes gradually increased pressure on the IP to change (Barber & Crisp, 1995). The first level is an explanation about the need for pressure from the drinker's environment in order for change to occur. The difference between pressure and nagging is discussed. The second level of pressure entails having CSOs identify their IP's typical drinking times, so that activities incompatible with drinking can be substituted. Level three involves having CSOs examine their usual responses to the drinking to ascertain whether they are inadvertently rewarding intoxicated behavior. CSOs also are taught how to give the IP feedback, and to be prepared to suggest treatment at optimal times. During the fourth level the CSOs attempt to negotiate a contract with their IP to abstain or moderate their drinking. Level five originally was a Johnson Institute confrontational session, but this was modified due to CSOs' discomfort with confrontational techniques. It now entails preparing CSOs to train others in their social network to implement the various levels of pressure (Barber & Gilbertson, 1997).

Empirical Support. The first PTC study involved individual PTC, group PTC, and a waiting list control. The results were noteworthy, as two-thirds of the drinkers with CSOs in one of the PTC conditions either entered treatment or substantially reduced their alcohol use. There were no comparable signs of improvement for drinkers associated with the control condition (Barber & Crisp, 1995). However, CSO functioning did not improve for any of the conditions. When a second study added a fourth group, Al-Anon, the results still favored the two PTC interventions in terms of the IPs' behavior (Barber & Gilbertson, 1996). CSO functioning improved this time as well, but only for CSOs assigned to either the individual PTC program or Al-Anon. A third study contrasted PTC counseling with a self-help version of it and a no-treatment control (Barber & Gilbertson, 1997). Both PTC conditions outperformed the control as far as the IPs' drinking or treatment engagement, and for the CSOs' level of depression.

In summary, the PTC program appears quite promising. However, one limitation of its reports is that the magnitude of success is sometimes unclear, due to the authors' tendency to combine the treatment entry and drinking reduction results. Also, the fact that the CSOs' own functioning did not consistently improve through their involvement in PTC is worth noting.

(c) ARISE

Description. A new unilateral treatment called ARISE (A Relational Intervention Sequence for Engagement) evolved from the Johnson Institute approach, but distinguishes itself in several ways. Importantly, ARISE informs IPs about the meetings between the therapist and the CSOs from the onset, and regularly invites them to attend. Also, rather than culminating in one intensive intervention, ARISE utilizes multiple, small confrontations that only build up to the more traditional intervention if the IP continues to offer resistance. Furthermore, the level of acceptable treatment for the IP is open to negotiation.

The seven basic assumptions of ARISE are: (1) by attempting to involve the IP in the intervention from the start, a message of respect and openness is conveyed, (2) a continuum of options for intervening is offered to each family, since this will allow them to draw upon their strengths, (3) the use of options is extended to IPs as well, as it decreases resistance, (4) the minimum amount of confrontation that is needed to be successful is used, (5) families can be highly influential in the change process, as they both care about and have extensive contact with the IP, (6) the strength of families enables them to heal themselves, and (7) the family requires support and assistance regardless of what happens with the IP (Garrett et al., 1998).

Empirical Support. Controlled studies are in progress, but none have been published. Promising reports were based on reviews of 350 randomly selected cases of treatment engaged IPs, but controls were unavailable (Landau et al., 2000; Loneck, Garrett, & Banks, 1996a).

In summary, the effectiveness of ARISE awaits sound empirical support. It is also not clear whether all of the IPs who become involved in ARISE are actually treatment refusers, since the least intrusive versions of the program sometimes simply entail telephone coaching of CSOs regarding how to invite their IP to attend treatment.

(d) Community Reinforcement and Family Training

Description. Community Reinforcement and Family Training (CRAFT) is an outgrowth of the Community Reinforcement Approach (CRA); a scientifically-supported program designed for use directly with the drinker/drug user (Hunt & Azrin, 1973; Meyers & Smith, 1995). In CRAFT, although CSOs are *not* seen as responsible for their loved one's drinking or drug problems, they can be very influential in affecting the IP's decision to seek treatment. It has three primary goals: (1) to decrease the IP's substance use, (2) to motivate the IP to enter treatment, and (3) to improve the quality of the CSO's life. CRAFT works through CSOs by teaching them skills to identify and utilize positive reinforcers ("rewards") for their IP's sober behavior. It further helps them recognize and reduce existing behaviors of their own that may have been unintentionally reinforcing the IP's substance use. While sharing some similarities with Thomas's UFT, CRAFT does not utilize "programmed confrontation," nor does it focus on educating CSOs about excessive use.

CRAFT begins with a violence assessment, as there is concern that risk may increase as CSOs alter their ways of interacting with the IP. CSOs learn to identify the precursors to violence, to develop new ways of responding in order to de-escalate the situation, and to have a safety plan. The assessment continues with CSOs outlining their loved one's typical using scenario, including the common antecedents as well as the positive and negative consequences for the IP. Throughout, CSOs examine the role they play in inadvertently making it easier for their IP to use.

In planning the behavioral change strategies, CSOs first generate a list of positive rewards (e.g., spending pleasant time with the IP) for sober behavior. These rewards are only utilized when the IP has *not* been using. CSOs next learn to allow the IP to experience the negative consequences of their drinking or drug use (e.g., deciding not to re-heat a meal for an intoxicated loved one who misses dinner). Additionally, training in communication skills is included, as positive communication is crucial for explaining the new behavioral change strategies being introduced by CSOs, and for decreasing the high levels of conflict in the CSO-IP relationship.

CSOs are coached to identify and take advantage of times when the IP might be most open to the idea of treatment. Time is devoted to preparing for this suggestion, and importantly, for the possibility that the IP may refuse treatment initially. Arrangements are made in advance for a rapid intake, so that the IP's fleeting motivation can be responded to quickly. The need for CSOs to be involved in therapy with their IP is discussed at length.

As noted, the third objective of CRAFT is to improve the quality of CSOs' lives regardless of what happens to their IP. Oftentimes CSOs' lives have become dominated by the many negative effects of their loved one's substance use. CRAFT helps CSOs develop strategies for increasing satisfaction, such as by reestablishing relationships with family and friends, and spending time on leisure interests that are independent of the IP. If a client's employment situation is not rewarding, the therapist discusses ways to improve it.

Empirical Support. The initial study by Sisson and Azrin (1986) compared Community Reinforcement Training (CRT), an early form of CRAFT, with a traditional 12-step program. The 12 female CSOs were family members of treatment-refusing drinkers. As far as treatment engagement, six of the seven alcoholic clients with CSOs in the CRT group initiated treatment, whereas none of those from the 12-step group did. On average this occurred after only seven CSO sessions. Interestingly, the CRT group alone showed a dramatic reduction in the drinker's frequency of use (approximately 50% reduction) *before* that individual even started treatment, while the CSO was receiving CRT.

The next study was one of three federally funded CRAFT research projects conducted at the University of New Mexico's Center on Alcoholism, Substance Abuse, and Addictions (CASAA; Miller et al., 1999). This sample of primarily white or Hispanic female CSOs included mostly spouses and parents of the IPs. These 130 CSOs were randomly assigned to Al-Anon facilitation therapy (Al-Anon FT), the Johnson Institute intervention, or CRAFT. Al-Anon FT, which was conducted as one-on-one therapy, paralleled the 12-step facilitation modality developed and tested in Project MATCH. CSOs who received CRAFT were successful at engaging 64% of the resistant drinkers. This was significantly better than the engagement rates for the Johnson Institute (30%) and Al-Anon FT (13%) approaches. Furthermore, CRAFT CSOs usually engaged their IPs after less than five CSO sessions. Importantly, IPs who entered treatment attended an average of 10.5 sessions. In terms of CSO functioning (e.g., depression, anger), significant improvement was found over time regardless of the intervention, and irrespective of whether the CSO's IP entered treatment.

In 1999 the CASAA team completed a pilot study to determine if CRAFT could be extended to work with CSOs of illicit drug using loved ones (Meyers, Miller, Hill, & Tonigan, 1999). The 62 CRAFT-trained CSOs had a 74% treatment engagement success rate. CSOs again showed improvement in their physical and emotional well-being that was independent of whether the IP entered treatment. The next drug study was a randomized trial that compared the early version of CRAFT; CRT, with a 12-step group condition for 32 CSOs of drug users (Kirby, Marlowe, Festinger, Garvey, & LaMonaca, 1999). CSOs who received the CRT intervention had 64% of their drug using IPs enter treatment, as compared to only 17% of those in the 12-step group. CSOs in both conditions again showed improvements in mood and social functioning.

The most recent randomized trial assigned 90 CSOs of illicit drug users to CRAFT, CRAFT plus aftercare group sessions (CRAFT + aftercare), and an Al-Anon/Nar-Anon Facilitation Therapy (Al-Anon/Nar-Anon FT) condition (Meyers et al., 2001). A significant difference in engagement rates by treatment condition was again found: 59% for CRAFT alone, 77% for CRAFT + aftercare, and 29% for Al-Anon/Nar-Anon FT. Each of the CRAFT groups differed statistically from Al-Anon/Nar-Anon FT. On average, fewer than five CSO sessions were required prior to IP engagement. Importantly, engaged IPs attended an average of more than eight sessions. Seven out of 19 variables measuring CSO functioning appeared to improve somewhat, and as with earlier studies, none of these improvements differed by treatment group.

In summary, these studies offer convincing evidence that CRAFT can powerfully impact the treatment engagement process; much more so than two more widely practiced approaches. Additionally, CRAFT works quickly, requiring few CSO sessions. Furthermore, engaged IPs tend to remain in treatment for reasonable periods of time. Finally, CRAFT's efficacy has been shown with a variety of types of CSOs (spouses, parents), for diverse ethnic groups, and for IPs with either alcohol or drug problems.

CONCLUSION

Concerned family members and friends do not need to stand by helplessly and wait for their substance-abusing loved ones to be ready to seek treatment. Instead, CSOs can take action by getting involved in one of several available empirically-supported interventions. But the first obstacle to overcome is identifying the potential CSOs, particularly in communities in which there are no specialized addiction programs. Based on the common psychological and physical symptoms manifested by these CSOs over time, ideas were offered in terms of *where* and *how* to locate these individuals. CSOs appear to be participants in a variety of public systems already, but without the basis for their symptomatology being known. If staff routinely asked patients about substance-abusing loved ones, conceivably many of these distressed CSOs could be identified and offered a program specifically designed to address both their needs and those of their IP.

Once the CSOs of substance-abusing individuals are located, a decision can be made about the type of intervention to utilize. Of course, this will depend on what is available in a community. The good news is that none of the programs require counselors with addiction training in order to work with CSOs, since CSOs do not usually have substance abuse problems. And the programs generally appear to be affordable, since the most efficacious ones only require a few CSO sessions before the treatment-refusing IP enters treatment. There are other considerations, however, such as whether the CSO is comfortable "detaching" from the IP and focusing on her/himself (i.e., Al-Anon), or in using a confrontational approach such as the Johnson Institute intervention. Within the third category of programs; those that teach CSOs skills to engage the IP in treatment *and* to enhance their own lives, there are choices as well. Although all of the interventions appear promising, some stand out as having more solid empirical backing and the potential to be more generalizeable, particularly in terms of their applicability to both alcohol and drug problems (e.g., CRAFT). Regardless of the choice made, it appears that the time has arrived to introduce an effective program that indirectly gains access to treatment-refusing individuals with alcohol and drug problems, while providing quality services for the concerned significant others as well.

REFERENCES

Al-Anon Family Groups. (1984). *Al-Anon faces alcoholism.* New York: Author.

Ananth, S. (1999). Alternative therapies for the medically underserved. *Health Forum Journal, 42,* 37–39.

Babor, T. F., & Higgins-Biddle, J. C. (2000). Alcohol screening and brief intervention: Dissemination strategies for medical practice and public health. *Addiction, 95,* 677–686.

Barber, J. G., & Crisp, B. R. (1995). The pressures to change approach to working with the partners of heavy drinkers. *Addictions, 90,* 271–278.

Barber, J. G., & Gilbertson, R. (1996). An experimental study of brief unilateral intervention for the partners of heavy drinkers. *Research on Social Work Practice, 6,* 325–336.

Barber, J. G., & Gilbertson, R. (1997). Unilateral interventions for women living with heavy drinkers. *Social Work, 42,* 69–77.

Brown, T. G., Kokin, M., Seraganian, P., & Shields, N. (1995). Models of helping and coping. *American Psychologist, 37,* 368–384.

Collins, R. L., Leonard, K., & Searles, J. (Eds.) (1990). *Alcohol and the family.* New York: Guilford Press.

Cook, R. F., Back, A. S., & Trudeau, J. (1996). Preventing alcohol use problems among blue-collar workers: A field test of the working people program. *Substance Use & Misuse, 31,* 255–275.

Council on Scientific Affairs. (1992). Violence against women: Relevance for medical practitioners. *Journal of the American Medical Association, 267,* 3184–3189.

Cryer, P. C., Jenkins, L. M., Cook, A. C., & Ditchburn, J. S. (1999). The use of acute and preventative medical services by a general population: Relationship to alcohol consumption. *Addiction, 94,* 1523–1532.

Cunningham, J. A., Sobell, L. C., Sobell, M. B., & Kapur, G. (1995). Resolution from alcohol treatment problems with and without treatment: Reasons for change. *Journal of Substance Abuse, 7,* 365–372.

Dittrich, J. E., & Traopold, M. A. (1984). A treatment program for the wives of alcoholics: An evaluation. *Bulletin of the Society of Psychologists in Addictive Behaviors, 3,* 91–102.

Garrett, J., Landau, J., Shea, R., Stanton, M. D., Baciewicz, G., & Brinkman-Sull, D. (1998). The ARISE intervention: Using family and network links to engage addicted persons in treatment. *Journal of Substance Abuse Treatment, 15,* 333–343.

Greenberg, R. (Winter 1999/2000). Substance abuse in families: Educational issues. *Childhood Education, 76,* 66–69.

Greenfeld, L. A. (1998). *Alcohol and crime: An analysis of national data on the prevalence of alcohol involvement in crime.* Report prepared for Assistant Attorney General's National Symposium on Alcohol Abuse and Crime. Washington, DC: U.S. Dept. of Justice.

Hohman, M. M., & Butt, R. L. (2001). How soon is too soon? Addiction recovery and family reunification. *Child Welfare, 80,* 53–67.

Holder, H. D., & Blose, J. O. (1986). Alcoholism treatment and total health care utilization and costs. *Journal of the American Medical Association, 256,* 1456–1460.

Hunt, G. M., & Azrin, N. H. (1973). A community-reinforcement approach to alcoholism. *Behavioral Research and Therapy, 11,* 91–104.

Institute of Medicine. (1990). *Treating Drug Problems, Vol. 1*. Washington, DC. National Academy Press.

Jacob, T., Krahn, G. L., & Leonard, K. (1991). Parent-child interactions in families with alcoholic fathers. *Journal of Consulting and Clinical Psychology, 59*, 176–181.

Johnson, V. E. (1986). *Intervention: How to help those who don't want help*. Minneapolis, MN: Johnson Institute.

Kirby, K. C., Marlowe, D. B., Festinger, D. S., Garvey, K. A., & LaMonaca, V. (1999). Community reinforcement training for family and significant others of drug abusers: a unilateral intervention to increase treatment entry of drug users. *Drug and Alcohol Dependence, 56*, 85–96.

Kyriacou, D. N., Anglin, D., Taliaferro, E., Stone, S., Tubb, T., Muelleman, R., Barton, E., & Kraus, J. F. (1999). Risk factors for injury to women from domestic violence. *New England Journal of Medicine, 341*, 1892–1898.

Landau, J., Garrett, J., Shea, R., Stanton, M. D., Baciewicz, G., & Brinkman-Sull, D. (2000). Strength in numbers: Using family links to overcome resistance to addiction treatment. *American Journal of Drug and Alcohol Abuse, 26*, 379–398.

Lapham, S. C., Chang, I., & Gregory, C. (2000). Substance abuse intervention for health care workers: A preliminary report. *Journal of Behavioral Health Services & Research, 27*, 131–143.

Larson, D. B., Hohmann, A. A., Kessler, L. G., Meador, K. G., Boyd, J. H., & McSherry, E. (1988). The couch and the cloth: The need for linkage. *Hospital and Community Psychiatry, 39*, 1064–1069.

Liepman, M. R., Nirenberg, T. D., & Begin, A. M. (1989). Evaluation of a program designed to help family and significant others to motivate resistant alcoholics into recovery. *American Journal of Drug and Alcohol Abuse, 15*, 209–221.

Logan, D. G. (1983). Getting alcoholics to treatment by social network intervention. *Hospital and Community Psychiatry, 34*, 360–361.

Loneck, B., Garret, J. A., & Banks, S. M. (1996a). A comparison of the Johnson intervention with four other methods of referral to outpatient treatment. *American Journal of Drug and Alcohol Abuse, 22*, 233–246.

Loneck, B., Garret, J. A., & Banks, S. M. (1996b). The Johnson Intervention and relapse during outpatient treatment. *The American Journal of Drug and Alcohol Abuse, 22*, 363–375.

Meyers, R. J., Miller, W. R., Hill, D. E., & Tonigan, J. S. (1999). Community reinforcement and family training (CRAFT): Engaging unmotivated drug users in treatment. *Journal of Substance Abuse, 10*, 1–18.

Meyers, R. J., Miller, W. R., Smith, J. E., & Tonigan, J. S. (2001). *A randomized trial of two methods for engaging treatment-refusing drug users through concerned significant others*. Manuscript submitted for publication.

Meyers, R. J., & Smith, J. E. (1995). *Clinical guide to alcohol treatment: The Community Reinforcement Approach*. New York: Guilford.

Miller, B. A., Wilsnack, S. C., & Cunradi, C. B. (2000). Family violence and victimization: Treatment issues for women with alcohol problems. *Alcoholism: Clinical and Experimental Research, 24*, 1287–1297.

Miller, W. R., Meyers, R. J., & Tonigan, J. S. (1999). Engaging the unmotivated in treatment for alcohol problems: A comparison of three strategies for intervention through family members. *Journal of Consulting and Clinical Psychology, 67*, 688–697.

Miller, W. R., & Rollnick, S. (1991). *Motivational interviewing: Preparing people to change addictive behavior*. New York: Guilford Press.

Paolino, T. J., & McCrady, B. S. (1977). *The alcoholic marriage: Alternative perspectives*. New York: Grune & Stratton.

Romijn, C. M., Platt, J. J., Schippers, G. M., & Schaap, C. P. (1992). Family therapy for Dutch drug users: The relationship between family functioning and success. *International Journal of Addictions, 27*, 1–14.

Sisson, R. W., & Azrin, N. H. (1986). Family-member involvement to initiate and promote treatment of problem drinkers. *Journal of Behavioral Therapy and Experimental Psychiatry, 17*, 15–21.

Snow, M. G., Prochaska, J. O., & Rossi, J. S. (1992). Stages of change for smoking cessation among former problem drinkers: A cross-sectional analysis. *Journal of Substance Abuse, 4*, 107–116.

Spear, S., & Mason, M. (1991). Impact of chemical dependency on family health status. *International Journal of Addictions, 26*, 179–187.

Stanton, M. D. (1982). Appendix A: Review of reports on drug abusers' family living arrangements and frequency of family contact. In M. D. Stanton, T. C. Todd, et al., *The family therapy of drug abuse and addiction* (pp. 427–432). New York: Guilford Press.

Terry, Y. M., VanderWaal, C. J., McBride, D. C., & Van Buren, H. (2000). Provision of drug treatment services in the juvenile justice system: A system reform. *The Journal of Behavioral Health Services & Research, 27*, 194–214.

Thomas, E. J., & Ager, R. D. (1993). Unilateral family therapy with spouses of uncooperative alcohol abusers. In T. G. O'Farrell (Ed.), *Treating alcohol problems; Marital and family interventions* (pp. 3–33). New York: Guilford Press.

Thomas, E., Santa, C., Bronson, D., & Oyserman, C. (1987). Unilateral family therapy with spouses of alcoholics. *Journal of Social Service Research, 10*, 145–163.

Titkin, S. N., & Mazorol III, E. J. (1999). Law and mediation. *Sage Family Studies Abstracts, 21*, 117.

Velleman, R., Bennett, G., Miller, T., Orford, J., Rigby, K., & Tod, A. (1993). The families of problem drug users: A study of 50 close relatives. *Addiction, 88*, 1281–1289.

Veroff, J., Kulks, R. A., & Douvan, E. (1981). *Mental health in America: Patterns of help seeking from 1957 to 1976*. New York: Basic Books.

Wechsler, H., Kelley, K., Weitzman, E. R., San Giovanni, J. P., & Seibring, M. (2000). What colleges are doing about student binge drinking. *Journal of American College Health, 48*, 219–226.

Whitfield, C. I. (1984). Co-alcoholism: Recognizing a treatable illness. *Family and Community Health, 7*, 16–27.

CHAPTER 17

Substance Abuse among Displaced and Indigenous Peoples

MIKYTA DAUGHERTY, WILLIAM H. JAMES, CRAIG T. LOVE, AND WILLIAM R. MILLER

On nearly every landmass of the earth there are indigenous peoples who have been displaced from what were once their native lands. Some have been relocated to designated reservations, often in isolated and resource-poor areas. Others have been dispersed into remote wilderness. Sometimes attempts have been made to exterminate them, or to strip away their native culture and assimilate them. Some populations have been removed from their homeland altogether, deported to foreign soil as prisoners or slaves. These displaced peoples are as diverse as humanity can be: the Maori of New Zealand, the Eskimos and Athabascans of Alaska, the black and colored peoples of South Africa, the Aboriginal people of Australia, African-Americans, Native Hawaiians, the Indians north and south of America's Rio Grande.

Yet there are some striking parallels in substance use patterns across these cultures that in most other respects would be considered to be quite diverse. That is the puzzle which we address in this chapter. Even for peoples on opposite sides of the earth, indigenous ethnic minority populations are commonly over-represented in rates of heavy drinking (and sometimes other drug use) and related problems, morbidity, and mortality. It seems unlikely that the diverse indigenous peoples discussed in this chapter share common genetic attributes that could account for the devastating effects of substance abuse in these populations (Phinney, 1996). Indeed, there is often more within-group than

MIKYTA DAUGHERTY AND WILLIAM R. MILLER • Department of Psychology, University of New Mexico, Albuquerque, New Mexico 87131 WILLIAM H. JAMES • College of Education, University of Washington, Seattle, Washington 98195 CRAIG T. LOVE • Center for Alcohol and Addiction Studies, Brown University, Providence, Rhode Island 02912

between-group variance regarding genes and their expression (Caetano, Clark, & Tam, 1998). To understand how such diverse populations came to such similar and destructive patterns of substance use, one must look beyond biological factors.

The heart of this chapter examines these cross-cultural patterns, reviewing research on substance use and its consequences among four particular displaced indigenous populations: Native Americans, Native Alaskans, the Maori of New Zealand, and Australian Aboriginals. For comparative purposes, we also reviewed two large U.S. populations that share a history of displacement: African Americans, and the homeless. It was the puzzling similarity among these diverse groups that led us to this chapter, which concludes with some reflections on why such parallel patterns may appear across otherwise distant and dissimilar populations.

NATIVE AMERICANS

Native Americans are descendants of many peoples who inhabited, prior to the arrival of Europeans, what it now the territory of the United States. (In U.S. political terminology, people from indigenous tribes south of the current U.S. border are classified as "Hispanic.") Many tribes were displaced from their native lands, and suffered sequential efforts first to exterminate and then to assimilate them. Some tribes disappeared. Others were relocated and confined to reservation lands, some of which are now recognized as sovereign nations within the United States.

Although the overall devastation related to alcohol among Native Americans is widely discussed, in fact the extent and type of alcohol problems among these peoples is as varied as their cultures (May, 1986; Weisner, Weibel-Orlando, & Long, 1984; Welty et al., 1995). Three million Native Americans comprise 577 recognized tribes. Still other tribes are not officially recognized and exist outside of the tribal structure in communities surrounding reservations or in major cities. Further, just over half of all Native Americans currently live in urban settings. Some tribes have pervasive levels of alcohol abuse and dependence, while others have very low rates (May, 1996). Among some plains tribes both men and women have high rates of drinking and related problems, whereas among the Navajo such problems are common for men but rare among women.

Clearly, the most common substance problem among Native Americans is alcohol (May, 1994). There are many indications that when alcohol is present in the community, Native Americans have a high rate of alcohol abuse (May, 1994; Beauvais, Oetting, & Edwards, 1985). Further, Native Americans show relatively higher prevalence of and mortality from liver dysfunction, diabetes, HIV/AIDS, and other health problems that are commonly caused or exacerbated by heavy drinking (CDC, 1998; Welty et al., 1995). A second significant substance abuse pattern among Native American youth is gasoline or glue sniffing (Herring, 1994; May, 1994). Inhalant abuse is most frequently seen among Native youth aged 7–15. A few tribes have reported problematic use of marijuana and stimulants, but the use of heroin and cocaine—common drugs of abuse in the U.S.—is still relatively rare among Native Americans (May, 1994). Both alcohol and gasoline are readily available, legally sold to adults, and relatively inexpensive.

The most common pattern of substance use among Native Americans is episodic binge drinking in groups (Welty et al., 1995), often fluctuating with the availability of alcohol. Drinking may begin on a payday and continue over a period of days, interrupted by unconsciousness, arrest, or lack of funds to purchase more alcohol. Such episodes are interspersed with extended periods of abstinence, a pattern that Jellinek (1960) referred to as "gamma alcoholism." Inhalant abuse may also extend over several days, most often in groups rather than in isolation.

Such episodic use is associated with a host of devastating social consequences, including automobile crashes, accidental injuries and deaths, physical and sexual abuse and victimization. The suicide rate among young Native Americans is nearly three times that of the general U.S. population, and alcohol is involved in most suicidal acts (May, 1994; 1996).

Abstinence rates among Native American tribal groups tend to be higher than in the general U.S. population. Among the Navajo, for example, 60 percent abstain completely from alcohol, as compared to 35 percent of the general population.

Alcohol-related annual death rates per 100,000 vary greatly among different tribal groups: from 6 among the Cherokee to 239 among the Cheyenne-Arapaho (Cohen, 1981). On average, however, alcohol-related deaths are quite high among Native Americans. A review of Indian Health Services (IHS) data from 1968 to 1988 for the 33 states with federally-recognized reservations indicated that 17% of all Indian deaths were alcohol related, as compared with the overall U.S. rate of 4.7% (May, 1989).

NATIVE ALASKANS

Alaska is geographically isolated from the rest of the United States, and much of its climate is arctic. As a result of this geographical difference, Native Alaskan villages are more isolated and seasonally inaccessible than those of any other indigenous group in the U.S. Indigenous Alaskans are comprised of two ethnic groups, generally known as Eskimo and Indian (Berger, 1995). Although they are distinguishable groups, they are usually combined in political considerations and in statistical reports. In fact, many reported statistics combine data from Alaskan Indians, Eskimos, and Native Americans in the other continental 48 states, in part because of small numbers in epidemiological and survey data. Unfortunately, this has diminished knowledge about the uniqueness of Alaskans (Peryhill-Paapke & Johnson, 1995).

The history of relocation and shifting political structures is more recent for Native Alaskans than for other Native Americans. Until 1971, the indigenous peoples of Alaska wintered in villages and towns across Alaska and spent summer months fishing and hunting in camps located in more remote sites across the state. The Alaska Native Claims Settlement Act of 1971 refuted the authority of tribal governments and established economic and political structures designed to assimilate Alaskan Natives into mainstream American society (Berger, 1995). These attempts to assimilate indigenous Alaskans failed, but left them with little or no land for subsistence. The result is impoverished peoples and bankrupt community corporations (Berger, 1995), though some groups hare fared better economically (Fairbanks Native Association, 1999).

Alcohol is the most prevalent substance used by Alaskan natives. Segal (1992) surveyed students in grades 7–12 and found that by age 14, 74% of Alaskan Native youth had used alcohol, 70% marijuana, and 25% inhalants. According to Segal, most substance abuse occurs during the young adult years (18–25), decreasing among adults over age 25. Patterns of use vary with availability. In more remote sites, access to alcohol and other drugs is limited, whereas Native Alaskans living in villages and towns have greater access. When the people move to fishing camps, they may spend 2–3 months in the wilderness with little or no access to alcohol or other drugs. Again, the pattern is of heavy episodic, availability-linked use in groups, not resembling steady use patterns often associated with the concept of alcohol dependence.

The consequences of use are reported mostly in combination with other Native populations, indicating that four of the ten leading causes of death are alcohol-related (Department of Health and Human Services, Bureau of Indian Affairs, 1995). The death rate from cirrhosis of the liver, for example, is five times higher among American Indians and Alaskan Natives than in the general U.S. population. Alcohol is involved in about 80% of homicides, suicides, and motor vehicle accidents.

THE MAORI

The Maori are the indigenous people who settled in Aoterearoa/New Zealand between 1000 and 1200 years ago. Like Native Americans, the Maori people are a heterogeneous group. Level of identification with traditional Maori practices varies, creating a continuum of Maori identities shaped by various social, economic, and cultural positions (Durie, 1999). As with many other indigenous populations, alcohol was not widely produced or consumed before the arrival of Europeans. Upon introduction, however, alcohol was rapidly incorporated into Maori culture and came to be associated with status and hospitality.

The Maori are rather consistently over-represented in a range of adverse health and social consequences stemming from alcohol use. Although they comprise 15% of the population of New Zealand, they constitute about 25% of those in treatment for substance use disorders (Durie, 1998). Another survey revealed that 32% of all Maori admissions to psychiatric hospitals and psychiatric wards in general hospitals were for substance use (primarily alcohol) disorders (Te Puni Kokiri, 1996). Of those admitted for drug and alcohol disorders, drug-related psychoses accounted for 21% of all Maori admissions, compared with 5% of "Pakeha" (majority group) admissions in New Zealand (Te Puni Kokiri, 1996). Furthermore, over the 10-year period of the survey (1984–1994), there was a 49% increase in female Maori first admission rates for drug and alcohol disorders.

By fusing information found in surveys and research reports, some general statements can be made regarding Maori patterns related to alcohol and drug use. The most frequently used drug is alcohol. Approximately 80% of Maori aged 14 to 25 have tried alcohol at some point during their lives. As in many populations, most of the drinking is done by young males. Half of all the alcohol consumed among the Maori is drunk by those aged 14–29, who comprise only a quarter of the population. Twelve cans of beer was reported as the median amount of weekly consumption for males, whereas for females the median amount was two cans per week. About 30% of males and 14% of women meet or surpass criteria for weekly heavy drinking (6 or more drinks in one session for men, or 4 or more drinks for women).

Drinking patterns among the Maori differ significantly from those of other New Zealanders. Maori are far more likely to be abstainers, but among those who do drink, the Maori are more likely to be heavy drinkers. Compared to their Pakeha counterparts, Maori drinkers drink less often, but consume about twice as much on average when they do drink (Kaunihera Whakatupato Waipiro o Aotearoa, 1995).

A significant number of Maori males (42%) and females (27%) experience some level of harmful consequences due to their substance use. The Maori suffer excessive morbidity and mortality from alcohol related causes (Public Health Commission, 1994). Between 1987 and 1992 Maori men were 2.7 times more likely to die of an alcohol related problem than non-Maori males, and among Maori females the same risk ratio was 1.6 (Kaunihera Whakatupato Waipiro o Aotearoa, 1995). Alcohol related-deaths from cirrhosis were 2.5 times greater in Maori males than non-Maori males. For fatal motor vehicle accidents, the 1991 Maori death rate in the 15–24 age group was 1.6 times higher than non-Maori. Of intoxicated drivers involved in fatal crashes in that same year, 43% were Maori (Kaunihera Whakatupato Waipiro o Aotearoa, 1995). Also, Maori make up about 15% of the population yet comprise over 50% of the prison population; and at least 60% of prison inmates have an alcohol or other drug problem (Kaunihera Whakatupato Waipiro o Aotearoa, 1995; Mason Durie, 1999).

ABORIGINAL AUSTRALIANS

The Aboriginal population of Australia is small and young, representing about 1.6% of the total Australian population, with 40% age 15 or younger (Commonwealth of Australia, 1994). About one-third live in small, remote areas with fewer than 1000 people, while a majority of Aboriginal people live in populated urban areas of Australia (Taylor, 1993). Although abstinence from alcohol is disproportionately high among Aboriginals (Perkins et al., 1994), a number of studies have indicated that Aboriginal people who do drink tend to be binge or episodic heavy drinkers. Aboriginal drinkers also frequently use alcohol at very harmful levels well beyond the National Health and Medical Research Council recommended limits of 14 standard drinks for women and 28 standard drinks for men per week (Pols & Hawks, 1992).

Among Aboriginal people, about 65% of males and 50% of females are current drinkers, with many drinking at hazardous levels. The proportion of heavy drinkers peaks in the 25–39 year age group (Perkins et al., 1994). In more remote Aboriginal communities, 92% of drinkers were found to be drinking at or above hazardous levels. In the Northern Territory, a kind of spiritual homeland for Aboriginals, 43% of males and 88% of females aged 15–20 were complete abstainers (Watson, Fleming, & Alexander, 1988).

Like other indigenous populations, Aboriginal people have suffered significant adverse consequences of heavy drinking. National surveys of Aboriginals reflect a high level of awareness and concern about the devastation caused by alcohol abuse (ABS, 1995; NATSIS, 1995), with 95% of urban Aboriginals perceiving alcohol to be a serious problem (CDHSH, 1994). There are well-documented elevated rates of alcohol-related mortality, hypertension, cirrhosis of the liver, cardiovascular disease, violence, motor vehicle crashes, other accidents, homicide, self-inflicted injuries, suicide, and mental health problems among Aboriginals (Blignault & Ryder, 1997; Bolger, 1991; Brady, 1992; Brady, 1993; Brady, Dawe, & Richmond, 1998; Brock, 1993; Burns, D'Abbs, & Currie, 1995). Alcohol is implicated in at least 10% of Aboriginal deaths nationwide, with higher rates in more remote areas (Weeramanthri, D'Abbs, & Matthews, 1994). Alcohol is related to about 75% of homicides among Aboriginals (Strang, 1992), is associated with spousal assault (Bolger, 1991; Brady, 1994; Hunter, 1993), and is strongly related to disproportionate rates of imprisonment and to deaths while in police or prison custody (D'Abbs et al., 1994; Johnson, 1991; Walker, 1992).

AFRICAN AMERICANS

African Americans were not indigenous to North America, but were forcibly imported as slaves. The first twenty African slaves were brought to Jamestown, Virginia in 1619 by a Dutch merchant vessel and traded for food and supplies. The African slave trade continued until the Emancipation Proclamation, which President Abraham Lincoln signed on January 1, 1863, freeing about three-fourths of slaves—those in states then controlled by the Union. The final abolition of slavery came with the passage of the 13th amendment to the U.S. Constitution in 1865 at the end of the American civil war. Currently African Americans constitute about 13% of the population of the United States. It is well accepted in the U.S. that the legacy of slavery has left its imprint on African Americans, for whom rates of poverty are much higher than in the general population.

Epidemiological studies consistently indicate that African Americans, particularly women, are strongly over-represented in the U.S. among alcohol abstainers, but are also over-represented among problem and binge drinkers; illicit drug users; and those in jails, prisons, and substance abuse treatment programs. Among U.S. women, rates of heavy drinkers are up to three times higher for African Americans than for Whites (Battle, 1990). The use of alcohol and illicit drugs among African Americans has been recognized as a serious and complex social and health problem that devastates many families (James and Johnson, 1996).

According to the 1999 National Household Survey on Drug Abuse (SAMHSA, 2000), an ongoing survey of the civilian non-institutionalized population of the United States, 12 years or older, the rates of illicit drug use (including marijuana) were high for various minority groups: 11.2% among persons reporting multiple race, 10.6% among the American Indian/ Alaska Native population, 7.7% for African-Americans, and 6.6% for Whites. Nevertheless, among African American youth, alcohol remains the drug most widely used, followed by tobacco and marijuana (Wallace et al., 1999).

Disparities in the burden of death and illness experienced by African Americans, as compared with the U.S. population as a whole, have existed since the government began tracking such statistics. At birth, the average life expectancy for African Americans is 71.8 years, compared to 77.4 years for whites. The age-adjusted death rate for the black population is 30 percent higher than for the non-Hispanic White population, and a significant part of this disparity can be linked to alcohol- and drug-related mortality. African Americans experience greater deleterious physical and mental health effects of alcohol and drug abuse, relative to other Americans (McNeece and DiNitto, 1998).

As with other populations discussed above, there is great variability in rates of substance use and related consequences among African American people. Elevated rates are substantially linked to poverty and educational disadvantage. When socioeconomic status is controlled, rates of alcohol and other drug abuse are not higher for African Americans. In fact, rates are lower among middle- and upper-class African Americans than for whites in those groups (Barr, Farrell, Barnes, & Welt, 1993; Herd, 1987). It is only in lower-income groups where rates are higher.

HOMELESS AMERICANS

Definitions of homelessness differ among studies, though usually include parts of the following criteria: (1) have limited or no shelter for any appreciable period of time, (2) stay in shelters or missions operated by religious or public agencies without rent paid, (3) stay in inexpensive hotels/motels, apartments, with family or friends, or rooms where the intended stay is temporary (Westerfelt & Bird, 1999; Gregoire, 1996). During the American great depression of the 1930s, the homeless population consisted primarily of older white males with alcohol problems. Since 1980, however the U.S. homeless population has grown substantially and become much more heterogeneous, including minorities, women, adolescents and children (Fisher, 1991). Ethnic minorities are significantly over-represented among the U.S. homeless.

Despite this heterogeneity, nearly all recent studies show that the homeless population has a high incidence of alcohol and drug use problems (30–60%, ranging between 2 and 7 times the rates in the general U.S. population (Benda & Vutchison, 1990; Fisher & Breakey, 1991; Johnson & Barret, 1992; Joseph, 1992; North et al., 1996; Susser et al., 1989; Vaillant, 1983). This pattern has been stable for decades. Among men admitted to New York shelters in 1985, 58% had a history of substance use and 27% used crack cocaine at least weekly (Susser et al., 1989).

Percentages of the homeless using illicit drugs within the past month range from 34% to 80%, although drug injection rates have been low (3–5%; Spinner & Leaf, 1992; Kahn et al., 1992; NYC Commission for the Homeless, 1992; Magura et al., 2000).

Lifetime rates of substance use disorders are still higher among the homeless. A California study found while half of the sample met criteria for current substance abuse or dependence, about 70% had met these criteria at some point in their lifetime. The most common current substance use disorders were with alcohol (38%), cocaine (24%) or crack cocaine (19%), marijuana (14%), stimulates (11%) and opiates (9%) (Robertson et al., 1997).

Not surprisingly, there is substantial diversity among the homeless. Gregoire (1996) reported a cluster analysis yielding subtypes that differed along dimensions such as alcohol and/or drug use, ethnicity, prior military service, imprisonment, employment status, family contact/support, physical health, and use of social agencies. In general, those with current alcohol or other drug use disorders had been homeless and unemployed for longer periods of time, were more transient and socially isolated, and had more physical problems than non-substance abusing homeless people (Brenda & Schroupfer, 1995). Homeless persons with more severe alcohol abuse are also more likely to suffer from all types of victimization (Lam & Rosenheck, 1998).

Mortality rates among the homeless vary greatly depending on geographic location and climate within the U.S. However, results from studies in three major cities report that homeless adults have an age-adjusted mortality rate 3.5–5.9 times higher than that of the general population (Hwang, 2000). Excess mortality is often related to substance use. Drug overdose has been reported the most common cause of death in some cities, with liver and pancreatic disease second and heart disease third (San Francisco Department of Public Health, 1999).

DISCUSSION

The six groups briefly reviewed above (Native Americans, Native Alaskans, the Maori, Aboriginal Australians, African Americans, and homeless Americans) are but a subset of the many displaced peoples of the world. Our review might have included Native Hawaiians, the black and colored peoples of South Africa, the Naskapi people of Quebec, Buganda peoples of Uganda, South Asian refugees, Mexican Mestizos, or the people of Tibet. For the six groups discussed here there happens to be an empirical literature regarding substance use and its consequences, which points to at least three clear parallels:

1. Rates of abstinence, particularly from alcohol, tend to be substantially higher than in the general population. People from displaced groups are more likely to abstain completely. Those who drink tend to have periods of abstinence between heavy episodes.
2. When drinking (and to a lesser extent, other drug use) does occur, it tends to be in episodes of heavy use, most often within groups of people from the same culture. Consequently, the phenomenon of light social drinking is relatively uncommon (Heath, 2000), and the rate of substance use disorders among non-abstainers is very high. This pattern seems to be clearest for groups with a more recent history of displacement.
3. Related to this pattern of heavy episodic use, displaced indigenous peoples tend to suffer disproportionately high adverse consequences of substance abuse, even though their rates of abstinence are often high, relative to the general population. Rates of substance-related morbidity and mortality are 3–7 times higher than in the majority population.

There is, of course, substantial variability in substance use patterns within and among these groups. Nevertheless, the parallels are noteworthy.

Why these similarities? The groups discussed in this chapter seem to have little else in common beyond their patterns of substance use (and non-use) and related consequences. They are racially and culturally diverse. Their histories as a people have evolved in almost complete isolation from one another. Not even with the wildest stretch of imagination would one expect a common genetic structure that distinguishes them from other peoples of the world.

DISPLACEMENT

One thing that they all do have in common is a history of massive displacement and sociocultural disintegration that historically preceded problematic substance use at a population level. Does population displacement (and its sequelae) constitute a common precipitating factor for the similar and devastating pattern of substance use in these diverse groups? There are several reasons for suspecting that it may. One of these is in the nature of historical time series. These extraordinarily diverse ethnic/cultural groups, with no significant prior history of substance abuse for centuries, developed parallel patterns of widespread binge use with devastating health and social consequences following cultural disruption and displacement.

There is also evidence that sociocultural displacement itself is often linked to binge drinking and adverse consequences. Even at an individual level, displacement events (e.g., homelessness, divorce) increase the incidence of substance abuse and problems. Perhaps the most-studied group of binge drinkers, U.S. college students show an abrupt acceleration of heavy episodic drinking, at the point of displacement to university study. This shift in drinking is much more pronounced among students who move to and live on campus, than among commuter students who continue to live at home (Schulenberg et al., 2001). Rapid acceleration of substance (including heroin) abuse and dependence was also apparent among U.S. soldiers in Vietnam. Upon returning home to the United States, however, most heroin-using Vietnam veterans abruptly discontinued use of the drug without treatment (Robins, Helzer, & Davis, 1975), although the prevalence of substance use disorders remains higher in this group than in the general U.S. population.

MEDIATING FACTORS

Displacement in itself is a broad phenomenon, and its apparent relationship to substance abuse may be mediated or moderated by various factors, including some of the common consequences of displacement. For example, when indigenous populations are displaced, they are often left impoverished as well. Poverty and associated desperation may themselves evoke or exacerbate substance abuse. Limited access to and resources to obtain substances would favor a pattern of sporadic use with interspersed abstinence, and within communal cultures, the sharing of supply when available. Adverse consequences of substance abuse also tend to be amplified by poverty. However, the acceleration of substance abuse among displaced peoples is by no means limited to the economically disadvantaged (e.g., White, 2001).

Stress

Poverty is one aspect of the more general stress associated with social adjustment after cultural displacement. Rapid social change and disruptions cause high stress levels that can evoke deviant behaviors (Caetano et al., 1998). This is a ubiquitous theme in research examining substance use patterns of indigenous populations adapting to a dominant culture. Al-Issa (1997) grouped these stressors into three categories. The first is *acculturative* stress, which is the stress of leaving one's homeland and adapting to a new society. The second is termed *minority* stress representing the disquietude that minorities endure from racism. The third is *socioeconomic* stress related to the poverty and disempowerment often experienced by ethnic minorities. Stress can also be related to unique aspects of the new context (e.g., combat stress, or the introduction of a money economy; Robbins, 1979). Relief and escape from distress is a commonly reported motivation for substance use, and is positively correlated with negative consequences of use. This may be exacerbated if the substance to which a group is exposed is not a familiar one for which the group has experience and established norms.

Changing Norms and Cultural Identity

The disruption of common social norms and controls is another possible mediating factor. An abrupt change in social norms is clearly a factor in substance use among college students and among soldiers in combat. A more general loss of cultural norms can also contribute to substance abuse. Durkheim (1933) posited that *anomie*—the absence within a society of common social norms and controls—is a significant source of social pathology. Under these conditions, people lack clear behavioral guidelines, which sometimes results in self-destructive tendencies. Others have postulated that a lack of clear cultural identification may contribute to substance abuse. Within this view, individuals who are clearly identified with one (or more) culture should show lower rates of substance abuse than those who have no clear cultural identity (Oetting & Beauvais, 1990–91). This would vary, however, with the substance use norms of the culture(s) with which one identifies. As people acculturate to a new society or subculture with heavier drinking norms, their own drinking tends to shift toward those norms. The degree of identification with a heavy-drinking culture, then, would be positively correlated with an individual's own alcohol use. For example, Venner (2001) found that among Mission Indians of California, high identification with Native American culture was associated with higher rather than lower rates of alcohol use and adverse consequences.

Relatedly, new substance use patterns can become a demarcation of group membership. Heavy binge drinking or drug use can become an outward and visible sign of what it means to be a member of a particular group (Indians, college students, a gang). Risky or harmful substance use may acquire a new significance within a community, demarcating a group's separateness and symbolizing rejection of the dominant culture's values. Using substances in disregard of legal and majority norms sets off the displaced culture from the dominant; the very act of using can become a form of social protest, a way of asserting a different identity.

Trauma

The effects of traumatic stress may endure for many years, perhaps even generations, after the acute stressors have subsided. There are clear and strong associations between traumatic stress and subsequent substance use disorders (Simpson & Miller, 2002). Childhood physical or sexual abuse predisposes to adult alcohol/drug problems. People with post-traumatic stress disorder have dramatically elevated rates of substance abuse (Jacobsen, Southwick, & Kosten, 2001).

At a societal level, some authors attribute the alcohol use of indigenous groups to the traumatic treatment they received during the invasion and occupation of their lands (Mason, 1985). Some postulate that the adverse sequelae of traumatic stress, including substance abuse, can be transmitted from one generation to the next, so that similar behavior patterns continue among generations that do not themselves experience the same level of trauma (Stewart, 1996).

While the above factors are plausible mediators of the link between cultural displacement and substance abuse, the relationship is by no means inexorable. As in the study of resilience in individuals, it may be informative to study exceptions to the pattern described above. As an historical people, Jews have been systematically persecuted, exterminated, and displaced for millennia, with dramatic examples continuing throughout the 20th century. More generally, peoples of the Middle East have suffered very high levels of stress, conflict, violence, and displacement. It would be unsurprising, then, if Jews and Palestinians showed extremely high rates of binge drinking and related consequences, but in fact these groups show precisely the opposite. If traumatic displacement exerts a large main effect on substance abuse, there must also be protective factors that moderate its effect.

There remains, then, a puzzle as to what aspects of cultural displacement produce such striking similarities in substance abuse across widely diverse populations. Certainly the similarities suggest looking beyond individual pathology or biological anomaly for the causes and remedies of substance abuse and related devastation among displaced peoples. To address problems of this scope effectively will require creativity and efforts well beyond the scope of treating affected individuals. Solving this puzzle may also provide important clues for effectively addressing the more general devastation of substance abuse among the diverse peoples of the world.

REFERENCES

ABS (Australian Bureau of Statistics) *National Aboriginal and Torres Strait Islander survey 1994* (1995). ABS catalogue no. 4190.0. Canberra: Australian Government Publishing Service.

Barr, K.E.M., Farrell, M.P., Barnes, G.M., & Welte, J.W. (1993). Race, class, and gender differences in substance abuse: Evidence of middle-class/underclass polarization among Black males. *Social Problems, 40*, 314–327.

Beauvais, F., Oetting, E.R., & Edwards, R.W. (1985). Trends in drug use of Indian adolescents living on reservations: 1975–1983. *American Journal of Drug and Alcohol Abuse, 11*, 209–229.

Benda, B. & Hutchison, E. (1995). Homelessness and alcohol. In Benda, B. & Schroepfer, T. (1995) Current drinking among the homeless according to past psychiatric and substance abuse treatment. *Alcoholism Treatment Quarterly, 12*, 1, 33–45.

Benda, B. & Schroepfer, T. (1995). Current drinking among the homeless according to past psychiatric and substance abuse treatment. *Alcoholism Treatment Quarterly, 12*, 1, 33–45.

Berger, T.R. (1995). *Village Journey: The Report of the Alaska Native Review Commission. (Rev. Ed.)* New York: Hill and Wang.

Berryhill-Paapke, E. & Johnson, M.E. (1995). Comparison of vlues of Alaska Native and Non-Native alcoholics and couselors. *The International Journal of the Additions, 30*, 481–488.

Blignault, I. & Ryder, C. (1997). Abstinence and alcohol use among urban Aboriginals in Western Australia. *Drug and Alcohol Review, 16*, 4, 365–371.

Bolger, A. (1991). *Aboriginal women and violence.* Darwin: ANU North Australia Research Unit.

Brady, M. (1993). Giving away the grog: An ethonography of Aboriginal drinkers who quit without help. *Drug and Alcohol Review, 12*, 4, 401–411.

Brady, M. (1992). Ethnography and understandings of aboriginal drinking. *Journal of Drug Issues, 22*, 3, 699–712.

Brady, M. (1994). *Alcohol use and its effects on Aboriginal women.* In: Broom, D (ed.) *Double bind. Women affected by alcohol and other drugs.* Sydney: Allen and Unwin, 53–63.

Brady, M., Dawe, S., & Richmond, R. (1998). Expanding knowledge among Aboriginal service providers on treatment options for excessive alcohol use. *Drug and Alcohol Review, 17*, 1, 69–76.

Brock, P. (1993). *Outback Ghettos: Aborigines, Institutionalization and Survival.* Cambridge University Press.

Burns, D., D'Abbs, P., & Currie, B. (1995). Patterns of petrol sniffing and other drug use in young men from an Australian Aboriginal community in Arnhem Land, Northern Territory. *Drug and Alcohol Review, 14*, 2, 159–169.

Caetano, R., Clark, C., & Tammy, T. (1998). Alcohol consumption among racial/ethnic minorities: theory and research. *Alcohol and health and Research World, 22*, 4, 233–241.

Center for Disease Control (1998). HIV/Aids among American Indians and Alaskan Natives-United States, 1981–1997. *Morbidity and Mortality Weekly Report, 47*, 154–161.

Cohen, S. Alcohol and the Indian. *Drug Abuse and Alcoholism Newsletter, 11*, 4, 1981.

Commonwealth of Australia. (1994). *Australia National Report on Population.* Canberra: Australian Government Publishing Service.

Commonwealth Department of Human Services and Health (1994). *National Drug Strategy Household Survey. Urban Aboriginal and Torres Strait Islander peoples supplement.* Canberra: Australian Government Printing Service.

D'Abbs, P., Hunter, E., Reser, J., & Martin, D. (1994). Alcohol misuse and violence. Alcohol related violence in Aboriginal and Torres Strait Islander communities: a literature review. *Report 8, National Symposium on Alcohol Misuse and Violence.* Canberra: Australian Government Publishing Services.

Durie, M. (1998). A maori development model for addressing alcohol misuse. *Journal of Alcohol Beverage Medical Research Foundation, 8*, 3, 51–60.

Durie, M. (1999). *Imprisonment, trapped lifestyles, and strategies for freedom.* Wellington: Foundation for Indigenous Research in Society and Technology.

Fairbanks Native Assocation (1999). *Annual Report.* Faribanks, AK: Fairbanks Native Association.

Fisher, P. (1991) *Alcohol, drug abuse, and mental health problems among homeless persons: a review of the literature.* Rockville, MD: Department of Health and Human Services.

Fisher, P. & Breakey, W. (1991). The epidemiology of alcohol, drug, and mental disorders among homeless persons. *American Psychology, 46*, 1115–1128.

Heath, D. (2000). *Drinking occasions: Comparative perspectives on alcohol and culture.* Ann Arbor, Michigan. Sheridan Books.

Herd, D. (1987). Rethinking Black drinking. *British Journal of Addiction, 82*, 219–223.

Herring, R.D. (1994) Substance use among Native American Indian youth: A selected review of causality. *Journal of Counseling and Development, 72*, 578–584.

Hunter, E. (1993). *Aboriginal Health and History: Power and Prejudice in Remote Australia.* Cambridge: University Press.

Hwang, S.W. (2000). Mortality among men using homeless shelters in Toronto, Ontario. *Journal of the American Medical Association, 283*, 16, 2152–2157.

Jacobsen, L., Southwick, S., & Kosten, T. (2001). Substance use disorders in patients with post-traumatic stress disorder: A review of the literature. *American Journal of Psychiatry Special Issue, 158*, 8, 1184–1190.

James, W. & Johnson, S. (1996). *Doin'Drugs: Patterns of Addiction in the African American Community.* Austin: University of Texas Press.

Johnston, E. (1991). *Royal Commision into Aboriginal deaths in custody, National Report Overview and Recommendation.* Canberra: Australian Government Publishing Service.

Kaunihera Whakatupatu Waipiro o Aotearoa. *Te Maori me te Waipiro Maori and Alcohol.* Wellington: Te Puni Kokiro and Alcohol advisory Council, 1995.

Lam, J. & Rosenheck, M. (1998). The effect of victimization on clinical outcomes of homeless persons with serious mental illness. *Psychiatric Services, 49*, 678–683.

Mac Marshall (1979). Belifs, behaviors, & alcoholic beverages: A Cross-Cultural Survey. Ann Arbor, MI: The University of Michigan Press.

Mason, V. (1985). *Relationship of Drug Use and Self Concept Among American Indian Youth.* Ph.D. Dissertation, University of New Mexico.

May, P.A. (1986). Alcohol and drug misuse prevention programs for Native Americans: Needs and opportunities. *International Journal of the Addictions, 17*, 118–1209.

May, P.A. (1989). Alcohol Abuse and alcoholism among Native Americans: An overview. In: T.D. Watts, R. Wright (eds.). *Alcoholism in Minority Populations*. Springfield, Illinois: Charles C. Thomas, pp. 95–119.

May, P.A. (1994). The epidemiology of alcohol abuse among American Indians: The mythical and real properties. *American Indian Culture and Research Journal, 18*, 121–143.

May, P.A. (1996) Overview of alcohol abuse epidemiology for American Indian populations. In G.D. Sandefur, R.R. Rundfuss, and B. Cohen (eds.), *Changing Numbers, Changing Needs: American Indian Demography and Public Health.* Washington, D.C.: Nationa Academy Press.

McNeese, C. & Ditto, D. (1998). *Chemical dependency: A systems approach.* Needham Heights, MA: Allyn & Bacon.

National Aboriginal Health Strategy Working Party (1989). *A national Aboriginal health strategy.* Canberra: Department of Aboriginal Affairs.

North, C., Thompson, S., & Pollio, D. (1997). A diagnostic comparison of homeless and nonhomeless patients in an urban mental health clinic. *Social Psychiatry & Psychiatric Epidiology, 32*(4), 236–240.

Perkins, J., Sansom-Fisher, R., Blunder, S., Lunnay, D., Redman, S., & Hensley, M. (1994). The prevalence of drug use in urban Aboriginal communities. *Addiction, 89*, 1319–1331.

Phinney, J.S. (1996). When we talk about American ethnic groups, what do we mean? *American Psychologist 51*, 918–927. In: Caetano, R., Clark, C., Tammy, T. (1998). Alcohol consumption among racial/ethnic minorities: theory and research. *Alcohol and health and Research World, 22*, 4, 233–241.

Pols, R. & Hawks, D. (1992). *Is there a safe level of daily consumption of alcohol for men and women? Recommendations regarding responsible drinking behaviour.* Canberra: Australian Government Publishing Service.

Public Health Commission. (1994). *Alcohol: The Public Health Commission's Advice to the Minister of Health.* Wellington: Public Health Commission.

Oetting, G. & Beauvais, F. (1990–91). Orthogonal cultural identification theory: The cultural identification of minority adolescents. *International Journal of the Addictions Special Issue: Use and misuse of alcohol and drugs: Ethnicity issues, 25*, 5a, 6a, 655–685.

Robertson, M., Zlotnick, C., & Westerfelt, A. (1997). Drug use disorders and treatment contract among homeless adults in Alameda County, California. *American Journal of Public Health, 87*, 2, 221–229.

Robins, L.N., Helzer, J.E., & Davis, D.H. (1975). Narcotic use in Southeast Asia and afterward. *Archives of General Psychiatry, 32*, 955–961.

San Francisco Department of Public Health. 1999 Deaths of Homeless San Franciscans Preliminary Results. http:www.dph.sf.ca.us/press/pr122299.htm/

Schulenberg, J., Maggs, J., Long, S., Sher, K., Gotham, H., Baer, J., Kivlahan, D., Marlatt, G., & Zucker, R. (2001). The problem of college drinking: Insights from a developmental perspective. *Alcoholism: Clinical & Experimental Research Special Issue, 25*, 3, 473–477.

Simpson, T. L. & Miller, W. R. (2002). Concomitance between childhood sexual and physical abuse and substance abuse: A review. *Clinical Psychology Review, 22*, 27–77.

Stewart, S.H. (1996). Alcohol abuse in individuals exposed to trauma: A critical review. *Psychological Bulletin, 120*, 83–112.

Strang, H. (1992). *Homicides in Australia 1990–91.* Canberra: Australian Institute of Criminology.

Susser, E., Struening, E., & Conover, S. (1989). Psychiatric problems in homeless men. *Archives of General Psychiatry, 46*, 845–850.

Taylor, J. (1993). *The relative economic status of indigenous Australians 1986–1991. Research monograph No. 5*, Centre for Aboriginal Economic Policy Research. Canberra: Australian National University.

Te Puni Kokiri. (1996). *Nga la o te Oranga Hinengaro Maori Trends in Maori Mental Health 1984–1993*. Wellington: Ministry of Maori Development.

U.S. Department of Health and Human Services (1995). *Trends in Indian Health*. Rockville, Md: Indian Health Service.

Venner, K. & Miller, W. (2001). Progression of alcohol problems in a Navajo sample. *Journal of Studies on Alcohol Special Issue, 62*, 2, 158–165.

Wallace, J., Forman, T., Gutherie, B., Bachman, J., O'Malley, & Johnson, L. (1999). The epidemiology of alcohol, tobacco and other drug use among Black youth. *Journal of Studies on Alcohol, 60*, 6, 800.

Walker, J. (1992). *Australian prisoners 1991. Results of the national prison census 30 June 1991*. Canberra: Australian Institute of Criminology.

Watson, C., Fleming, J., & Alexander, K. (1988). *A survey of drug using patterns in Northern Territory Aboriginal communities: 1986–1987*. Northern Territory Department of Health and Community Services, Drug and Alcohol Bureau.

Weeramanthri, T., D'Abbs, P., & Matthews, J. (1994). Towards a direct definition of an alcohol-related death: an analysis of Aboriginal adults. *Australian Journal of Public Health, 18*, 71–78.

Weisner, T.S., Weibel-Orlando, J.C., & Long (1984). "Serious drinking," "White man's drinking" and "teetotaling" Dirnking levels and styles in an urban American Indian population. *Journal of Studies on Alcohol, 45*, 237–250.

Welty, T.K., Lee, E.T., Yeh, J., Cowan, L.D., Go, O., Fabsitz, R.R., Le, N., Oopik, A.J., Robbins, D.C., & Howard, B.V. (1995). Cadiovascular disease risk factors among American Indians: The strong heart study. *American Journal of Epidemiology, 142*, 269–287.

White, R. (2001). Heroin use, ethnicity and the environment: The case of the London Bangladeshi community. *Addiction, 96*, 1815–1824.

PART E

Conclusions

CHAPTER 18

Integrated Care

The Need for Evidence-Based Policy, Prevention, and Treatment

WILLIAM R. MILLER AND CONSTANCE WEISNER

Throughout the world, substance use disorders are inextricably intertwined with a broad array of other health and social problems. It is a chicken-and-egg question as to which causes which, but in practicality one cannot effectively address addictions in isolation from these broader concerns. Furthermore, only a small minority of people with active substance use disorders are engaged with specialist addiction treatment programs. Instead, they frequent health care, social service, and correctional systems, constituting at least a large minority of those seen in these settings, and often present some of the most complex and expensive challenges to care (see Chapters 1, 9, 11).

LIMITATIONS OF SPECIALIST TREATMENT

Some regional and national care systems rely upon referral to specialist programs for treating substance use disorders. While there remains a role for specialist treatment (as discussed later in this chapter) there are several persuasive reasons why this is not an optimal strategy upon which to rely in addressing addictions. First, many cases are lost in the referral process; they simply don't engage in treatment, even if it is low-cost or free. There are often substantial barriers to addiction treatment, not the least of which is social stigma. Many people with addictive disorders do not regard themselves as needing specialist treatment, and whatever concerns they may have regarding

---

WILLIAM R. MILLER • Department of Psychology, University of New Mexico, Albuquerque, New Mexico 87131 CONSTANCE WEISNER • Department of Psychiatry, University of California, San Francisco, San Francisco, California 94143

their substance use are intertwined with and often quite secondary to their health and social concerns. When a window of opportunity opens up, rapid access to specialist treatment may be barred by waiting lists, bureaucracy, or practicalities such as transportation, child care, and safety.

A care map that relies on identification-and-referral also poses a rather high threshold for care. Health and social service professionals are likely to identify only the more severe cases, and for various reasons (cost, skepticism, stigma, preservation of ongoing care relationship) may be reluctant even then to refer. A refer-out orientation also discourages integrated care. In such systems, it is common for people to be referred back and forth between addiction treatment, health care, and social service systems, each seeing the person as more suitable for care elsewhere because of concomitant problems (Shavelson, 2001).

Furthermore, fragmented care is not particularly effective. People with concomitant substance use disorders are less "reliable" users of health and social services. They are less likely to adhere to care plans or return dependably for appointments. Similarly, people with concomitant psychological, health and social problems usually show poorer retention and adherence in specialist addiction treatment programs. What does seem to work is integrated care. Retention and adherence can be improved by addressing the person's problems together (Chapter 10). This is also, we believe, likely to improve the overall quality of care.

The chapters of this volume further question an acute-treatment model for addressing addictions. Substance use disorders are more akin to chronic diseases, not bacterial infections (Chapter 3). There are obvious flaws in thinking that one can remove the person to a specialist program, deliver treatment, and then return him or her cured to the natural environment. More apt is a model of ongoing care and support for the person's matrix of health and social problems. A specialist-expert model of treatment also, we believe, focuses far too little attention on broader sociocultural factors that promote the development and maintenance of substance abuse, reducing attention to prevention and relevant social policy issues and to natural processes of change (Chapter 2).

OPPORTUNITIES FOR INTEGRATED CARE

Once one steps back from a specialist-treatment-referral model, the opportunities for integrated care are many. In most health care and social service systems, the density of substance use disorders is far higher than in the general population. The opportunity is there to see a far larger number of cases than would ever be found in specialist treatment. Indeed, they are *already* being seen and cared for in health and social service systems, but for other problems. There is no way in such care systems *not* to serve a large number of people with substance abuse and dependence. The question is how well these problems are being identified and addressed in care.

It is also possible to initiate care far *earlier* in many cases than would occur (if ever) through referral to specialist treatment. Health and social problems emerge throughout the development of addictive disorders, usually well before the person perceives a need to address substance use. There is an opportunity, then, to explore this aspect of care and to enhance motivation for change before problems reach the level of severity usually associated with referral for specialist treatment, where they often require the most expertise and are most expensive to treat.

There are also significant ways in which it is better to address the full range of people's concerns. Mental health and substance abuse concerns, for example, are often so intertwined as to require integrated care, just on pragmatic grounds (Chapter 10). People also tend to experience their own problems as interrelated, and often prefer integrative care that takes this bigger view of the whole person, rather than a specialist focus.

Substantial gains have already been made in some nations in addressing tobacco and alcohol use through routine health care. Screening and low-threshold brief interventions are being developed (Rollnick, Mason & Butler, 1999), but there are many opportunities yet to be explored.

Health Care

Many of the pioneering efforts to address smoking and problem drinking through health care have focused on doctors, but physician time is increasingly precious and pressured. Other health professionals such as nurses, home visitors, and pharmacists (Chapter 7) may have longer and/or more frequent contact with patients. Such health professionals can be prepared to recognize and address substance abuse as part of health care. Other health professionals, such as dentists and ophthalmologists, are likely to observe recognizable acute and chronic effects of substance use, and could be prepared to address these in helpful ways. Trauma centers and emergency departments regularly see people whose injury or illness is directly related substance abuse, often at a teachable moment of opportunity (Chapter 5). Beyond tobacco (Chapter 8) and alcohol, very little has been done to address other drugs of abuse through routine health care.

Behavioral Health

The concept of "behavioral health" is a confluence of mental health and addictions care. Although this merger has occurred partially in response to economic pressures, it also recognizes the inter-related nature of these problems and the need for integrated care. Unfortunately, mental health professionals have seldom been encouraged to think of substance use disorders as part of their mission, or given sufficient training and expertise to address them. In the U.S., "substance abuse counselors" have historically focused exclusively or primarily on addictive behaviors, with little training and expertise to address psychological disorders. Yet nearly all psychologists, social workers, psychiatrists and counselors will encounter substance use disorders throughout their careers. Those who treat substance use disorders should be more broadly qualified to address behavioral health issues, and mental health professionals should be trained to address addictions as part of their routine expertise. In other words, there is emerging, appropriately, a broader behavioral health specialty to treat both addiction and mental health problems in an integrated fashion. There is, of course, a danger of substance use disorders being overlooked when such services are combined (see Chapter 15).

Social Services

Whereas some progress has been made to address addictions through health care, there have been fewer models and examples of such integrated care through social service systems. Yet substance use disorders are highly prevalent among the clientele of programs to address social problems such as unemployment, domestic violence, child protective services, school and work problems, crime, poverty, and family welfare (Chapters 11–15). A refer-out policy is common, in part because of limited time, resources, and training of social service staff to address the complexity of addictions. Yet when left unaddressed, substance abuse compromises adherence and impoverishes outcomes of social services, contributing to a high-cost revolving-door pattern that further depletes resources and demoralizes staff. The needs and opportunities for integrated care are legion.

OPPORTUNITIES FOR SPECIALIST TREATMENT

Providing care for substance dependence, particularly in its more advanced stages, is a complex task, warranting a high degree of professional expertise. Not all addiction problems can be handled through routine health care and social service systems. There will be a continuing role for centers of specialist expertise to treat addictions, as for the care of diabetes, heart disease, and cancer. There is ample evidence that addictions can be treated effectively, and that focused treatment is warranted (Chapter 3). We believe, however, that some important and fundamental changes are needed in the way such treatment is provided within nations that can afford specialist care systems.

Rapid Access

While substance use disorders are properly understood as chronic conditions prone to recurrence, the windows of opportunity to initiate treatment are often acute. Motivation for change waxes and wanes, and when a moment of readiness occurs it is unwise to delay access to care. There is evidence that the longer people are on a “waiting list” for addiction treatment, the less likely they are to initiate it, and the more retention and outcomes are compromised. It seems to be far better to see people quickly, even if briefly, than to consign them to a waiting list. At one specialist treatment center (the University of New Mexico Center on Alcoholism, Substance Abuse, and Addictions; CASAA), we redesigned the intake process so that the first contact was an hour with a skilled counselor who listened to the person's concerns, enhanced motivation for change, and obtained the minimal information required. This replaced an arduous gauntlet of assessment through which the client previously had to pass before seeing a treatment professional. We tried to deliver at least this much service to everyone within a day or two of contact, so that even if this were the only service they received we would have given them something likely to help them. This approach is also used in some large U.S. health plans, such as Kaiser Permanente, where initial intakes to specialist substance abuse programs can occur on a "drop-in" non-appointment basis, and individuals are given at least an interview and the opportunity to attend part of the program on the same day. Immediate access to care ought to be the norm, rather than requiring a pre-selection endurance test for entry to treatment.

Evidence-Based Treatment

There is now a substantial literature of outcome research differentiating treatment methods most likely to be effective for substance use disorders. There is also a widely-recognized gap between research and practice in this field, so that the treatment methods often delivered in specialist programs are often not optimally effective. It seems an obvious humanitarian policy to deliver the treatment methods with the best evidence of efficacy and cost-effectiveness, but this is surprisingly rare in practice, which tends to be guided instead by personal belief and tradition. Where public resources are used to fund treatment, or when the force of law is applied to coerce people into treatment, there is a special obligation to ensure that the services delivered are likely to be beneficial.

A key to change here lies with those who fund treatment. So long as providers are permitted to use whatever methods they choose to treat addictions, there is no contingency for improved care. When reimbursement policy requires the delivery of evidence-based treatment, practice begins to change in the right direction. The policy of any particular treatment system, however, need not await the imposition of such controls from above. In the 1990s, the above-mentioned program adopted the following policy with regard to treatment delivery:

> CASAA shall operate only those treatments, services, and programs for which there exists reasonable evidence of efficacy in the current scientific literature. Services with unproven efficacy will be designated as experimental procedures and offered only within the context of appropriately designed research to determine their efficacy.

Although this seems a sensible policy, it proved surprisingly controversial among treatment staff. It is also challenging to ensure that evidence-based methods are, in fact, being applied behind closed doors. To support such policy requires considerable staff training, support, and ongoing supervision (Chapter 6).

An additional problem in implementing such an evidence-based policy is that many of the most commonly-used treatments have not been adequately studied. Funding for clinical trials is often "investigator-initiated," meaning that the treatments are those which most interest researchers, or which may be easier to study. Issues of concern to clinicians (e.g., cultural relevance, the importance of childcare, gender-specific programs, and integrated "program" approaches) are often more difficult to study, and may not have had the opportunity to meet an evidence-based standard. Much substance abuse treatment in the U.S. occurs in the context of group therapy, and many treatments have not been adequately tested in group format. It is important, therefore, for the international research community to take note of the treatments used in real-life agencies and study them, thus building the population base of interventions on which rigorous studies have been conducted.

Professional Qualification

The standards required for treating substance use disorders have varied widely across nations and time. In the U.S., little more than a personal history of substance abuse and recovery was required of counselors in the 1970s and 1980s, and even in the 1990s states struggled to increase minimum requirements to include a college education. This, of course, reflects public and political conceptions of the level and kind of expertise required to treat addictions competently. It is our view that those who treat people with substance use disorders should be professionally qualified and more generally trained health practitioners who meet national standards for licensure in their profession (e.g., physician, nurse, psychologist, social worker), and that those who deliver *specialist* treatment should ideally have had additional professional training in the addiction field. This is to say that, in our view, the era of the addiction-only counselor is past. It is time to understand substance abuse as one aspect of broader health care. In doing so, it is important to rely in training upon state-of-the-art, research-based methods for identifying, assessing, treating, and preventing substance use disorders.

Integrated Care

Similarly, specialist addiction treatment needs to be closely connected and integrated with health care and social services. Models for such integration are slowly emerging. As much a possible, it makes sense to co-locate addiction treatment programs with larger health care and social service systems. This facilitates patient transition and access to the various kinds of services needed. If an addiction treatment program is just down the hall, referrals are more likely to be made and completed. Location in a routine health care facility may also diminish perceived stigma in receiving care.

When addiction treatment is provided in a separate location, consideration should be given to providing more comprehensive on-site services, given the common need for more general health care and social services among people with substance use disorders (McLellan et al., 1994; Weisner, Mertens, Parthasarathy, Moore, & Lu, 2001). In short, addiction treatment should be seen as an integral part of a larger health care system.

Continuing Care

Specialist systems should also be redesigned toward a continuing care model that matches the normal course of treatment and recovery. Addiction problems (like chronic diseases) are seldom resolved through a single episode of acute treatment. Programs can *expect* to care for clients over time, rather than viewing any return for care as some sort of failure. The historic term "aftercare"—a term and model rarely used in addressing, say, diabetes or hypertension—carries the implication that primary care was provided during an acute treatment episode. Continuing care (Donovan, 1998) extends from the first contact, with periodic visits over a prolonged span of time as need arises. It may include regularly scheduled check-ups of decreasing frequency as recovery progresses. This is quite a different approach from fixed-model standard-duration acute treatment programming.

In nations where mutual-help networks (such as 12-step programs) are available, these can form an important part of ongoing support. While continuing care should not rely entirely on mutual-help networks, there is good evidence that involvement in such programs is associated with more stable sobriety (e.g., Tonigan, Connors, & Miller, in press). Such mutual support networks may be particularly important for individuals whose current social support networks favor substance abuse rather than abstinence (Project MATCH Research Group, 1997).

CHALLENGES OF INTEGRATED CARE

We hope that we have documented the need for integrated care, and for the placement of specialist addiction treatment within a broader spectrum of health care and social services. We believe that this is the present and future direction of addiction treatment. Yet most service systems are ill-prepared for this transition, important thought it be. We close this chapter and book with some thoughts on what is needed to prepare for truly integrated care.

Professional Attitude and Training

First and foremost, it is important for those who deliver health and social services to perceive substance abuse as part of their own realm of concern and competence. For many if not most generalist health and behavioral health professionals, aware of it or not, substance use disorders will be among the three most common diagnoses they will encounter throughout their life work. It is important, in the future training of professionals, to convey that these concerns are a natural part of practice, and one that can be addressed effectively with broad benefit. This is in contrast to a "don't ask, don't tell" approach, viewing addictions as an annoyance, a refer-out policy when problems are detected, and cynicism about the chances of favorable outcome. Similarly, as we have discussed, it is important to train alcohol and drug professionals in the importance of assessing the other health, mental health, and social functioning problems of those they treat in specialist care.

It is always a challenge, of course, to fit one more competency into the already-overcrowded curricula of professional training programs. A focus on substance use disorders is warranted by their sheer prevalence, relative to less common conditions to which considerably more curricular time is currently devoted in the training of physicians, psychologists, etc., but need alone often does not change practice. An attractive advantage here is that brief counseling methods that are beneficial in addressing substance abuse within health care are more generally useful in behavior change consultations that arise with regard to many other concerns in everyday practice (Rollnick et al., 1999).

Proactive Inquiry

It would seem to go without saying that substance use should be among the areas covered in a comprehensive health screen, yet it is still surprisingly rare to find meaningful inquiry as routine practice. Substance use disorders are vastly under-identified, although they have quite serious potential health and social consequences. Even to *ask* about substance use (let alone implement a standardized screening) has been uncommon in health care and social services. This is due in part, no doubt, to a lack of training in simple and comfortable ways to raise the subject with patients and clients (Rollnick et al., 1999), and in part to uncertainty about what to do if the person screens positive. Inquiry about smoking is, perhaps, most common, and the use of tobacco has come to be seen as a legitimate health concern to be addressed within the scope of routine care (Chapter 8). The same needs to occur with regard to alcohol and other drug use. One way may be to take a more parsimonious approach by paying attention to the medical and social conditions that have higher prevalence among heavy drinkers and substance abusers than among other individuals (Sikkink & Fleming, 1991; Weisner et al., 2001). It is also sensible to be proactive through special efforts in the many contexts where substance abuse is especially likely to be involved (e.g., domestic violence, child protective services, emergency department). Professional training should routinely include methods for raising the topic and inquiring about it without fostering defensiveness.

There are also excellent opportunities to identify addiction problems and intervene through significant others. The family members of people with substance use disorders have elevated rates of utilization of health care and social services. There are now proactive approaches for working through significant others to enhance motivation and behavior change (Chapter 16).

Care Maps

Health care and social service systems should develop clear care maps—a shared system-wide plan for how to provide care for a particular problem, in this case a substance use disorder. The very development of such a plan by a health care system or social service agency announces the importance and relevance of substance abuse to the program's mission. Such a care map can include screening, brief interventions compatible with normal service delivery, and interface with specialist care systems.

Concomitant Care

Substance abuse ordinarily comes as part of a cluster of behavioral, health and social problems. Models are needed, therefore, to address these problems in the context of one another. Important steps in this direction have occurred in research on the treatment of "dual diagnosis," but models for concomitant care are still in early stages (Chapter 10). Treatment research has often focused on a single diagnosis, seeking to reduce the noise in outcomes by eliminating cases with other significant problems. The reality of practice, however, suggests a need for studies of the treatment of X *and* Y, of commonly concomitant problems. Where concomitant care cannot be provided by the same professional or team, better models and care maps are needed for the coordination of care by multiple specialists.

Concomitant care also involves simultaneous attention to substance use disorders and other concerns. The requirement, "First take care of your ______ and then we'll treat you" is one source of people being bounced from agency to agency, and is exacerbated by the idea that an acute treatment episode is the appropriate treatment for addictions. Although there is sometimes a logic for addressing one problem before another, often it is possible and even fruitful to work on various parts of a problem cluster simultaneously (Chapter 10). Again, this can be done through integrated intervention with the same professional or team, or by coordinated care from separate professionals or teams treating different components of a complex problem cluster.

Prevention and Policy

Finally, it is important to think well beyond the treatment of already-established addiction problems. It is understandable that tertiary care is the focus of specialist treatment programs, but within the broader context of health care and social services it makes sense to address primary (universal) and secondary (targeted) prevention. Public health problems are not effectively addressed solely by treating one affected case at a time. It is important to examine the larger sociocultural environment, and consider what can be done to decrease the occurrence of new cases (Chapter 17).

Here, too, it is important to take an evidence-based approach. Far too often, substance abuse "prevention" programs are not founded on a scientifically sound approach. The U.S. Drug Abuse Resistance Education (DARE) program is but one of the most recent examples of a widely practiced approach that, upon careful evaluation, appears to exert no preventive effect (Clayton et al., 1996; Ennet et al., 1994; Lynam et al., 1999). When large numbers of people are being exposed to any "prevention" program through community-based (e.g., Chapter 12), school-based (Chapter 13), correctional (Chapter 14) or workplace programs (Chapter 15), there is both a public interest and a moral obligation to ensure that the program's effects are likely to be beneficial. The desire to "do something" must be tempered by the evidence base that one is actually doing something helpful and not harmful.

As empirical evidence continues to accumulate, it can be transferred into social and system policy to guide practice. There is a natural human tendency to implement in practice (e.g., treatment, prevention) that which seems rational, sensible, and consistent with one's own understanding of how and why problems occur. There is also a long history of seemingly sensible ideas that have failed, or have even generated counterintuitive harm in trying to address substance abuse. Evidence-based policy places some governing constraints on our human biases, slowly steering social and system efforts in the direction of effective change.

REFERENCES

Clayton, R. R., Cattarello, A. M., & Johnstone, B. M. (1996). The effectiveness of Drug Abuse Resistance Education (Project DARE): 5-year follow-up results. *Preventive Medicine, 25*, 307–318.

Donovan, D. (1998). Continuing care: Promoting the maintenance of change. In W. R. Miller & N. Heather (Eds.), *Treating addictive behaviors* (2nd ed., pp. 317–336).

Ennet, S. T., Tobler, N. S., Ringwalt, C. L., & Flewelling, R. L. (1994). How effective is drug abuse resistance education? A meta-analysis of Project DARE outcome evalutions. *American Journal of Public Health, 81*, 1394–1401.

Lynam, D. R., Milich R., Zimmerman, R., Novak, S. P., Logan, T. K., Martin, C., Leukefeld, C., & Clayton, R. (1999). Project DARE: no effects at 10-year follow-up. *Journal of Consulting and Clinical Psychology, 67*, 590–593.

McLellan, A. T., Alterman, A. I., Metzger, D. S., Grissom, G. R., Woody, G. E., Luborsky, L., & O'Brien, C. P. (1994). Similarity of outcome predictors across opiate, cocaine, and alcohol treatments: Role of treatment services. *Journal of Consulting and Clinical Psychology, 62*, 1141–1158.

Project MATCH Research Group (1997). Project MATCH secondary a priori hypotheses. *Addiction, 92*, 1671–1698.

Rollnick, S., Mason, P., & Butler, C. (1999). *Health behavior change: A guide for practitioners*. New York: Churchill Livingstone.

Shavelson, L. (2001). *Hooked: Five addicts challenge our misguided drug rehab system*. New York: New Press.

Tonigan, J. S., Connors, G., & Miller, W. R. (in press). Participation and involvement in Alcoholics Anonymous. In T. F. Babor & F. K. DelBoca (Eds.), *Treatment matching in alcoholism*. Cambridge, UK: Cambridge University Press.

Sikkink J. & Fleming, M. (1991). Adverse health effects and medical complications of alcohol, nicotine, and drug use. In M. F. Fleming & K. L. Barry (Eds.), *Addictive disorders* (pp. 145–168). St. Louis, MO: Mosby-Year Books.

Weisner C., Mertens J., Parthasarathy S., Moore C., & Lu Y. (2001). Integrating primary medical care with addiction treatment: A randomized controlled trial. *Journal of the American Medical Association, 286*: 1715–1723.

Index